Lippincott Williams & Wilkins

atlas of

ANATOMY

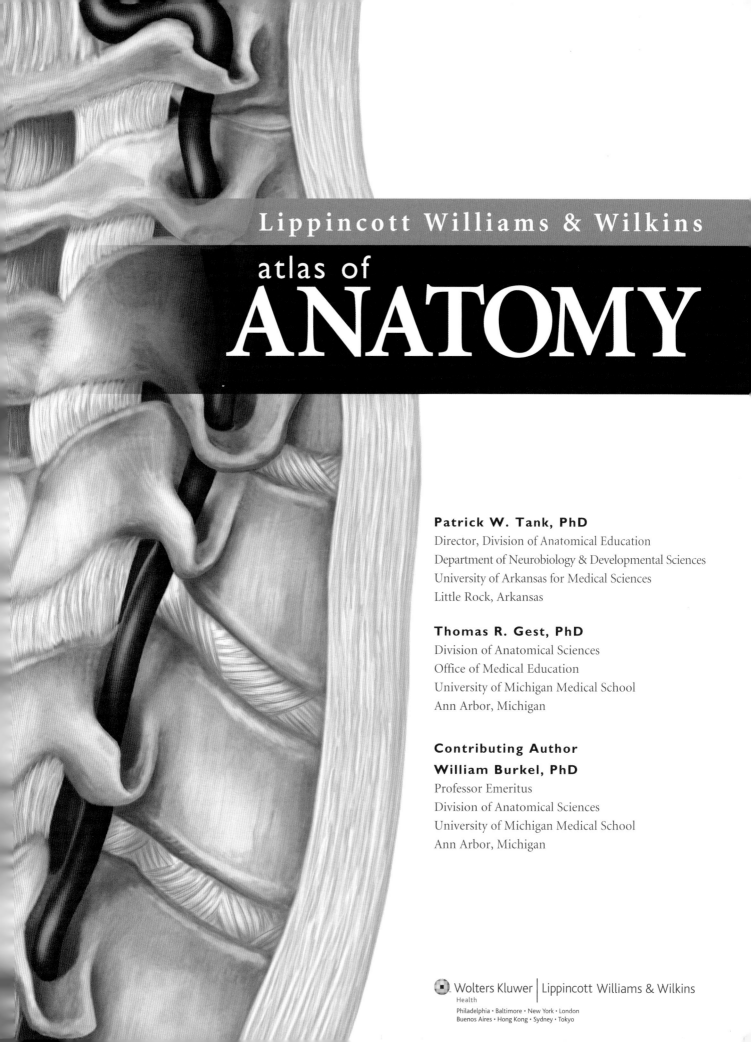

Lippincott Williams & Wilkins

atlas of
ANATOMY

Patrick W. Tank, PhD

Director, Division of Anatomical Education
Department of Neurobiology & Developmental Sciences
University of Arkansas for Medical Sciences
Little Rock, Arkansas

Thomas R. Gest, PhD

Division of Anatomical Sciences
Office of Medical Education
University of Michigan Medical School
Ann Arbor, Michigan

Contributing Author
William Burkel, PhD

Professor Emeritus
Division of Anatomical Sciences
University of Michigan Medical School
Ann Arbor, Michigan

Wolters Kluwer | Lippincott Williams & Wilkins
Health
Philadelphia · Baltimore · New York · London
Buenos Aires · Hong Kong · Sydney · Tokyo

Acquisitions Editor: **Betty Sun**
Developmental Editor: **Kathleen H. Scogna**
Creative Director: **Susan Hermansen**
Art Director: **Andrea La Bon-Dominguez**
Marketing Manager: **Valerie Sanders**
Production Editor: **Julie Montalbano**
Design: **Andrea La Bon-Dominguez**
Illustration Coordinators: **Lik Kwong and Dawn Scheuerman**
Compositor: **Circle Graphics, Inc.**
Additional art services: **Urszula Adamowska and Sean McCabe**

351 West Camden Street   530 Walnut Street
Baltimore, MD 21201   Philadelphia, PA 19106

Printed in China

9 8 7 6 5 4 3

Library of Congress Cataloging-in-Publication Data

Tank, Patrick W., 1950-
  Lippincott Williams & Wilkins atlas of anatomy / Patrick W. Tank, Thomas R. Gest ;
contributing author William Burkel.
     p. ; cm.
  Includes index.
  ISBN 978-0-7817-8505-1
  1. Anatomy—Atlases. I. Gest, Thomas R. II. Burkel, William E. III.
Lippincott Williams & Wilkins. IV. Title. V. Title: Lippincott Williams and Wilkins atlas
of anatomy. VI. Title: Atlas of anatomy.
  [DNLM: 1. Anatomy—Atlases. QS 17 T1651 2009]
  QM25.T36 2009
  611.0022'3—dc22

                                                        2008001527

Dedicated to the memory of

Russell T. Woodburne, PhD

whose descriptions of anatomy are as valid and accurate today

as they were when first written over 50 years ago.

The opportunity to create a new anatomical atlas could not be described as even a once-in-a-lifetime opportunity. Original atlases simply are not produced often enough to make that statement accurate. As anatomical educators of medical students with nearly 60 years of classroom experience between us, we are familiar with all of the anatomical atlases that are currently on the market, and it is a very esteemed group. Our experience with these existing atlases has helped us formulate strong ideas of how to present anatomical images more concisely and in a more logical sequence. The intent of this new atlas is to make images easier and faster for the student to use. Speed and ease of use have become critical needs in the era of compressed anatomical curricula.

The development of this atlas required the combined efforts of a large group of people and the good fortune to have all of these resources available simultaneously. First, we had the complete support of Lippincott Williams & Wilkins (LWW). This support came in many forms, from editorial and production assistance and project funding to art direction and expert market analysis as well as many words of encouragement.

Second, we had the exceptional talents of the creative team at the Anatomical Chart Company (ACC). ACC produces the thousands of anatomical and diagnostic charts that are displayed in clinics and doctors' offices all over the world. The ACC creative team recruited a small army of the best medical illustrators in the country, kept this army organized, and guided them throughout the project. The ACC design team created a truly inspired design and oversaw the construction of pages. Working with the LWW production team, ACC also guided this complex atlas through the production phase.

Third, the authors have been friends and colleagues for many years. The result of our combined efforts to develop educational material has always been greater than the sum of our individual efforts. To this project we have brought the ability and desire to work as a team.

Using these resources to the maximum extent, we have developed an atlas that stands out among contemporary atlases in several areas.

Teaching Perspective

The *LWW Atlas of Anatomy* is organized regionally. However, the atlas is not simply a series of flat anatomical drawings with every structure labeled. Every aspect of the atlas, from the selection and organization of the plates, to the coloring, style, and labeling of the individual images is grounded in a teaching perspective. The organization follows a teacher's logic, in that it begins with surface anatomy and superficial features, then proceeds into deeper structures with plate groupings that support regional dissection sequences. The labels are carefully selected and placed to tell a story and direct the attention of the viewer to important relationships.

A New Art Style

A new art style was created for the *LWW Atlas of Anatomy*. The illustrations use a vibrant palette, new surface textures, effective use of shading to add depth, and a clean, uncluttered labeling approach. The main illustrations are designed to depict the most common anatomical features (i.e., "average" anatomy) that a student is likely to encounter in dissections or clinical practice. Common important anatomical variations are also depicted in supporting illustrations.

Careful Selection of Images

There are fewer illustrations in the *LWW Atlas of Anatomy* than in other atlases. In today's shrinking anatomy curriculum, more is not necessarily better. We carefully considered the number of illustrations necessary to get the job done, with no superfluous figures or concepts. Illustrations are placed in logical dissection order, followed by summary illustrations (systemically organized illustrations of vessels and nerves) that help the student assemble the parts into a whole.

Consistent Perspective

To aid the novice, the images in the *LWW Atlas of Anatomy* use consistent viewpoints: Directly anterior, directly posterior, directly lateral, or directly medial. The specimen is always placed in the anatomical position. Oblique views and quartering views are not used. Positioning of the limbs or the head in other than the anatomical position has been strictly avoided.

Effective Use of Color

Images in the *LWW Atlas of Anatomy* use color to draw the viewer's attention to the important part of the figure. Many figures have highly detailed peripheral anatomy rendered in gray to provide context for the illustration without distracting the viewer from the central theme. Summary illustrations use this color technique to particular advantage to show systemic anatomy of body regions.

Ghosted Structures

Many illustrations in the *LWW Atlas of Anatomy* employ a ghosting technique to allow the viewer to look into the illustration in greater depth. In some illustrations, the viewer looks through ghosted structures to see important anatomical relationships. In other illustrations, a solid object is rendered as a ghost where it passes behind another solid object. By use of these ghosting techniques, we are able to illustrate the relationships of deep structures to more superficial structures and allow students to see connections and associations that previously they had to imagine.

Limited Labeling

We have intentionally limited the number of labels per illustration in the *LWW Atlas of Anatomy*. We deliberately selected only those structures most likely to be taught in modern curricula and to provide labels for those structures. We did not label everything in each illustration. Many additional structures could have been labeled, but at a loss of the didactic impact of the image.

Effective Label Placement

We have juxtaposed labels to increase the pedagogical impact of the illustration. These label placements encourage the student to notice important relationships. We also have used lists of labels to reinforce the relationship of parts of structures to the whole. The arrangement of labels, combined with the use of color, leaves little doubt as to the intent of the illustration.

No Captions

The *LWW Atlas of Anatomy* has no captions or text to explain the figures. Market analysis indicates that students and faculty are sharply divided on whether or not this type of material is useful. It is our feeling that an atlas is a supplement to a textbook. We feel that students consult an atlas for visual identification, not description, and that lengthy discussion of the illustrations is not necessary if the illustrations are designed and organized properly and used in the context of text materials.

Complete Product Package

We are also offering with the text a set of supporting products designed to help students learn anatomy. All of the images are available electronically in an interactive atlas that can be accessed on thePoint (Lippincott Williams & Wilkins's website). The interactive atlas has several useful features, including a search function and zoom and compare features. Students can also test their knowledge of anatomy with a unique drag-and-drop labeling exercise available for each image. Instructors also receive an image bank that provides each image in a file suitable for multimedia presentations and an extensive repository of anatomy-oriented test questions

The *LWW Atlas of Anatomy* has taken many years to complete, and its creation took full advantage of electronic communication and imaging. It has not been an easy feat, as the artists, editors, authors, and publisher are spread all over the country. Approximately 7500 versions of the illustrations were reviewed and critiqued during the course of the project. We all suffered moments of fatigue but the result is well worth the time invested. The experience has been both exhausting and exhilarating.

We hope that you enjoy the outcome.

PT & TG

Lik Kwong, MFA
Medical Illustration
University of Michigan
Ann Arbor, Michigan

Dawn Scheuerman, MAMS
Biomedical Visualization
University of Illinois at Chicago
Chicago, Illinois

Karen Bucher, MA
Medical and Biological Illustration
Johns Hopkins University School of Medicine
Baltimore, Maryland

Anne D. Rains, MS
Medical Illustration
Medical College of Georgia
Augusta, Georgia

Jonathan Dimes, MFA
Medical Illustration
University of Michigan
Ann Arbor, Michigan

Megan E. Bluhm Foldenauer, MA
Medical and Biological Illustration
Johns Hopkins University School of Medicine
Baltimore, Maryland

Liana Bauman, MAMS
Biomedical Visualization
University of Illinois at Chicago
Chicago, Illinois

Christopher Rufo, MA
Medical Illustration
Johns Hopkins University School of Medicine
Baltimore, Maryland

William Scavone, MA, CMI
Medical and Biological Illustration
Johns Hopkins University School of Medicine
Baltimore, Maryland

Alison E. Burke, MA
Medical Illustration
Johns Hopkins University School of Medicine
Baltimore, Maryland

Denise Wurl, MS
Biomedical Visualization
University of Illinois at Chicago
Chicago, Illinois

Jennifer C. Darcy, MS
Medical Illustration
Medical College of Georgia
Augusta, Georgia

Jaye Schlesinger, MFA
Medical Illustration
University of Michigan
Ann Arbor, Michigan

The authors and publisher would like to gratefully acknowledge the following individuals who reviewed illustrations and provided critical feedback during the development of this atlas:

Marc Abel, PhD
Rosalind Franklin University of Medicine and Science
Chicago, Illinois

Androniki Abelidis
Hull York Medical School
Hull and York, England

Diana Alagna
Branford Hall Career Institute at Southington
Southington, Connecticut

Maryanne Arienmughare
Jefferson Medical College
Philadelphia, Pennsylvania

Fredric Bassett, PhD
Rose State College
Midwest City, Oklahoma

Sonny Batra
Stanford University
Stanford, California

Paulette Bernd, PhD
SUNY Brooklyn College of Medicine
Brooklyn, NY

Neil Boaz, MD, PhD
Ross University
Edison, New Jersey

Anna Brassington
Hull York Medical School
Hull and York, England

Eric Brinton
University of Utah School of Medicine
Salt Lake City, Utah

Ashlee Brown
University of Missouri School of Medicine
Columbia, Missouri

David Brown
University of California at Irvine
Irvine, California

Craig Canby, PhD
Des Moines University Osteopathic Medical Center
Des Moines, Iowa

Walter Castelli, DDS
University of Michigan Medical School
Ann Arbor, Michigan

Silvia Chiang
Case Western Reserve University
Cleveland, Ohio

Matthew Comstock
Oklahoma State University College of Osteopathic Medicine
Tulsa, Oklahoma

Gerald Cortright, PhD
University of Michigan Medical School
Ann Arbor, Michigan

Eugene Daniels, MSc, PhD
McGill University
Montreal, Quebec, Canada

David L. Davies, PhD
University of Arkansas for Medical Sciences
Little Rock, Arkansas

Megan Duffy
Catholic Healthcare West
San Francisco, California

Norm Eizenberg, MB
University of Melbourne
Victoria, Australia

Matt Gardiner
University College London
London, England

Niggy Gouldsborough, BSc, PhD
University of Manchester
Manchester, England

Lauren Graham
Johns Hopkins School of Medicine
Baltimore, Maryland

ACKNOWLEDGMENTS

Santina Grant
University of Illinois at Chicago College of Medicine
Chicago, Illinois

Bill Gross
Medical College of Wisconsin
Milwaukee, Wisconsin

Robert Hage, MD, PhD
St. Georges University
Grenada, West Indies

Felicia Hawkins-Troupe
Loyola University Medical School
Chicago, Illinois

Keels Hillebart de Jong, PhD
Academic Medical Center of the University of Amsterdam
Amsterdam, The Netherlands

Alireza Jalali, MD, LMCC
University of Ottawa
Ottawa, Ontario, Canada

Jennifer Jenkins
Brown University
Providence, Rhode Island

Subramaniam Krisnan
University of Malaya
Kuala Lumpur, Malaysia

Randy Kulesza, PhD
Lake Erie College of Osteopathic Medicine
Erie, Pennsylvania

Anton Kurtz
University of Vermont
Burlington, Vermont

Scherly Leon
State University of New York at Stony Brook
Stony Brook, New York

Jing Xi Li
University of Ottawa—Downtown
Ottawa, Ontario, Canada

Ryan Light
Eastern Virginia Medical School
Norfolk, Virginia

Darren Mack
Medical College of Georgia
Augusta, Georgia

Linda McLoon, PhD
University of Minnesota at Minneapolis
Minneapolis, Minnesota

Jodi McQuillen
University of Vermont College of Medicine
Burlington, Vermont

Nonna Morozova
Asa Institute of Business and Computer Technology
Brooklyn, New York

Karuna Munjal
Baylor College of Medicine
Houston, Texas

Barbara Murphy, PhD
University of Nebraska at Omaha
Omaha, Nebraska

Bruce W. Newton, PhD
University of Arkansas for Medical Sciences
Little Rock, Arkansas

Lily Ning
University of Medicine and Dentistry of New Jersey
Newark, New Jersey

Gezzer Ortega
Howard University College of Medicine
Washington, D.C.

Steve Palazzo, DC
University of Bridgeport
Bridgeport, Connecticut

Lynn Palmeri
Georgetown University School of Medicine
Washington, D.C.

Jilma Patrick
Meharry Medical College
Nashville, Tennesee

Kevin D. Phelan, PhD
University of Arkansas for Medical Sciences
Little Rock, Arkansas

John Polk, PhD
University of Illinois at Urbana
Urbana, Illinois

Omid Rahimi, PhD
University of Texas Health Science Center
San Antonio, Texas

Christopher Rodrique
Louisiana State University
Baton Rouge, Louisiana

Dario Roque
University of Florida
Gainesville, Florida

Heiko Schoenfuss, MS, PhD
St. Cloud State University
St. Cloud, Minnesota

Simant Shah
University of Medicine and Dentistry of New Jersey
Newark, New Jersey

Shahin Sheibani-Rad
Rosalind Franklin University of Medicine and Science
Chicago, Illinois

Parikshat Sirpal
Nova Southeastern University College of Medicine
Fort Lauderdale, Florida

Jan Smit
Queen's University Belfast
Belfast, Northern Ireland

Maria Sosa, PhD
University of Puerto Rico
San Juan, Puerto Rico

Rayapati Sreenathan, MSC, PhD
St. Matthews University Medical School
Grand Cayman, British West Indies

Lisal Stevens
Loma Linda University
Loma Linda, California

Rob Stoeckart, PhD
Erasmus University Rotterdam
Rotterdam, The Netherlands

Stuart Sumida, MA, PhD
California State University at San Bernardino
San Bernardino, California

Frans Thors, PhD
Akademisch Ziekenhuis Maastricht
Maastricht, The Netherlands

Grace Tsuei
University of Texas Southwestern Medical School
Dallas, Texas

Linda Walters, PhD
Midwestern University
Arizona College of Osteopathic Medicine
Glendale, Arizona

Daniel Weber
Michigan State University College of Osteopathic Medicine
East Lansing, Michigan

Benjamin Weeks
University of Arkansas
Fayetteville, Arkansas

William Woo
Drexel University College of Medicine
Philadelphia, Pennsylvania

Floris Wouterlood, PhD
Vu Medisch Centrum
Amsterdam, The Netherlands

Jill Zackrisson
Virginia Commonwealth University School of Medicine
Medical College of Virginia Campus
Richmond, Virginia

Michael Zumpano, PhD
New York Chiropractic College
Seneca Falls, New York

Contents

Lippincott Williams & Wilkins

atlas of
ANATOMY

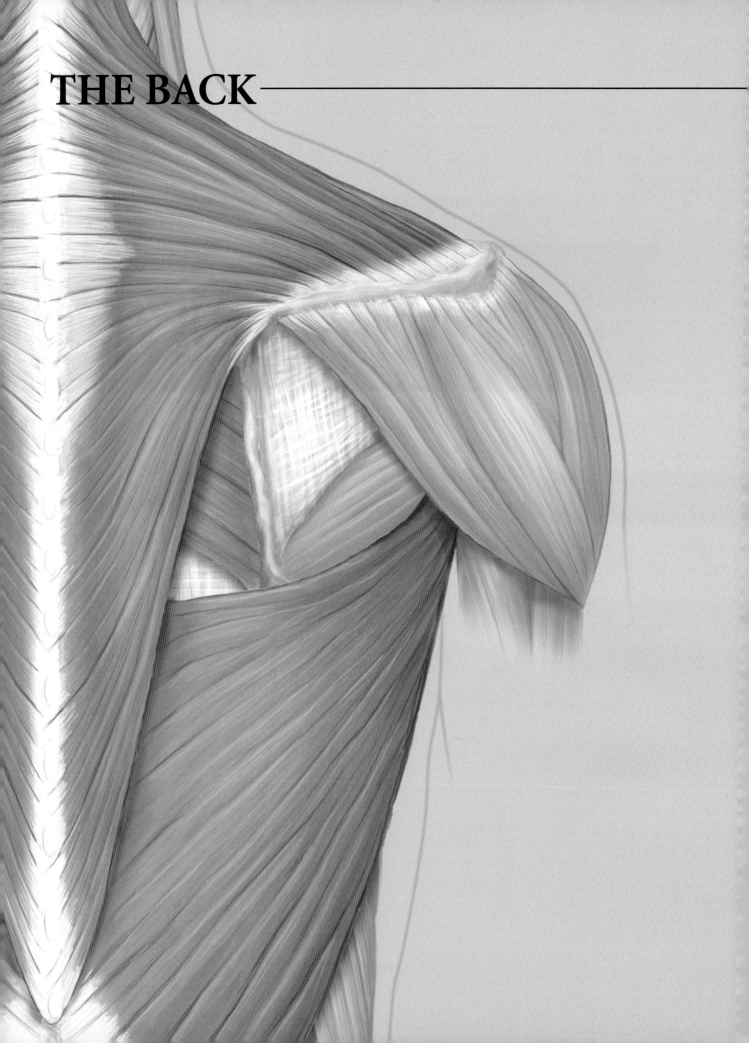

THE BACK

Palpable bony structures

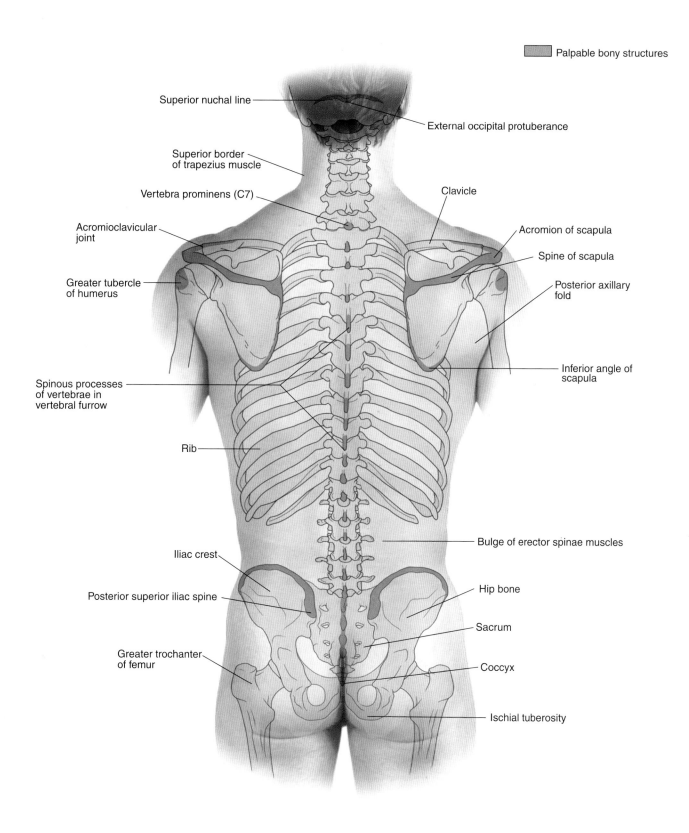

Superior nuchal line

External occipital protuberance

Superior border of trapezius muscle

Clavicle

Vertebra prominens (C7)

Acromion of scapula

Acromioclavicular joint

Spine of scapula

Greater tubercle of humerus

Posterior axillary fold

Spinous processes of vertebrae in vertebral furrow

Inferior angle of scapula

Rib

Bulge of erector spinae muscles

Iliac crest

Posterior superior iliac spine

Hip bone

Sacrum

Greater trochanter of femur

Coccyx

Ischial tuberosity

PLATE I-02   **Vertebral Column, Lateral View**

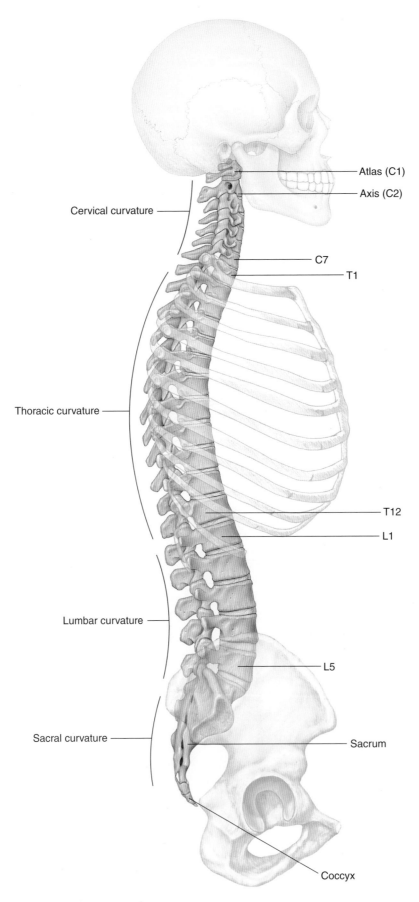

Atlas (C1)

Axis (C2)

Cervical curvature

C7

T1

Thoracic curvature

T12

L1

Lumbar curvature

L5

Sacral curvature

Sacrum

Coccyx

A. Atlas (C1), superior view

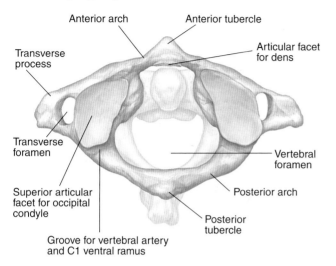

Anterior arch
Anterior tubercle
Articular facet for dens
Transverse process
Transverse foramen
Vertebral foramen
Posterior arch
Superior articular facet for occipital condyle
Posterior tubercle
Groove for vertebral artery and C1 ventral ramus

B. Atlas (C1), inferior view

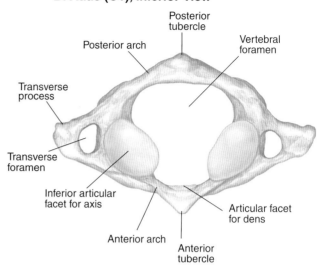

Posterior tubercle
Posterior arch
Vertebral foramen
Transverse process
Transverse foramen
Inferior articular facet for axis
Anterior arch
Anterior tubercle
Articular facet for dens

C. Axis (C2), superior view

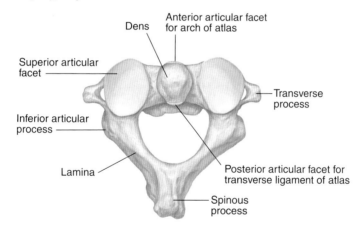

Dens
Anterior articular facet for arch of atlas
Superior articular facet
Transverse process
Inferior articular process
Lamina
Posterior articular facet for transverse ligament of atlas
Spinous process

D. Cervical vertebra (C4), superior view

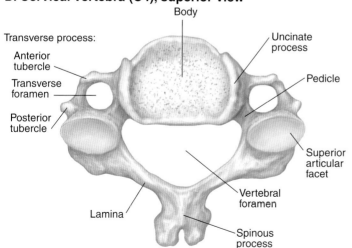

Body
Uncinate process
Transverse process:
Anterior tubercle
Pedicle
Transverse foramen
Posterior tubercle
Superior articular facet
Lamina
Vertebral foramen
Spinous process

E. Cervical vertebra (C4), lateral view

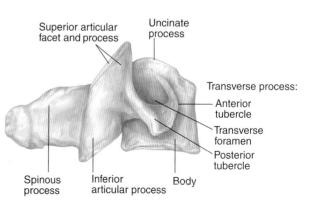

Superior articular facet and process
Uncinate process
Transverse process:
Anterior tubercle
Transverse foramen
Posterior tubercle
Spinous process
Inferior articular process
Body

PLATE I-04   Articulated Cervical Vertebrae

A. Lateral view

B. Radiograph of cervical vertebrae, lateral view

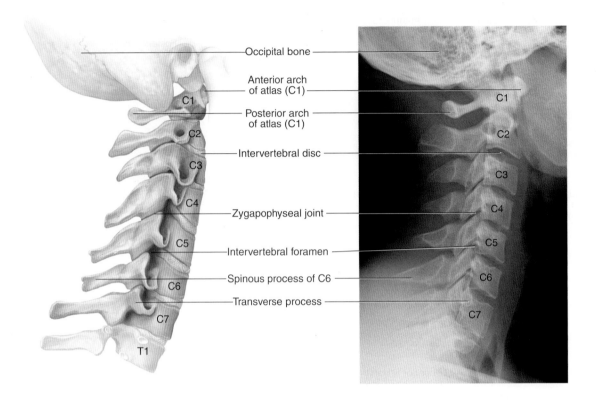

Occipital bone

Anterior arch of atlas (C1)

Posterior arch of atlas (C1)

Intervertebral disc

Zygapophyseal joint

Intervertebral foramen

Spinous process of C6

Transverse process

C. Posterior view

D. Radiograph of cervical vertebrae, posterior view

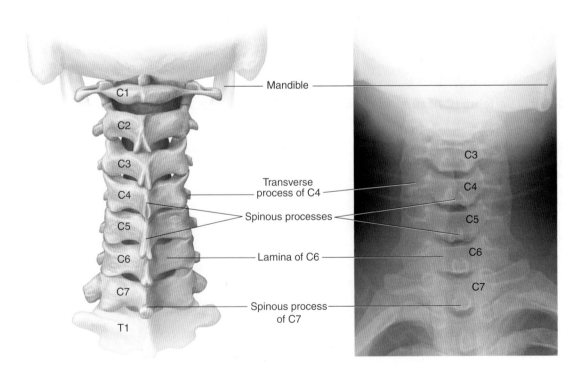

Mandible

Transverse process of C4

Spinous processes

Lamina of C6

Spinous process of C7

A. Thoracic vertebra (T6), superior view

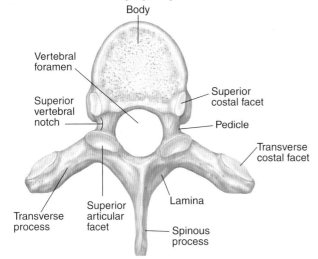

Body

Vertebral foramen

Superior vertebral notch

Superior costal facet

Pedicle

Transverse costal facet

Transverse process

Superior articular facet

Lamina

Spinous process

B. Thoracic vertebra (T6), lateral view

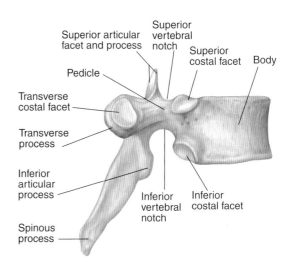

Superior articular facet and process

Superior vertebral notch

Superior costal facet

Body

Pedicle

Transverse costal facet

Transverse process

Inferior articular process

Inferior vertebral notch

Inferior costal facet

Spinous process

C. Intervertebral disc, superior view

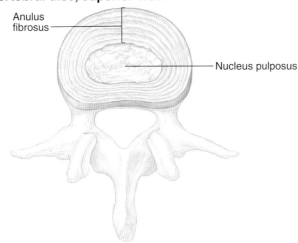

Anulus fibrosus

Nucleus pulposus

D. Lumbar vertebra (L3), superior view

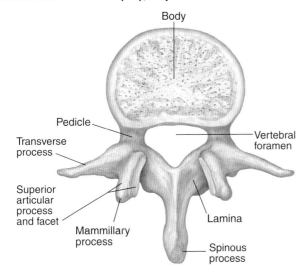

Body

Pedicle

Transverse process

Vertebral foramen

Superior articular process and facet

Mammillary process

Lamina

Spinous process

E. Lumbar vertebra (L3), lateral view

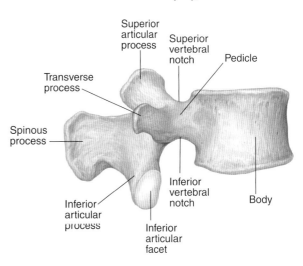

Superior articular process

Superior vertebral notch

Pedicle

Transverse process

Spinous process

Inferior articular process

Inferior vertebral notch

Body

Inferior articular facet

PLATE I-06   Articulated Thoracic Vertebrae

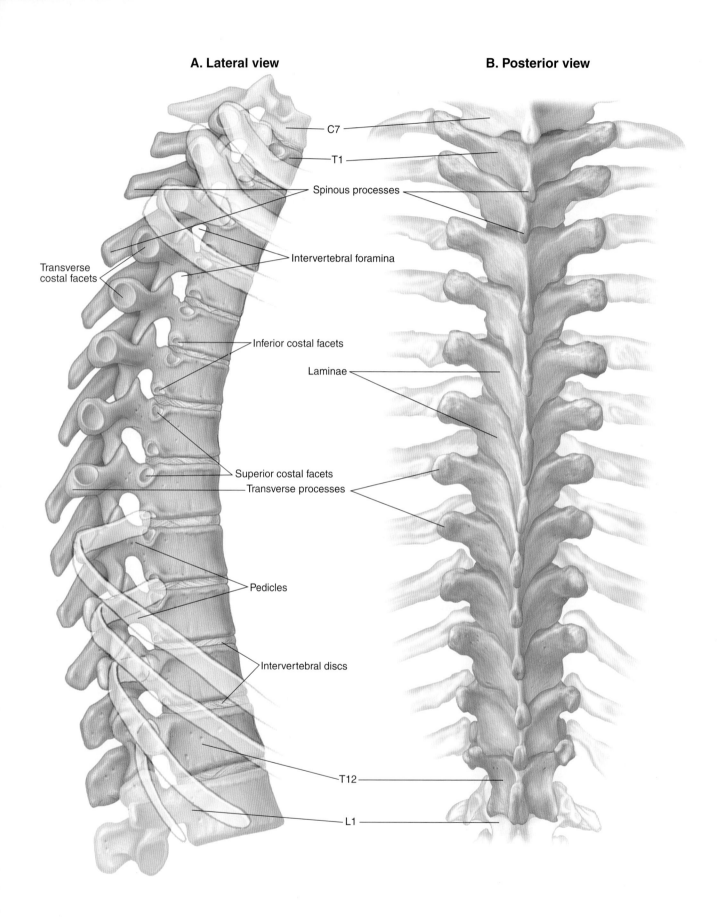

A. Lateral view

B. Posterior view

C7

T1

Spinous processes

Transverse
costal facets

Intervertebral foramina

Inferior costal facets

Laminae

Superior costal facets

Transverse processes

Pedicles

Intervertebral discs

T12

L1

A. Lateral view

B. Radiograph of lumbar vertebrae, lateral view

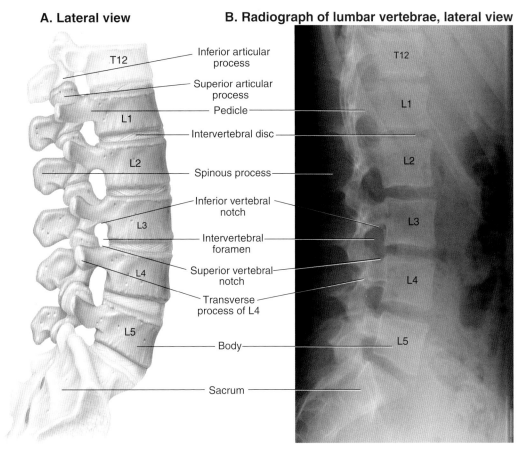

T12
Inferior articular process
Superior articular process
Pedicle
L1
Intervertebral disc
L2
Spinous process
Inferior vertebral notch
L3
Intervertebral foramen
Superior vertebral notch
L4
Transverse process of L4
L5
Body
Sacrum

T12
L1
L2
L3
L4
L5

C. Posterior view

D. Radiograph of lumbar vertebrae, posterior view

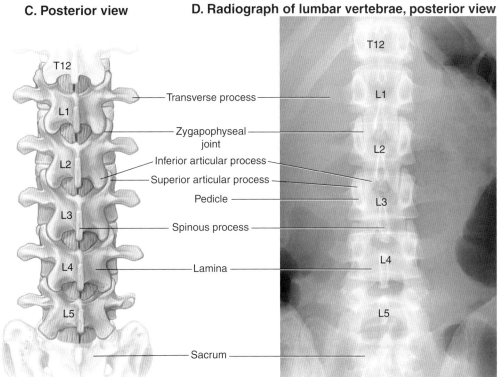

T12
L1
Transverse process
Zygapophyseal joint
L2
Inferior articular process
Superior articular process
Pedicle
L3
Spinous process
L4
Lamina
L5
Sacrum

T12
L1
L2
L3
L4
L5

PLATE 1-08 | **Sacrum and Coccyx**

A. Anterior view

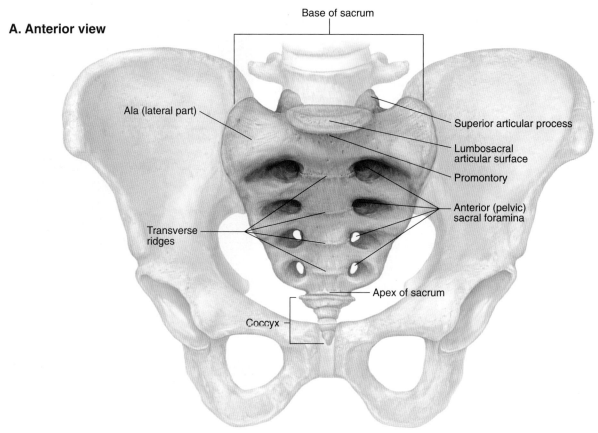

Base of sacrum

Ala (lateral part)

Superior articular process

Lumbosacral articular surface

Promontory

Anterior (pelvic) sacral foramina

Transverse ridges

Apex of sacrum

Coccyx

B. Posterior view

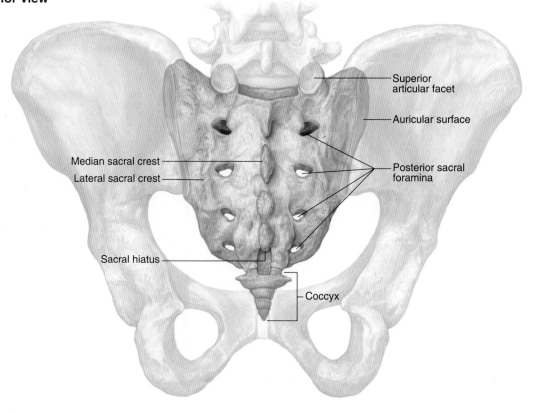

Superior articular facet

Auricular surface

Median sacral crest

Lateral sacral crest

Posterior sacral foramina

Sacral hiatus

Coccyx

A. Lateral view

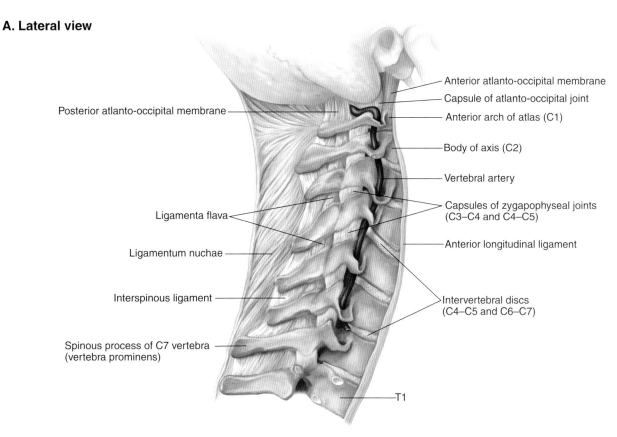

Anterior atlanto-occipital membrane

Capsule of atlanto-occipital joint

Posterior atlanto-occipital membrane

Anterior arch of atlas (C1)

Body of axis (C2)

Vertebral artery

Capsules of zygapophyseal joints (C3–C4 and C4–C5)

Ligamenta flava

Anterior longitudinal ligament

Ligamentum nuchae

Interspinous ligament

Intervertebral discs (C4–C5 and C6–C7)

Spinous process of C7 vertebra (vertebra prominens)

T1

B. Posterior view

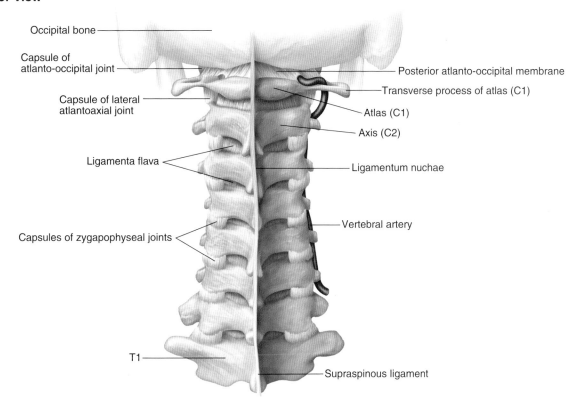

Occipital bone

Capsule of atlanto-occipital joint

Posterior atlanto-occipital membrane

Transverse process of atlas (C1)

Capsule of lateral atlantoaxial joint

Atlas (C1)

Axis (C2)

Ligamenta flava

Ligamentum nuchae

Capsules of zygapophyseal joints

Vertebral artery

T1

Supraspinous ligament

PLATE I-10   Ligaments of the Thoracic Vertebrae

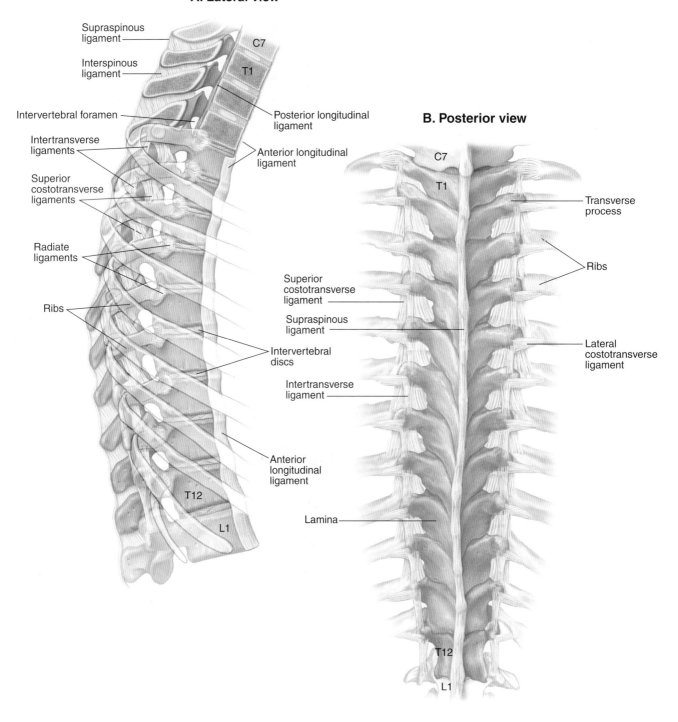

A. Lateral view

Supraspinous ligament

Interspinous ligament

Intervertebral foramen

Intertransverse ligaments

Superior costotransverse ligaments

Radiate ligaments

Ribs

C7

T1

Posterior longitudinal ligament

Anterior longitudinal ligament

Intervertebral discs

Anterior longitudinal ligament

T12

L1

B. Posterior view

C7

T1

Transverse process

Ribs

Superior costotransverse ligament

Supraspinous ligament

Intertransverse ligament

Lateral costotransverse ligament

Lamina

T12

L1

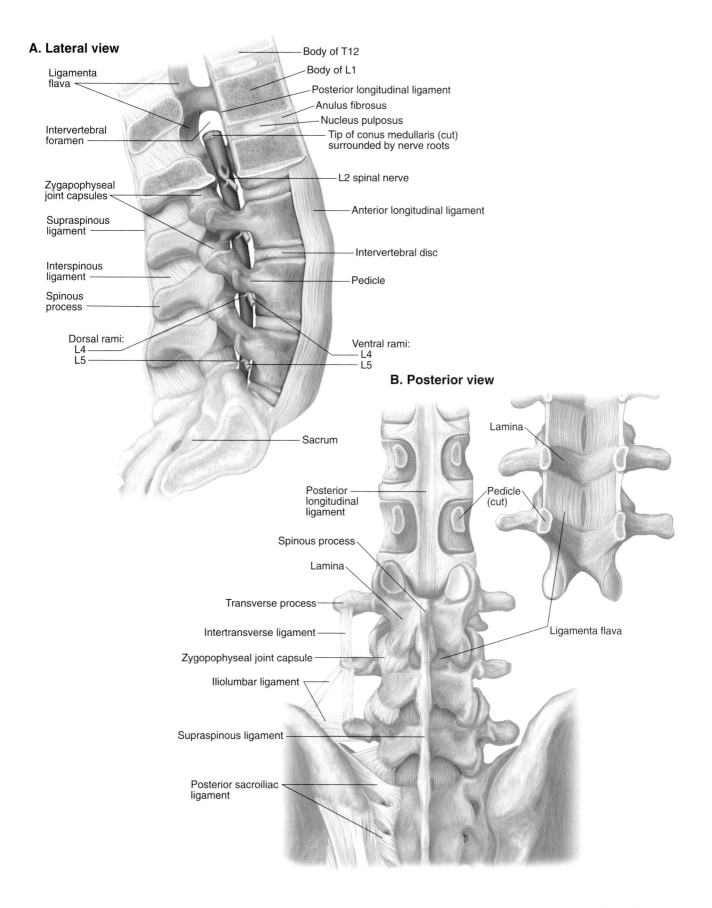

A. Lateral view

Ligamenta flava

Intervertebral foramen

Zygapophyseal joint capsules

Supraspinous ligament

Interspinous ligament

Spinous process

Dorsal rami:
L4
L5

Body of T12

Body of L1

Posterior longitudinal ligament

Anulus fibrosus

Nucleus pulposus

Tip of conus medullaris (cut) surrounded by nerve roots

L2 spinal nerve

Anterior longitudinal ligament

Intervertebral disc

Pedicle

Ventral rami:
L4
L5

Sacrum

B. Posterior view

Posterior longitudinal ligament

Spinous process

Lamina

Transverse process

Intertransverse ligament

Zygopophyseal joint capsule

Iliolumbar ligament

Supraspinous ligament

Posterior sacroiliac ligament

Lamina

Pedicle (cut)

Ligamenta flava

PLATE 1-12   **Cutaneous Innervation of the Back**

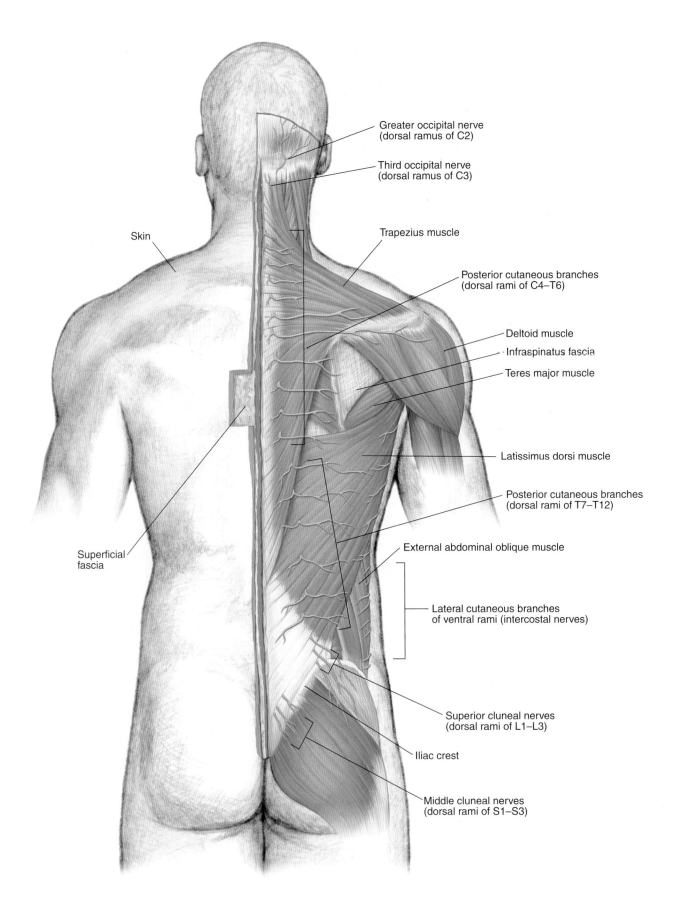

Greater occipital nerve
(dorsal ramus of C2)

Third occipital nerve
(dorsal ramus of C3)

Trapezius muscle

Skin

Posterior cutaneous branches
(dorsal rami of C4–T6)

Deltoid muscle

Infraspinatus fascia

Teres major muscle

Latissimus dorsi muscle

Posterior cutaneous branches
(dorsal rami of T7–T12)

External abdominal oblique muscle

Lateral cutaneous branches
of ventral rami (intercostal nerves)

Superficial
fascia

Superior cluneal nerves
(dorsal rami of L1–L3)

Iliac crest

Middle cluneal nerves
(dorsal rami of S1–S3)

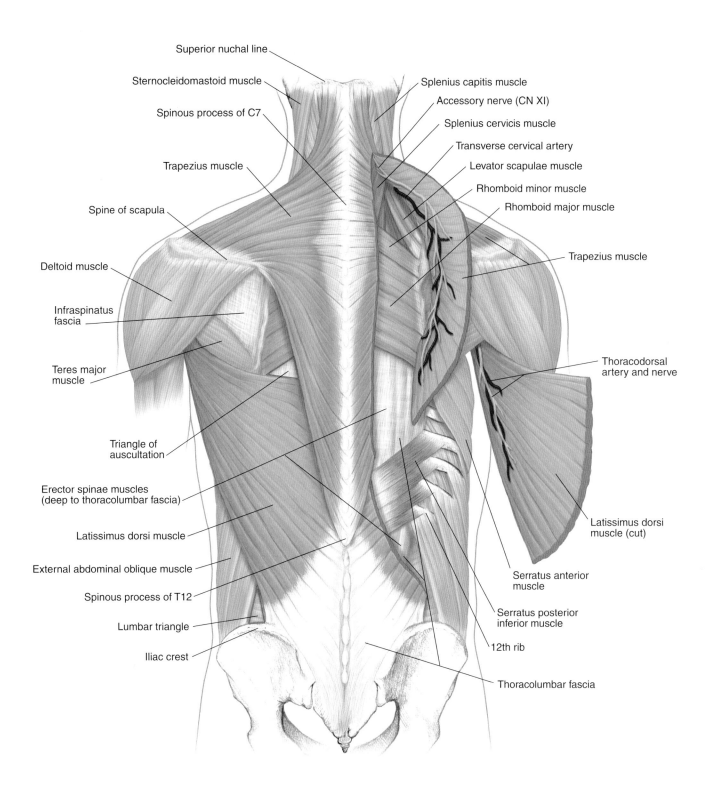

Superior nuchal line

Sternocleidomastoid muscle

Spinous process of C7

Trapezius muscle

Spine of scapula

Deltoid muscle

Infraspinatus fascia

Teres major muscle

Triangle of auscultation

Erector spinae muscles (deep to thoracolumbar fascia)

Latissimus dorsi muscle

External abdominal oblique muscle

Spinous process of T12

Lumbar triangle

Iliac crest

Splenius capitis muscle

Accessory nerve (CN XI)

Splenius cervicis muscle

Transverse cervical artery

Levator scapulae muscle

Rhomboid minor muscle

Rhomboid major muscle

Trapezius muscle

Thoracodorsal artery and nerve

Latissimus dorsi muscle (cut)

Serratus anterior muscle

Serratus posterior inferior muscle

12th rib

Thoracolumbar fascia

PLATE 1-14   **Deep Back Muscles, Superficial Dissection**

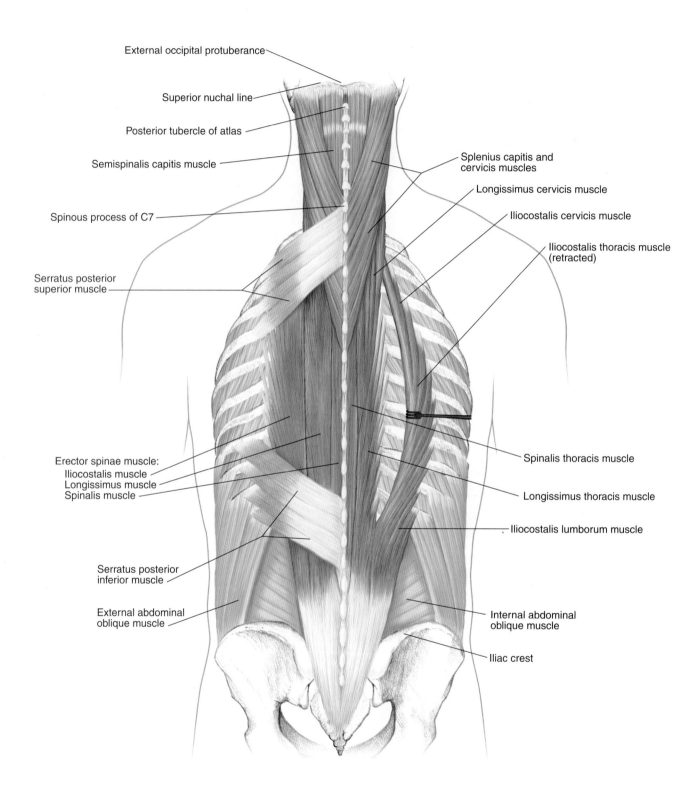

External occipital protuberance

Superior nuchal line

Posterior tubercle of atlas

Semispinalis capitis muscle

Spinous process of C7

Serratus posterior
superior muscle

Erector spinae muscle:
Iliocostalis muscle
Longissimus muscle
Spinalis muscle

Serratus posterior
inferior muscle

External abdominal
oblique muscle

Splenius capitis and
cervicis muscles

Longissimus cervicis muscle

Iliocostalis cervicis muscle

Iliocostalis thoracis muscle
(retracted)

Spinalis thoracis muscle

Longissimus thoracis muscle

Iliocostalis lumborum muscle

Internal abdominal
oblique muscle

Iliac crest

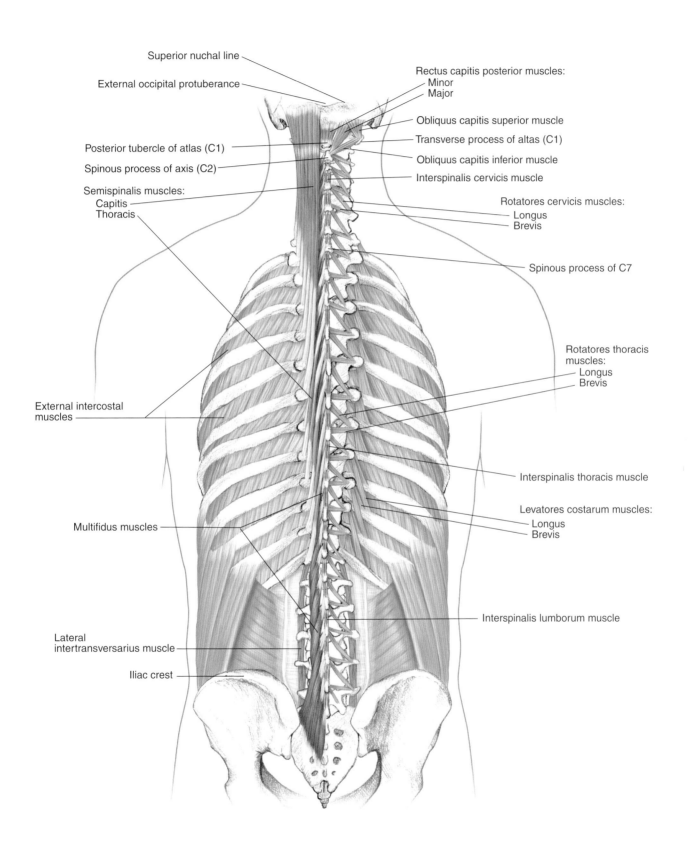

Superior nuchal line

External occipital protuberance

Rectus capitis posterior muscles:
Minor
Major

Obliquus capitis superior muscle

Transverse process of altas (C1)

Posterior tubercle of atlas (C1)

Obliquus capitis inferior muscle

Spinous process of axis (C2)

Interspinalis cervicis muscle

Semispinalis muscles:
Capitis
Thoracis

Rotatores cervicis muscles:
Longus
Brevis

Spinous process of C7

Rotatores thoracis muscles:
Longus
Brevis

External intercostal muscles

Interspinalis thoracis muscle

Levatores costarum muscles:
Longus
Brevis

Multifidus muscles

Interspinalis lumborum muscle

Lateral intertransversarius muscle

Iliac crest

PLATE 1-16   **Suboccipital Region**

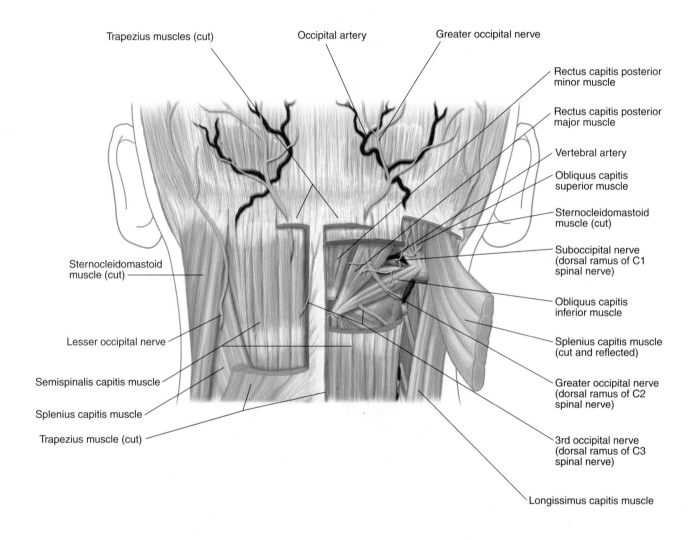

Trapezius muscles (cut)

Occipital artery

Greater occipital nerve

Rectus capitis posterior
minor muscle

Rectus capitis posterior
major muscle

Vertebral artery

Obliquus capitis
superior muscle

Sternocleidomastoid
muscle (cut)

Suboccipital nerve
(dorsal ramus of C1
spinal nerve)

Obliquus capitis
inferior muscle

Splenius capitis muscle
(cut and reflected)

Greater occipital nerve
(dorsal ramus of C2
spinal nerve)

3rd occipital nerve
(dorsal ramus of C3
spinal nerve)

Longissimus capitis muscle

Sternocleidomastoid
muscle (cut)

Lesser occipital nerve

Semispinalis capitis muscle

Splenius capitis muscle

Trapezius muscle (cut)

A. Orientation

B. Oblique section

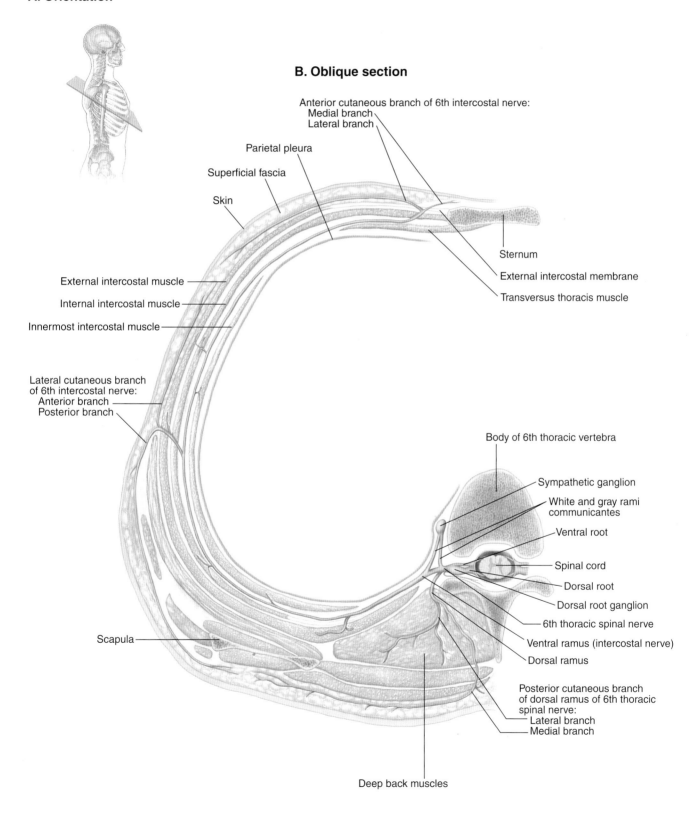

Anterior cutaneous branch of 6th intercostal nerve:
Medial branch
Lateral branch

Parietal pleura

Superficial fascia

Skin

Sternum

External intercostal membrane

Transversus thoracis muscle

External intercostal muscle

Internal intercostal muscle

Innermost intercostal muscle

Lateral cutaneous branch
of 6th intercostal nerve:
Anterior branch
Posterior branch

Body of 6th thoracic vertebra

Sympathetic ganglion

White and gray rami
communicantes

Ventral root

Spinal cord

Dorsal root

Dorsal root ganglion

6th thoracic spinal nerve

Ventral ramus (intercostal nerve)

Dorsal ramus

Scapula

Posterior cutaneous branch
of dorsal ramus of 6th thoracic
spinal nerve:
Lateral branch
Medial branch

Deep back muscles

PLATE I-18   Spinal Cord, Posterior View

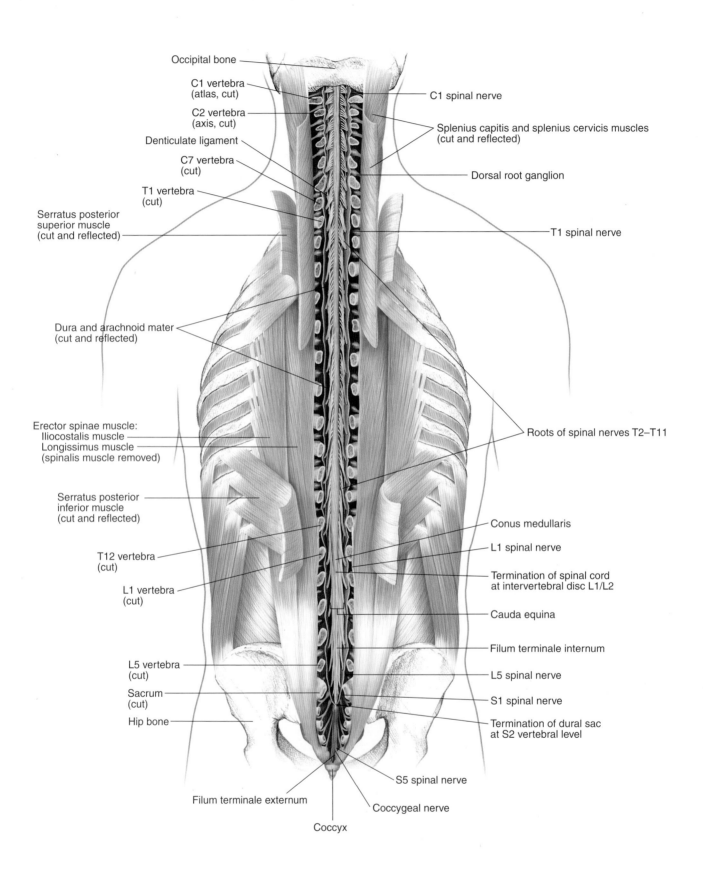

Occipital bone

C1 vertebra (atlas, cut)

C2 vertebra (axis, cut)

Denticulate ligament

C7 vertebra (cut)

T1 vertebra (cut)

Serratus posterior superior muscle (cut and reflected)

Dura and arachnoid mater (cut and reflected)

Erector spinae muscle: Iliocostalis muscle Longissimus muscle (spinalis muscle removed)

Serratus posterior inferior muscle (cut and reflected)

T12 vertebra (cut)

L1 vertebra (cut)

L5 vertebra (cut)

Sacrum (cut)

Hip bone

Filum terminale externum

Coccyx

C1 spinal nerve

Splenius capitis and splenius cervicis muscles (cut and reflected)

Dorsal root ganglion

T1 spinal nerve

Roots of spinal nerves T2–T11

Conus medullaris

L1 spinal nerve

Termination of spinal cord at intervertebral disc L1/L2

Cauda equina

Filum terminale internum

L5 spinal nerve

S1 spinal nerve

Termination of dural sac at S2 vertebral level

S5 spinal nerve

Coccygeal nerve

A. Orientation

B. Dissection

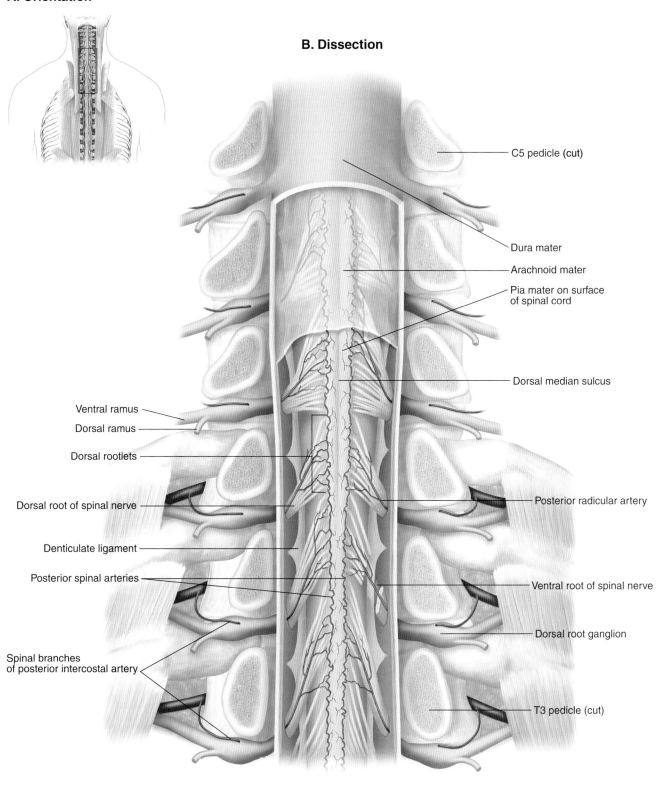

C5 pedicle (cut)

Dura mater

Arachnoid mater

Pia mater on surface of spinal cord

Dorsal median sulcus

Ventral ramus

Dorsal ramus

Dorsal rootlets

Posterior radicular artery

Dorsal root of spinal nerve

Denticulate ligament

Ventral root of spinal nerve

Posterior spinal arteries

Dorsal root ganglion

Spinal branches of posterior intercostal artery

T3 pedicle (cut)

PLATE 1-20   Inferior Portion of the Spinal Cord

A. Orientation

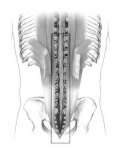

B. Dissection

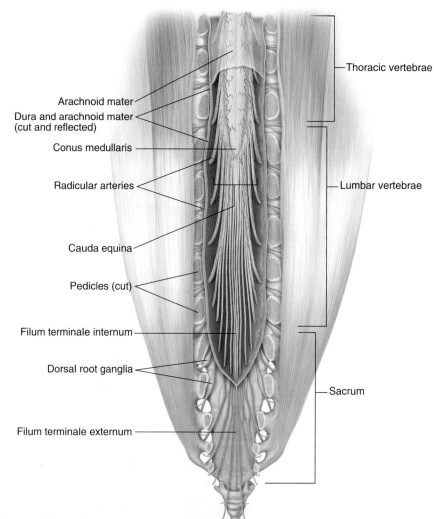

Arachnoid mater

Dura and arachnoid mater
(cut and reflected)

Conus medullaris

Radicular arteries

Cauda equina

Pedicles (cut)

Filum terminale internum

Dorsal root ganglia

Filum terminale externum

Thoracic vertebrae

Lumbar vertebrae

Sacrum

C. MRI (T2 weighted), sagittal view

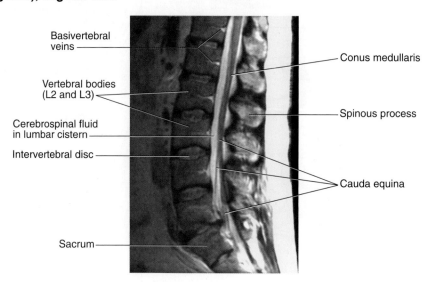

Basivertebral
veins

Vertebral bodies
(L2 and L3)

Cerebrospinal fluid
in lumbar cistern

Intervertebral disc

Sacrum

Conus medullaris

Spinous process

Cauda equina

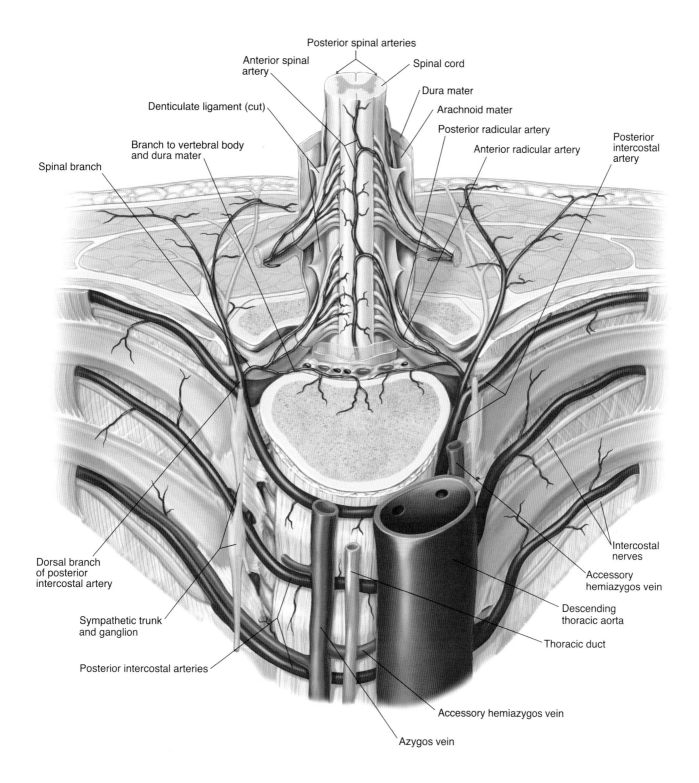

Posterior spinal arteries

Anterior spinal artery

Spinal cord

Dura mater

Denticulate ligament (cut)

Arachnoid mater

Posterior radicular artery

Branch to vertebral body and dura mater

Anterior radicular artery

Posterior intercostal artery

Spinal branch

Intercostal nerves

Accessory hemiazygos vein

Dorsal branch of posterior intercostal artery

Descending thoracic aorta

Sympathetic trunk and ganglion

Thoracic duct

Posterior intercostal arteries

Accessory hemiazygos vein

Azygos vein

PLATE 1-22 **Venous Drainage of the Vertebral Column and Spinal Cord**

A. Sagittal view

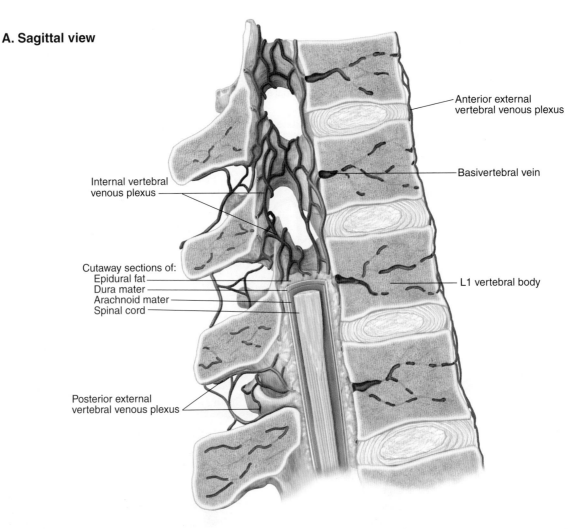

Anterior external
vertebral venous plexus

Internal vertebral
venous plexus

Basivertebral vein

Cutaway sections of:
Epidural fat
Dura mater
Arachnoid mater
Spinal cord

L1 vertebral body

Posterior external
vertebral venous plexus

B. Superior view

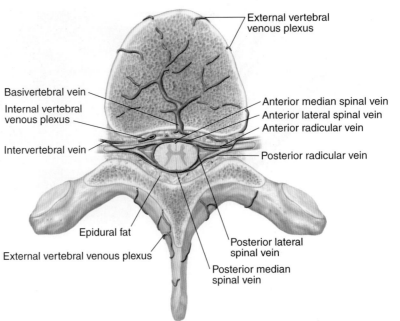

External vertebral
venous plexus

Basivertebral vein

Internal vertebral
venous plexus

Intervertebral vein

Anterior median spinal vein
Anterior lateral spinal vein
Anterior radicular vein

Posterior radicular vein

Epidural fat

External vertebral venous plexus

Posterior lateral
spinal vein

Posterior median
spinal vein

A. Anterior view

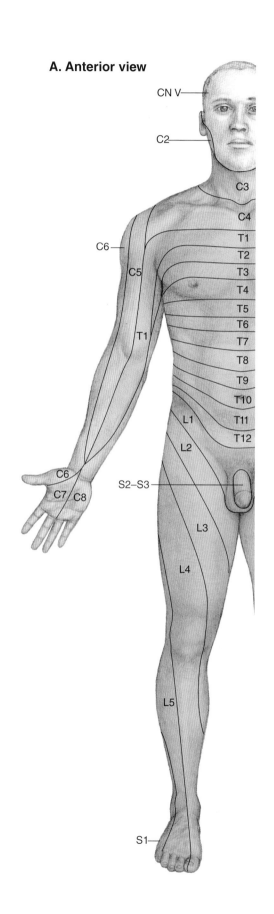

CN V
C2
C3
C4
C6
C5
T1
C6
C7 C8
T1
T2
T3
T4
T5
T6
T7
T8
T9
T10
T11
T12
L1
L2
S2–S3
L3
L4
L5
S1

B. Posterior view

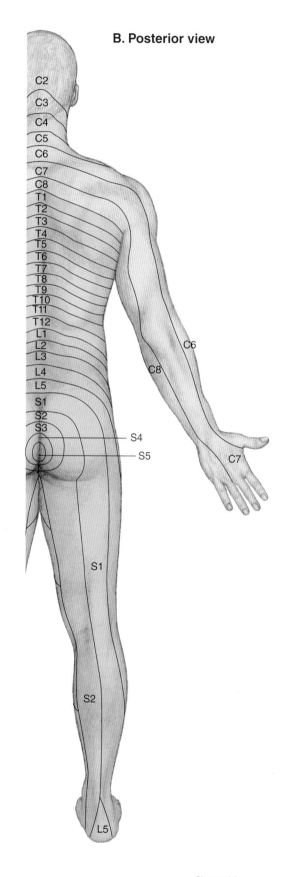

C2
C3
C4
C5
C6
C7
C8
T1
T2
T3
T4
T5
T6
T7
T8
T9
T10
T11
T12
L1
L2
L3
L4
L5
S1
S2
S3
S4
S5
C6
C8
C7
S1
S2
L5

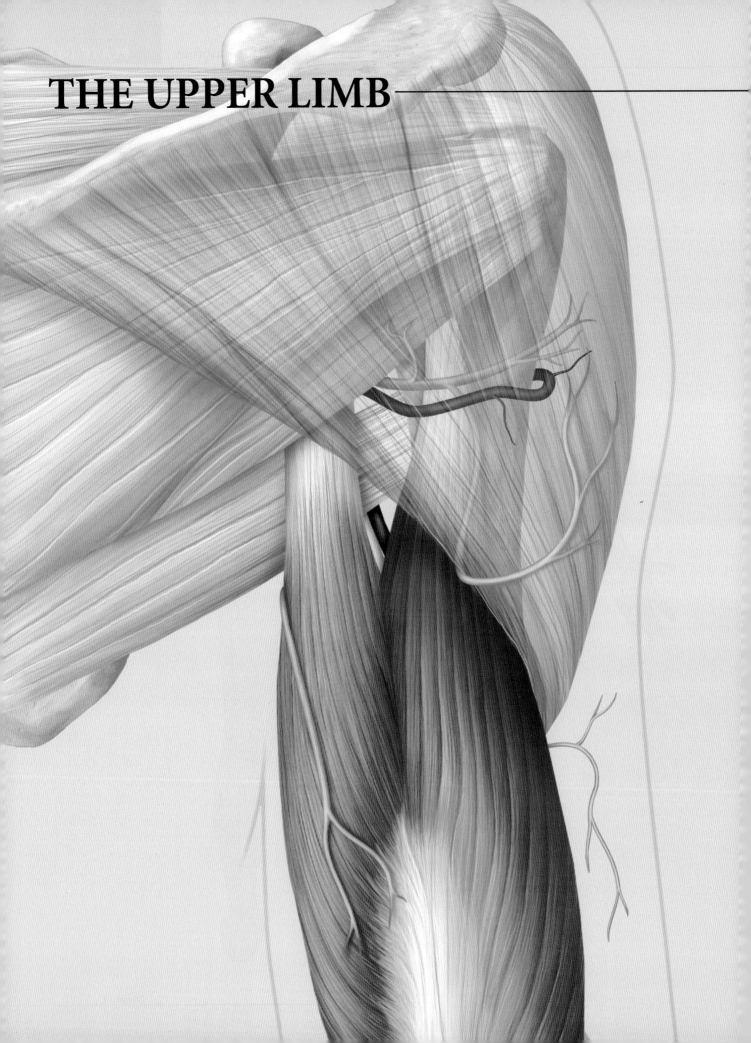

THE UPPER LIMB

PLATE 2-01 **Palpable Features of the Upper Limb**

A. Anterior view

B. Posterior view

Palpable bony structures

Coracoid process
of scapula

Superior border of clavicle

Acromioclavicular joint

Jugular notch

Acromion of scapula

Acromion of scapula

Greater tubercle
of humerus

Greater tubercle
of humerus

Lesser tubercle
of humerus

Scapular spine

Medial (vertebral)
border of scapula

Inferior angle
of scapula

Olecranon

Lateral epicondyle
of humerus

Lateral epicondyle
of humerus

Medial epicondyle
of humerus

Head of radius

Posterior border of ulna

Distal lateral
border of radius

Distal lateral
border of radius

Dorsal radial
tubercle

Radial styloid
process

Head of ulna

Styloid process

Tubercle of
scaphoid

Ulnar styloid process

Capitate

Pisiform

Tubercle of
trapezium

Hook of hamate

Heads of metacarpals

Bases, shafts, and
heads of phalanges

Posterior aspects of
metacarpals and phalanges

A. Anterior view

Supraclavicular nerves

Superior lateral brachial cutaneous nerve

Inferior lateral brachial cutaneous nerve

Brachial fascia

Lateral antebrachial cutaneous nerve

Antebrachial fascia

Cephalic vein

Superficial branch of radial nerve

Palmar branch of median nerve

Medial brachial cutaneous nerve

Intercostobrachial nerve

Medial antebrachial cutaneous nerve

Median cubital vein

Dorsal branch of ulnar nerve

Palmar branch of ulnar nerve

B. Posterior view

Supraclavicular nerve

Superior lateral brachial cutaneous nerve

Posterior brachial cutaneous nerve

Inferior lateral brachial cutaneous nerve

Brachial fascia

Posterior antebrachial cutaneous nerve

Antebrachial fascia

Cephalic vein

Superficial branch of radial nerve

Dorsal branch of ulnar nerve

Dorsal venous network

Dorsal metacarpal veins

Basilic vein

PLATE 2-03   Skeleton of the Proximal Upper Limb

A. Anterior view

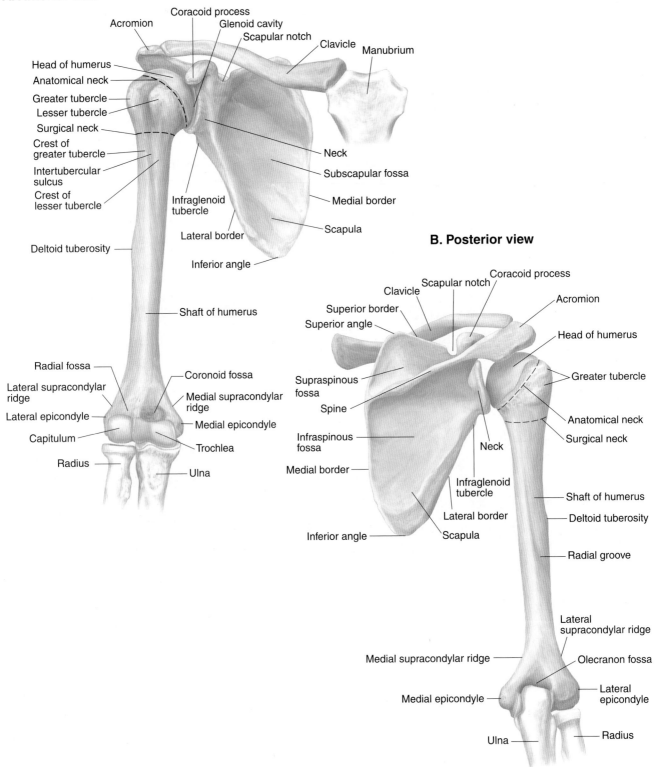

Coracoid process
Acromion
Glenoid cavity
Scapular notch
Clavicle
Manubrium
Head of humerus
Anatomical neck
Greater tubercle
Lesser tubercle
Surgical neck
Crest of greater tubercle
Intertubercular sulcus
Crest of lesser tubercle
Infraglenoid tubercle
Neck
Subscapular fossa
Medial border
Scapula
Lateral border
Deltoid tuberosity
Inferior angle
Shaft of humerus

B. Posterior view

Coracoid process
Scapular notch
Clavicle
Acromion
Superior border
Superior angle
Head of humerus
Supraspinous fossa
Spine
Greater tubercle
Infraspinous fossa
Anatomical neck
Surgical neck
Medial border
Neck
Infraglenoid tubercle
Shaft of humerus
Lateral border
Deltoid tuberosity
Inferior angle
Scapula
Radial groove

Radial fossa
Coronoid fossa
Lateral supracondylar ridge
Medial supracondylar ridge
Lateral epicondyle
Medial epicondyle
Capitulum
Trochlea
Radius
Ulna

Lateral supracondylar ridge
Medial supracondylar ridge
Olecranon fossa
Lateral epicondyle
Medial epicondyle
Ulna
Radius

A. Anterior view

B. Posterior view

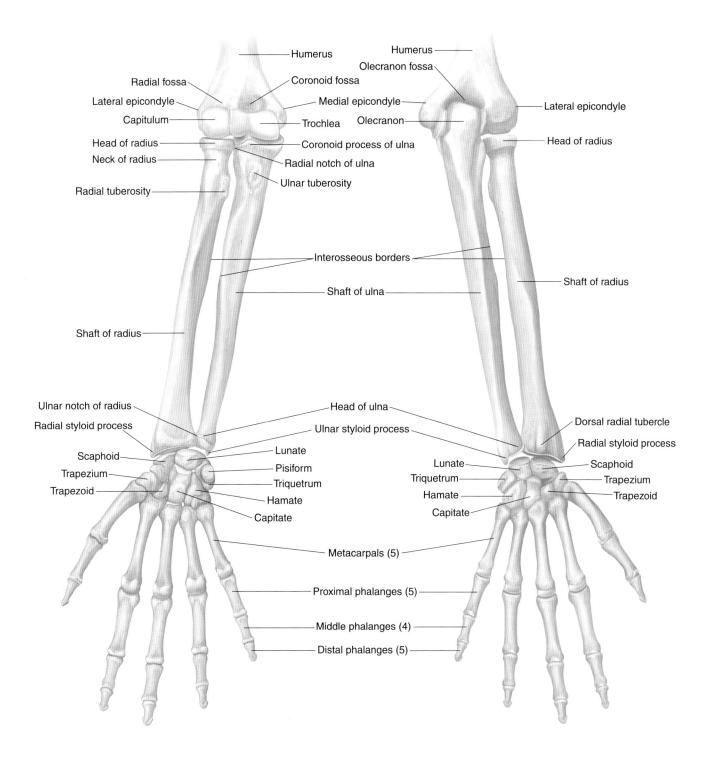

Humerus

Radial fossa

Lateral epicondyle

Capitulum

Head of radius

Neck of radius

Radial tuberosity

Coronoid fossa

Medial epicondyle

Trochlea

Coronoid process of ulna

Radial notch of ulna

Ulnar tuberosity

Humerus

Olecranon fossa

Olecranon

Lateral epicondyle

Head of radius

Interosseous borders

Shaft of ulna

Shaft of radius

Shaft of radius

Ulnar notch of radius

Radial styloid process

Scaphoid

Trapezium

Trapezoid

Head of ulna

Ulnar styloid process

Lunate

Pisiform

Triquetrum

Hamate

Capitate

Dorsal radial tubercle

Radial styloid process

Scaphoid

Trapezium

Trapezoid

Lunate

Triquetrum

Hamate

Capitate

Metacarpals (5)

Proximal phalanges (5)

Middle phalanges (4)

Distal phalanges (5)

PLATE 2-05   **Radiographs of the Upper Limb**

A. Right shoulder, anterior view

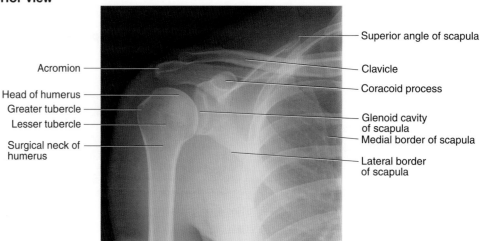

Acromion

Head of humerus
Greater tubercle
Lesser tubercle

Surgical neck of
humerus

Superior angle of scapula

Clavicle

Coracoid process

Glenoid cavity
of scapula
Medial border of scapula

Lateral border
of scapula

B. Right elbow, anterior view

Lateral supracondylar ridge

Lateral epicondyle
Capitulum
Head of radius
Neck of radius

Radial tuberosity

Medial supracondylar ridge
Coronoid fossa
Medial epicondyle
Olecranon
Trochlea
Coronoid process
of ulna

C. Right wrist and hand, anterior view

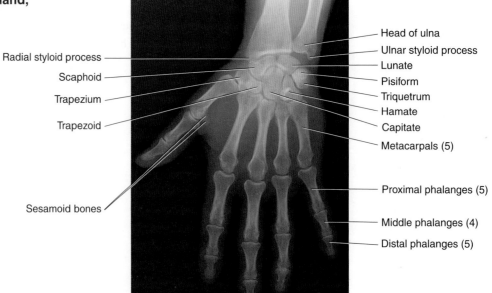

Radial styloid process
Scaphoid
Trapezium
Trapezoid

Sesamoid bones

Head of ulna
Ulnar styloid process
Lunate
Pisiform
Triquetrum
Hamate
Capitate
Metacarpals (5)

Proximal phalanges (5)

Middle phalanges (4)

Distal phalanges (5)

A. Anterior view

Biceps brachii muscle (long head)

Trapezius muscle

Deltoid muscle

Pectoralis minor muscle

Omohyoid muscle

Coracobrachialis muscle and biceps brachii muscle (short head) shared origin

Supraspinatus muscle

Subscapularis muscle

Pectoralis major muscle

Latissimus dorsi muscle

Teres major muscle

Serratus anterior muscle

Deltoid muscle

Coracobrachialis muscle

Subscapularis muscle

Triceps brachii muscle (long head)

Brachialis muscle

Brachioradialis muscle

Extensor carpi radialis longus muscle

Common extensor tendon

Pronator teres muscle (humeral head)

Common flexor tendon

B. Posterior view

Brachialis muscle

Biceps brachii muscle

Biceps brachii muscle (long head)

Supraspinatus muscle

Levator scapulae muscle

Rhomboid minor muscle

Trapezius muscle

Deltoid muscle

Supraspinatus muscle

Infraspinatus muscle

Teres minor muscle

Triceps brachii muscle (lateral head)

Teres minor muscle

Infraspinatus muscle

Rhomboid major muscle

Triceps brachii muscle (long head)

Deltoid muscle

Teres major muscle

Brachialis muscle

Latissimus dorsi muscle*

Triceps brachii muscle (medial head)

Triceps brachii muscle

Common flexor tendon

Common extensor tendon

Anconeus muscle

Muscle attachments

Origins

Insertions

*Small slip of origin in 53% of cases

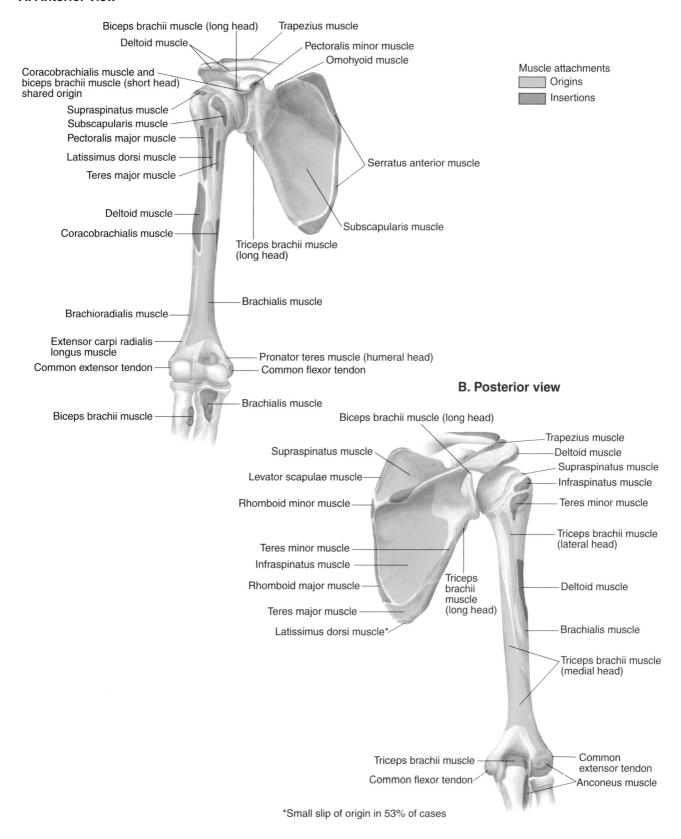

PLATE 2-07 | **Superficial Muscles of the Back**

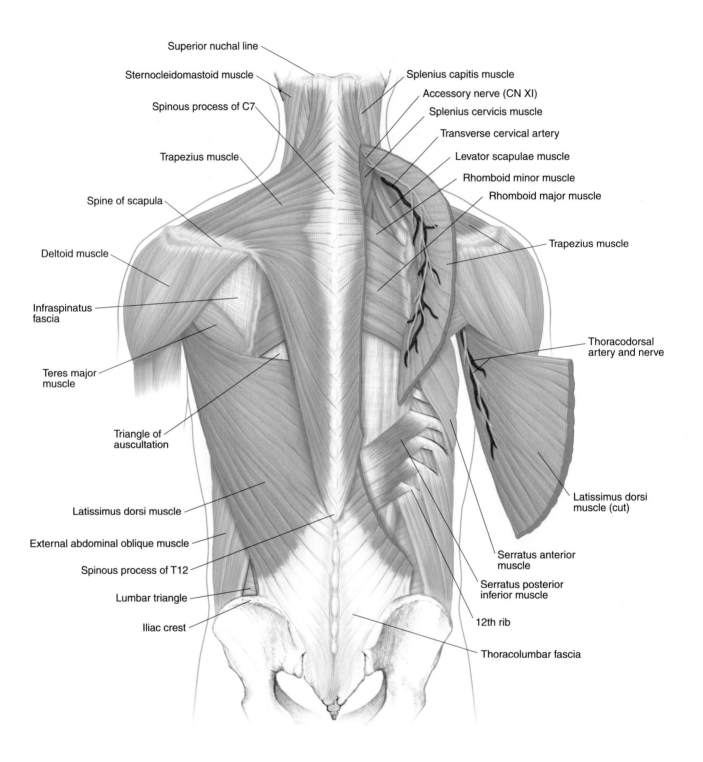

Superior nuchal line

Sternocleidomastoid muscle

Spinous process of C7

Trapezius muscle

Spine of scapula

Deltoid muscle

Infraspinatus fascia

Teres major muscle

Triangle of auscultation

Latissimus dorsi muscle

External abdominal oblique muscle

Spinous process of T12

Lumbar triangle

Iliac crest

Splenius capitis muscle

Accessory nerve (CN XI)

Splenius cervicis muscle

Transverse cervical artery

Levator scapulae muscle

Rhomboid minor muscle

Rhomboid major muscle

Trapezius muscle

Thoracodorsal artery and nerve

Latissimus dorsi muscle (cut)

Serratus anterior muscle

Serratus posterior inferior muscle

12th rib

Thoracolumbar fascia

A. Superficial view

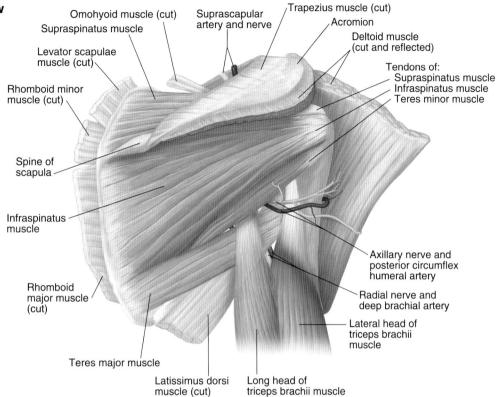

Omohyoid muscle (cut)

Supraspinatus muscle

Suprascapular artery and nerve

Trapezius muscle (cut)

Acromion

Deltoid muscle (cut and reflected)

Tendons of:
Supraspinatus muscle
Infraspinatus muscle
Teres minor muscle

Levator scapulae muscle (cut)

Rhomboid minor muscle (cut)

Spine of scapula

Infraspinatus muscle

Rhomboid major muscle (cut)

Axillary nerve and posterior circumflex humeral artery

Radial nerve and deep brachial artery

Lateral head of triceps brachii muscle

Teres major muscle

Latissimus dorsi muscle (cut)

Long head of triceps brachii muscle

B. Deep view

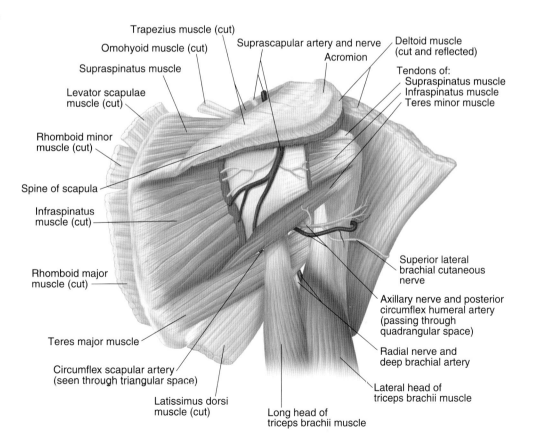

Trapezius muscle (cut)

Omohyoid muscle (cut)

Suprascapular artery and nerve

Acromion

Deltoid muscle (cut and reflected)

Supraspinatus muscle

Tendons of:
Supraspinatus muscle
Infraspinatus muscle
Teres minor muscle

Levator scapulae muscle (cut)

Rhomboid minor muscle (cut)

Spine of scapula

Infraspinatus muscle (cut)

Superior lateral brachial cutaneous nerve

Rhomboid major muscle (cut)

Axillary nerve and posterior circumflex humeral artery (passing through quadrangular space)

Teres major muscle

Radial nerve and deep brachial artery

Circumflex scapular artery (seen through triangular space)

Lateral head of triceps brachii muscle

Latissimus dorsi muscle (cut)

Long head of triceps brachii muscle

PLATE 2-09   **Blood Supply to the Shoulder**

A. Arteries

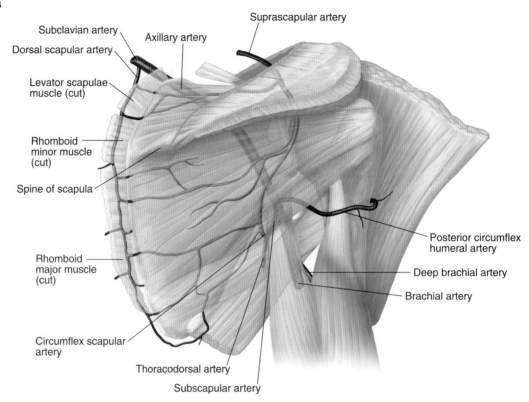

Subclavian artery

Dorsal scapular artery

Levator scapulae muscle (cut)

Rhomboid minor muscle (cut)

Spine of scapula

Rhomboid major muscle (cut)

Circumflex scapular artery

Axillary artery

Suprascapular artery

Posterior circumflex humeral artery

Deep brachial artery

Brachial artery

Thoracodorsal artery

Subscapular artery

B. Angiogram

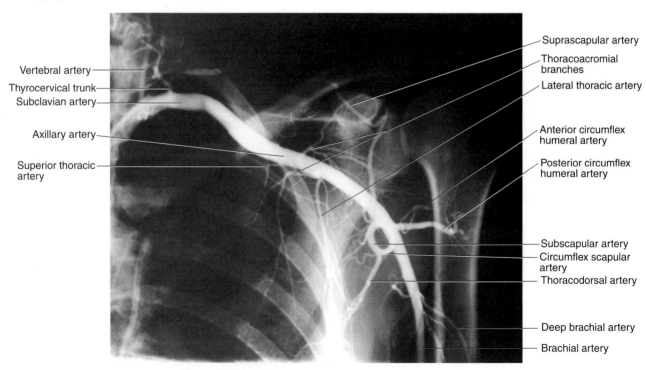

Vertebral artery

Thyrocervical trunk

Subclavian artery

Axillary artery

Superior thoracic artery

Suprascapular artery

Thoracoacromial branches

Lateral thoracic artery

Anterior circumflex humeral artery

Posterior circumflex humeral artery

Subscapular artery

Circumflex scapular artery

Thoracodorsal artery

Deep brachial artery

Brachial artery

A. Anterior view

Pectoralis major muscle, deep to pectoral fascia

Areolar glands

Axillary tail

Suspensory ligaments

Serratus anterior muscle

External abdominal oblique muscle

Lobes

Fat

Lactiferous sinus

Lactiferous ducts

Nipple

Areola

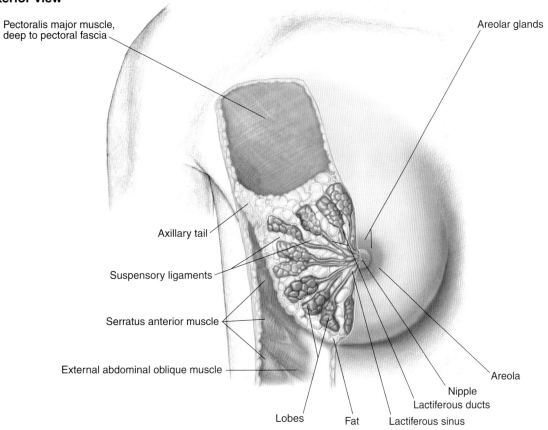

B. Sagittal section

Clavicle

Pectoralis major muscle

Pectoral fascia

2nd rib

Intercostal vessels and nerves

Intercostal muscles

Pectoralis minor muscle

Lung

6th rib

Suspensory ligaments

Lactiferous ducts

Lactiferous sinus

Fat (superficial fascia)

Lobes

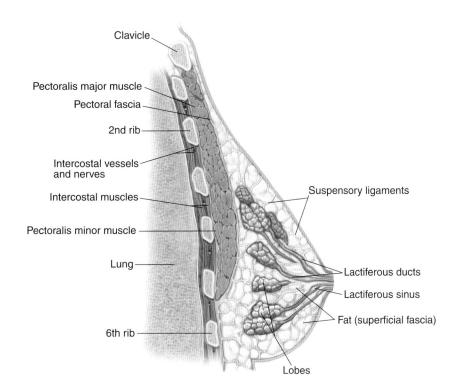

PLATE 2-11 **Blood Supply and Lymphatic Drainage of the Breast**

A. Arteries

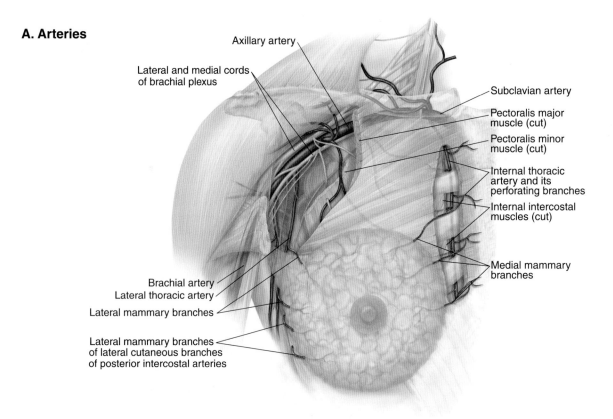

Axillary artery

Lateral and medial cords of brachial plexus

Subclavian artery

Pectoralis major muscle (cut)

Pectoralis minor muscle (cut)

Internal thoracic artery and its perforating branches

Internal intercostal muscles (cut)

Medial mammary branches

Brachial artery

Lateral thoracic artery

Lateral mammary branches

Lateral mammary branches of lateral cutaneous branches of posterior intercostal arteries

B. Lymphatic drainage

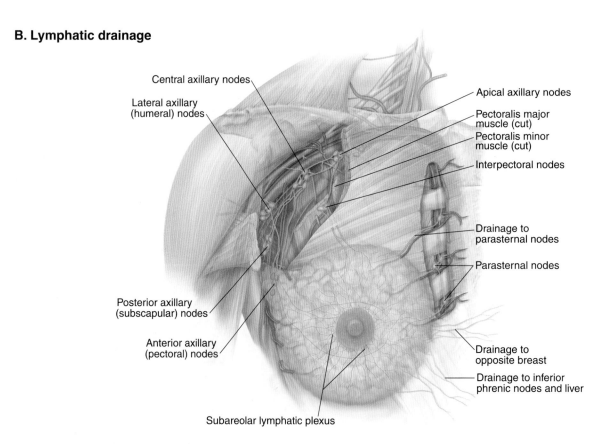

Central axillary nodes

Lateral axillary (humeral) nodes

Apical axillary nodes

Pectoralis major muscle (cut)

Pectoralis minor muscle (cut)

Interpectoral nodes

Drainage to parasternal nodes

Parasternal nodes

Posterior axillary (subscapular) nodes

Anterior axillary (pectoral) nodes

Drainage to opposite breast

Drainage to inferior phrenic nodes and liver

Subareolar lymphatic plexus

A. Superficial dissection

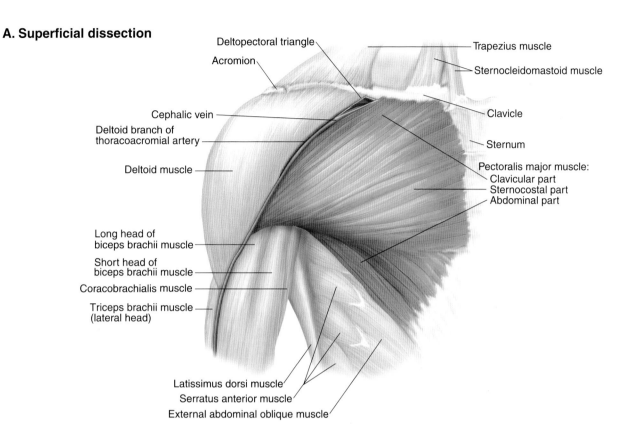

Deltopectoral triangle

Acromion

Cephalic vein

Deltoid branch of thoracoacromial artery

Deltoid muscle

Long head of biceps brachii muscle

Short head of biceps brachii muscle

Coracobrachialis muscle

Triceps brachii muscle (lateral head)

Latissimus dorsi muscle

Serratus anterior muscle

External abdominal oblique muscle

Trapezius muscle

Sternocleidomastoid muscle

Clavicle

Sternum

Pectoralis major muscle:
Clavicular part
Sternocostal part
Abdominal part

B. Deep dissection

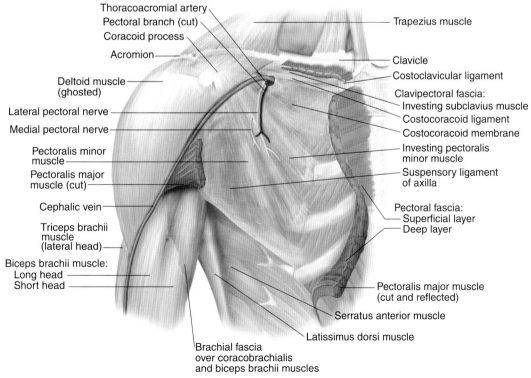

Thoracoacromial artery

Pectoral branch (cut)

Coracoid process

Acromion

Deltoid muscle (ghosted)

Lateral pectoral nerve

Medial pectoral nerve

Pectoralis minor muscle

Pectoralis major muscle (cut)

Cephalic vein

Triceps brachii muscle (lateral head)

Biceps brachii muscle:
Long head
Short head

Brachial fascia over coracobrachialis and biceps brachii muscles

Trapezius muscle

Clavicle

Costoclavicular ligament

Clavipectoral fascia:
Investing subclavius muscle
Costocoracoid ligament
Costocoracoid membrane

Investing pectoralis minor muscle

Suspensory ligament of axilla

Pectoral fascia:
Superficial layer
Deep layer

Pectoralis major muscle (cut and reflected)

Serratus anterior muscle

Latissimus dorsi muscle

PLATE 2-13   **Brachial Plexus and Nerves of the Axilla**

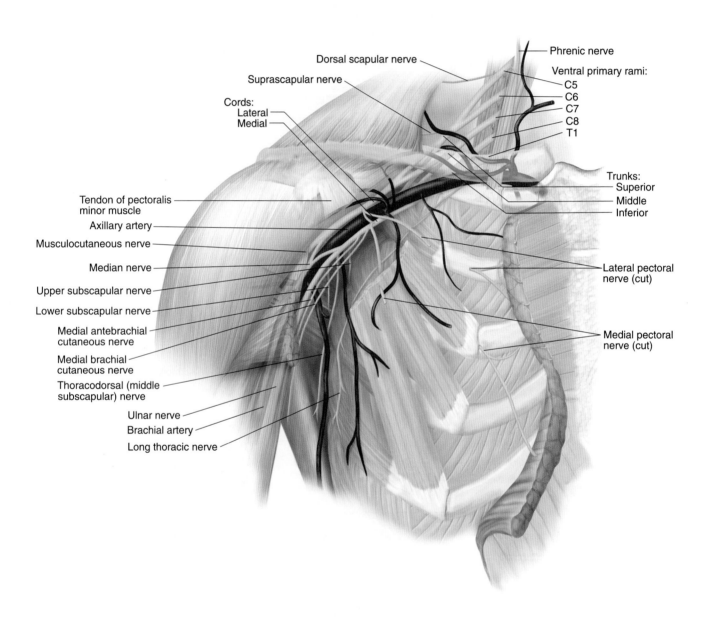

Dorsal scapular nerve

Suprascapular nerve

Cords:
Lateral
Medial

Tendon of pectoralis
minor muscle

Axillary artery

Musculocutaneous nerve

Median nerve

Upper subscapular nerve

Lower subscapular nerve

Medial antebrachial
cutaneous nerve

Medial brachial
cutaneous nerve

Thoracodorsal (middle
subscapular) nerve

Ulnar nerve

Brachial artery

Long thoracic nerve

Phrenic nerve

Ventral primary rami:
C5
C6
C7
C8
T1

Trunks:
Superior
Middle
Inferior

Lateral pectoral
nerve (cut)

Medial pectoral
nerve (cut)

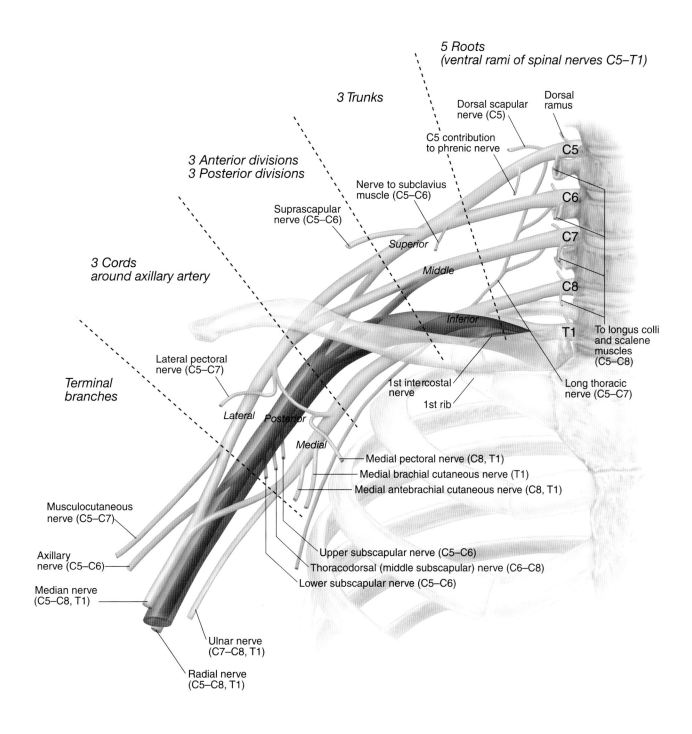

5 Roots
(ventral rami of spinal nerves C5–T1)

3 Trunks

Dorsal scapular
nerve (C5)

Dorsal
ramus

C5 contribution
to phrenic nerve

C5

3 Anterior divisions
3 Posterior divisions

Nerve to subclavius
muscle (C5–C6)

C6

Suprascapular
nerve (C5–C6)

C7

Superior

3 Cords
around axillary artery

Middle

C8

Inferior

T1

To longus colli
and scalene
muscles
(C5–C8)

Lateral pectoral
nerve (C5–C7)

1st intercostal
nerve

Long thoracic
nerve (C5–C7)

Terminal
branches

1st rib

Lateral   Posterior

Medial

Medial pectoral nerve (C8, T1)

Medial brachial cutaneous nerve (T1)

Medial antebrachial cutaneous nerve (C8, T1)

Musculocutaneous
nerve (C5–C7)

Upper subscapular nerve (C5–C6)

Thoracodorsal (middle subscapular) nerve (C6–C8)

Axillary
nerve (C5–C6)

Lower subscapular nerve (C5–C6)

Median nerve
(C5–C8, T1)

Ulnar nerve
(C7–C8, T1)

Radial nerve
(C5–C8, T1)

PLATE 2-15   **Axillary Artery and Its Branches**

A. Axillary artery, dissection

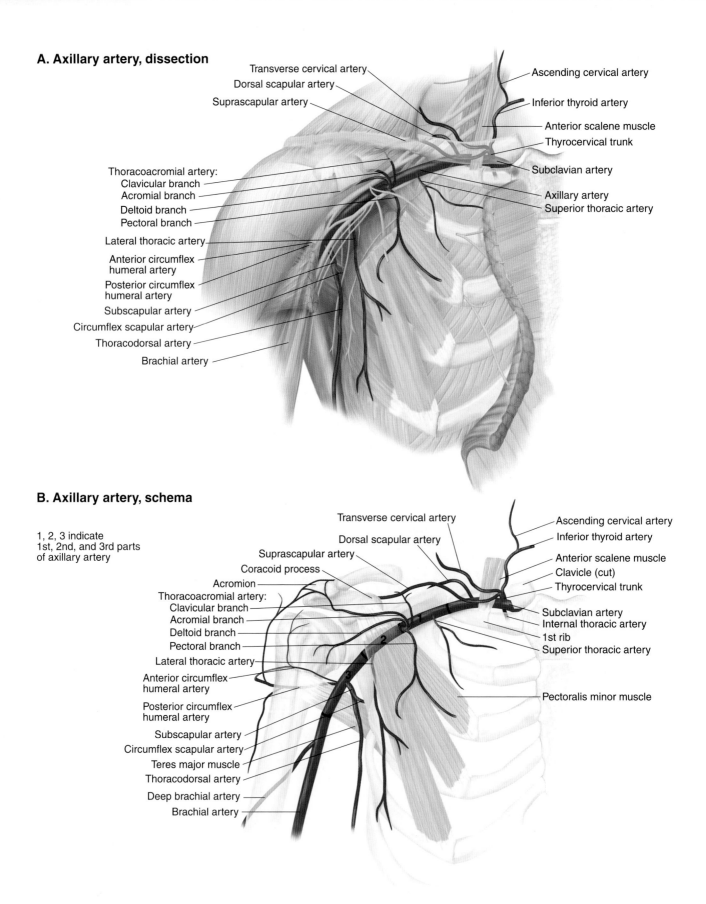

Transverse cervical artery
Dorsal scapular artery
Suprascapular artery

Ascending cervical artery
Inferior thyroid artery
Anterior scalene muscle
Thyrocervical trunk
Subclavian artery
Axillary artery
Superior thoracic artery

Thoracoacromial artery:
Clavicular branch
Acromial branch
Deltoid branch
Pectoral branch
Lateral thoracic artery
Anterior circumflex humeral artery
Posterior circumflex humeral artery
Subscapular artery
Circumflex scapular artery
Thoracodorsal artery
Brachial artery

B. Axillary artery, schema

1, 2, 3 indicate
1st, 2nd, and 3rd parts
of axillary artery

Transverse cervical artery
Dorsal scapular artery
Suprascapular artery
Coracoid process
Acromion
Thoracoacromial artery:
Clavicular branch
Acromial branch
Deltoid branch
Pectoral branch
Lateral thoracic artery
Anterior circumflex humeral artery
Posterior circumflex humeral artery
Subscapular artery
Circumflex scapular artery
Teres major muscle
Thoracodorsal artery
Deep brachial artery
Brachial artery

Ascending cervical artery
Inferior thyroid artery
Anterior scalene muscle
Clavicle (cut)
Thyrocervical trunk
Subclavian artery
Internal thoracic artery
1st rib
Superior thoracic artery
Pectoralis minor muscle

A. Posterior view

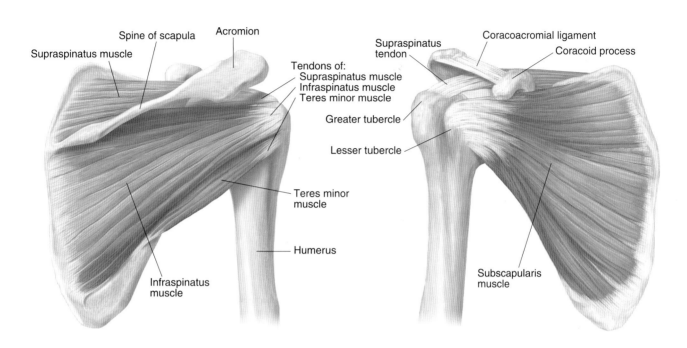

Spine of scapula

Acromion

Supraspinatus muscle

Tendons of:
Supraspinatus muscle
Infraspinatus muscle
Teres minor muscle

Greater tubercle

Lesser tubercle

Teres minor muscle

Humerus

Infraspinatus muscle

B. Anterior view

Supraspinatus tendon

Coracoacromial ligament

Coracoid process

Subscapularis muscle

C. Superolateral view

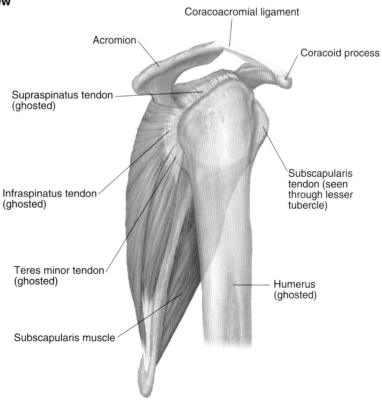

Coracoacromial ligament

Acromion

Coracoid process

Supraspinatus tendon (ghosted)

Infraspinatus tendon (ghosted)

Subscapularis tendon (seen through lesser tubercle)

Teres minor tendon (ghosted)

Humerus (ghosted)

Subscapularis muscle

PLATE 2-17   **Muscles of the Anterior Arm**

A. Superficial view

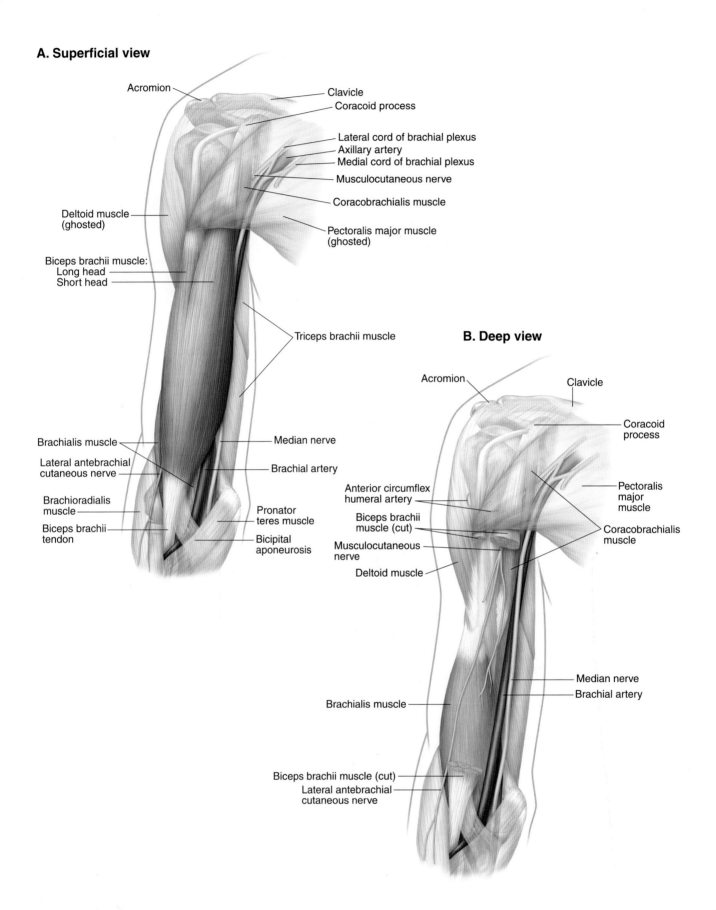

Acromion

Clavicle

Coracoid process

Lateral cord of brachial plexus

Axillary artery

Medial cord of brachial plexus

Musculocutaneous nerve

Coracobrachialis muscle

Deltoid muscle (ghosted)

Pectoralis major muscle (ghosted)

Biceps brachii muscle:
Long head
Short head

Triceps brachii muscle

B. Deep view

Acromion

Clavicle

Coracoid process

Pectoralis major muscle

Anterior circumflex humeral artery

Coracobrachialis muscle

Biceps brachii muscle (cut)

Musculocutaneous nerve

Deltoid muscle

Brachialis muscle

Lateral antebrachial cutaneous nerve

Brachioradialis muscle

Biceps brachii tendon

Median nerve

Brachial artery

Pronator teres muscle

Bicipital aponeurosis

Median nerve

Brachial artery

Brachialis muscle

Biceps brachii muscle (cut)

Lateral antebrachial cutaneous nerve

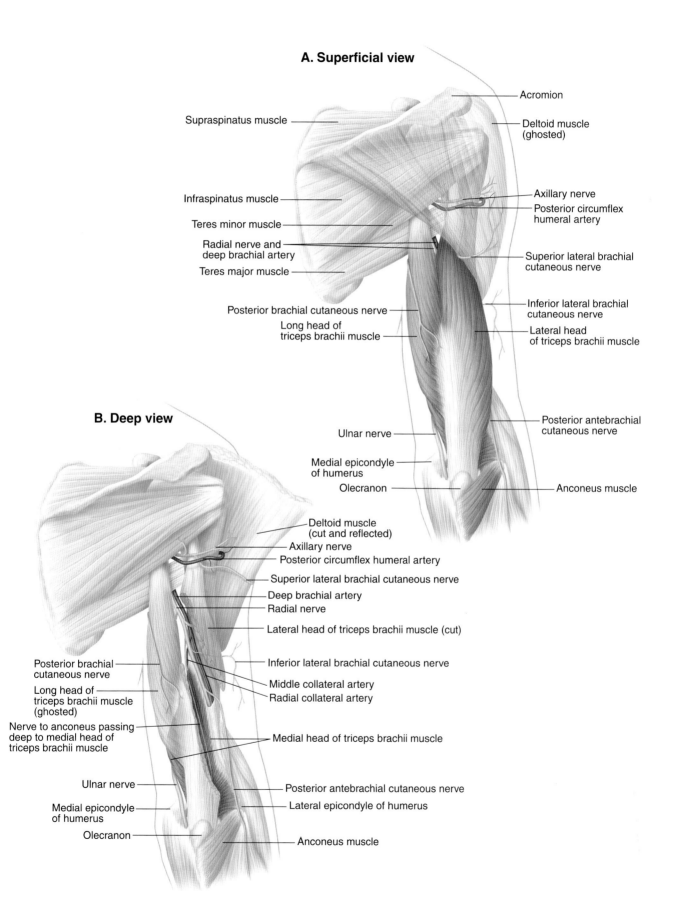

A. Superficial view

Supraspinatus muscle

Infraspinatus muscle

Teres minor muscle

Radial nerve and
deep brachial artery

Teres major muscle

Posterior brachial cutaneous nerve

Long head of
triceps brachii muscle

Ulnar nerve

Medial epicondyle
of humerus

Olecranon

Acromion

Deltoid muscle
(ghosted)

Axillary nerve

Posterior circumflex
humeral artery

Superior lateral brachial
cutaneous nerve

Inferior lateral brachial
cutaneous nerve

Lateral head
of triceps brachii muscle

Posterior antebrachial
cutaneous nerve

Anconeus muscle

B. Deep view

Deltoid muscle
(cut and reflected)

Axillary nerve

Posterior circumflex humeral artery

Superior lateral brachial cutaneous nerve

Deep brachial artery

Radial nerve

Lateral head of triceps brachii muscle (cut)

Inferior lateral brachial cutaneous nerve

Middle collateral artery

Radial collateral artery

Posterior brachial
cutaneous nerve

Long head of
triceps brachii muscle
(ghosted)

Nerve to anconeus passing
deep to medial head of
triceps brachii muscle

Medial head of triceps brachii muscle

Ulnar nerve

Medial epicondyle
of humerus

Olecranon

Posterior antebrachial cutaneous nerve

Lateral epicondyle of humerus

Anconeus muscle

PLATE 2-19   **Arteries of the Arm**

A. Orientation

B. Schema

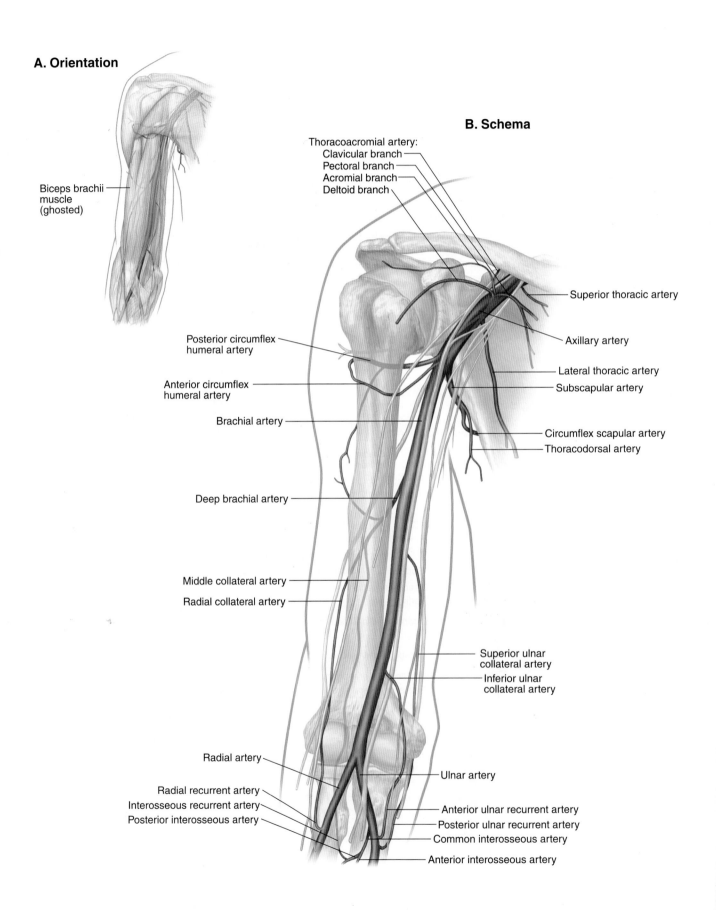

Biceps brachii muscle (ghosted)

Thoracoacromial artery:
Clavicular branch
Pectoral branch
Acromial branch
Deltoid branch

Superior thoracic artery

Axillary artery

Posterior circumflex humeral artery

Lateral thoracic artery

Anterior circumflex humeral artery

Subscapular artery

Brachial artery

Circumflex scapular artery
Thoracodorsal artery

Deep brachial artery

Middle collateral artery

Radial collateral artery

Superior ulnar collateral artery

Inferior ulnar collateral artery

Radial artery

Ulnar artery

Radial recurrent artery

Anterior ulnar recurrent artery

Interosseous recurrent artery

Posterior ulnar recurrent artery

Posterior interosseous artery

Common interosseous artery

Anterior interosseous artery

A. Orientation

Biceps brachii
muscle
(ghosted)

B. Schema

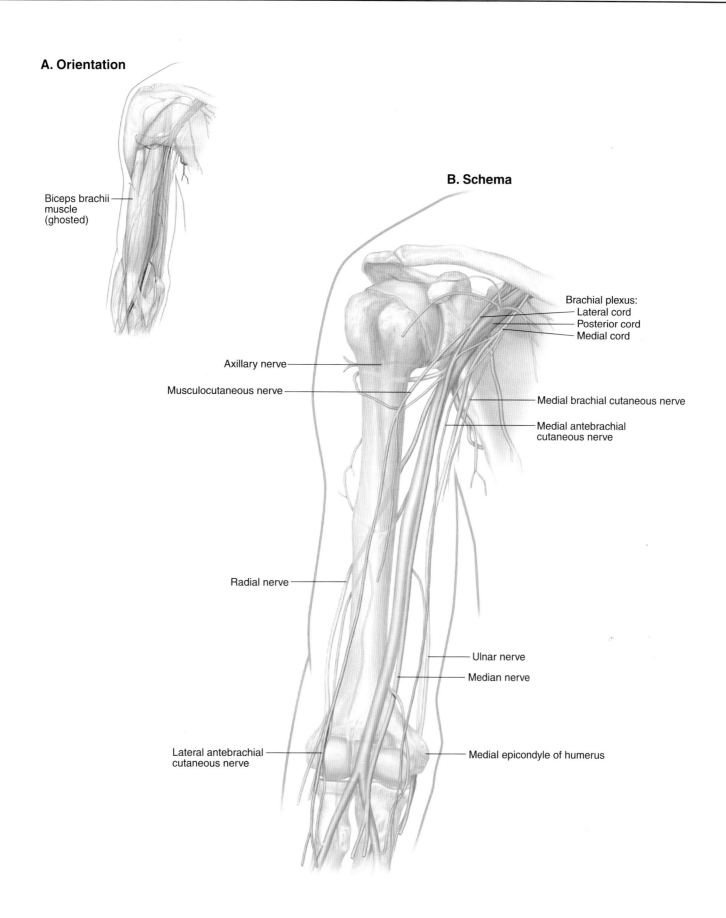

Brachial plexus:
Lateral cord
Posterior cord
Medial cord

Axillary nerve

Musculocutaneous nerve

Medial brachial cutaneous nerve

Medial antebrachial
cutaneous nerve

Radial nerve

Ulnar nerve

Median nerve

Lateral antebrachial
cutaneous nerve

Medial epicondyle of humerus

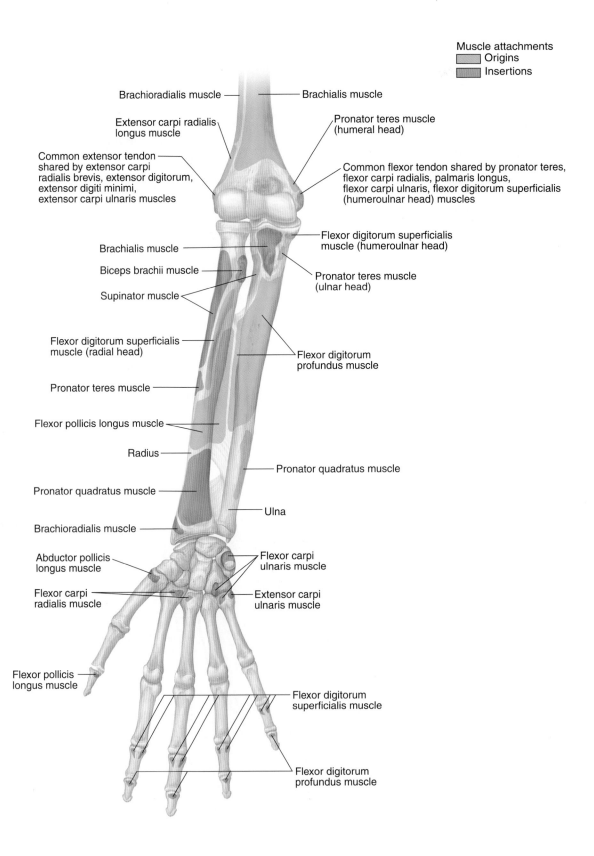

Muscle attachments
Origins
Insertions

Brachioradialis muscle

Brachialis muscle

Extensor carpi radialis longus muscle

Pronator teres muscle (humeral head)

Common extensor tendon shared by extensor carpi radialis brevis, extensor digitorum, extensor digiti minimi, extensor carpi ulnaris muscles

Common flexor tendon shared by pronator teres, flexor carpi radialis, palmaris longus, flexor carpi ulnaris, flexor digitorum superficialis (humeroulnar head) muscles

Brachialis muscle

Flexor digitorum superficialis muscle (humeroulnar head)

Biceps brachii muscle

Pronator teres muscle (ulnar head)

Supinator muscle

Flexor digitorum superficialis muscle (radial head)

Flexor digitorum profundus muscle

Pronator teres muscle

Flexor pollicis longus muscle

Radius

Pronator quadratus muscle

Pronator quadratus muscle

Ulna

Brachioradialis muscle

Abductor pollicis longus muscle

Flexor carpi ulnaris muscle

Flexor carpi radialis muscle

Extensor carpi ulnaris muscle

Flexor pollicis longus muscle

Flexor digitorum superficialis muscle

Flexor digitorum profundus muscle

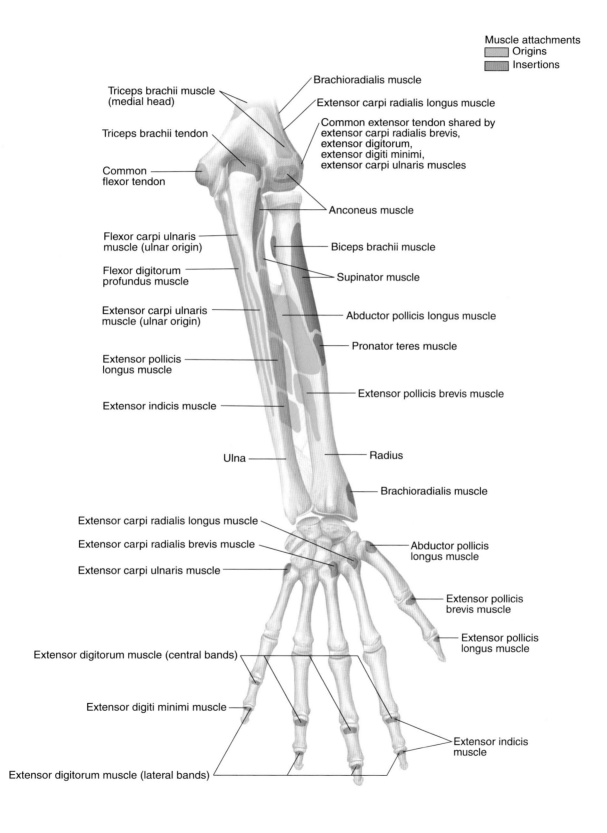

Muscle attachments
▢ Origins
▢ Insertions

Triceps brachii muscle (medial head)

Triceps brachii tendon

Common flexor tendon

Flexor carpi ulnaris muscle (ulnar origin)

Flexor digitorum profundus muscle

Extensor carpi ulnaris muscle (ulnar origin)

Extensor pollicis longus muscle

Extensor indicis muscle

Ulna

Extensor carpi radialis longus muscle

Extensor carpi radialis brevis muscle

Extensor carpi ulnaris muscle

Extensor digitorum muscle (central bands)

Extensor digiti minimi muscle

Extensor digitorum muscle (lateral bands)

Brachioradialis muscle

Extensor carpi radialis longus muscle

Common extensor tendon shared by extensor carpi radialis brevis, extensor digitorum, extensor digiti minimi, extensor carpi ulnaris muscles

Anconeus muscle

Biceps brachii muscle

Supinator muscle

Abductor pollicis longus muscle

Pronator teres muscle

Extensor pollicis brevis muscle

Radius

Brachioradialis muscle

Abductor pollicis longus muscle

Extensor pollicis brevis muscle

Extensor pollicis longus muscle

Extensor indicis muscle

PLATE 2-23   **Muscles of the Anterior Forearm, Superficial Dissection**

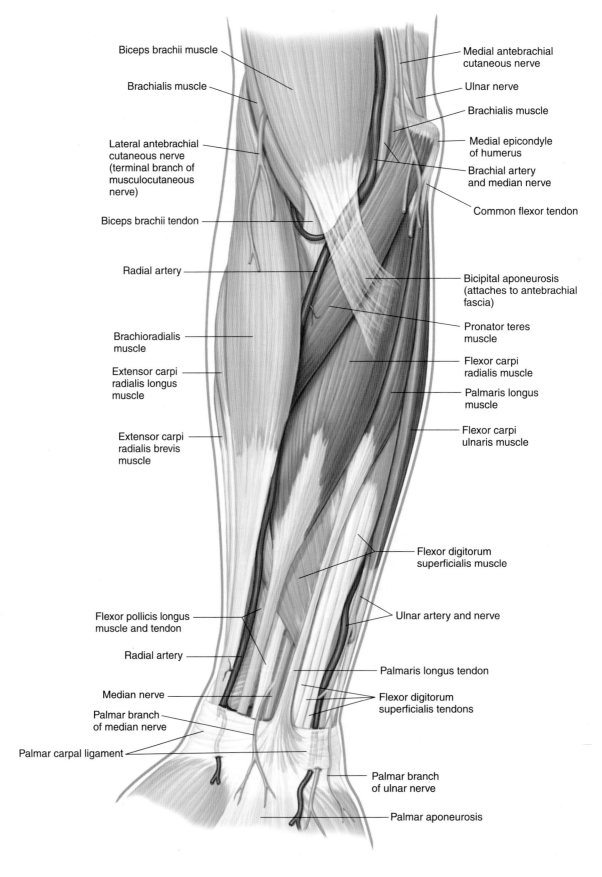

Biceps brachii muscle

Brachialis muscle

Lateral antebrachial
cutaneous nerve
(terminal branch of
musculocutaneous
nerve)

Biceps brachii tendon

Radial artery

Brachioradialis
muscle

Extensor carpi
radialis longus
muscle

Extensor carpi
radialis brevis
muscle

Flexor pollicis longus
muscle and tendon

Radial artery

Median nerve

Palmar branch
of median nerve

Palmar carpal ligament

Medial antebrachial
cutaneous nerve

Ulnar nerve

Brachialis muscle

Medial epicondyle
of humerus

Brachial artery
and median nerve

Common flexor tendon

Bicipital aponeurosis
(attaches to antebrachial
fascia)

Pronator teres
muscle

Flexor carpi
radialis muscle

Palmaris longus
muscle

Flexor carpi
ulnaris muscle

Flexor digitorum
superficialis muscle

Ulnar artery and nerve

Palmaris longus tendon

Flexor digitorum
superficialis tendons

Palmar branch
of ulnar nerve

Palmar aponeurosis

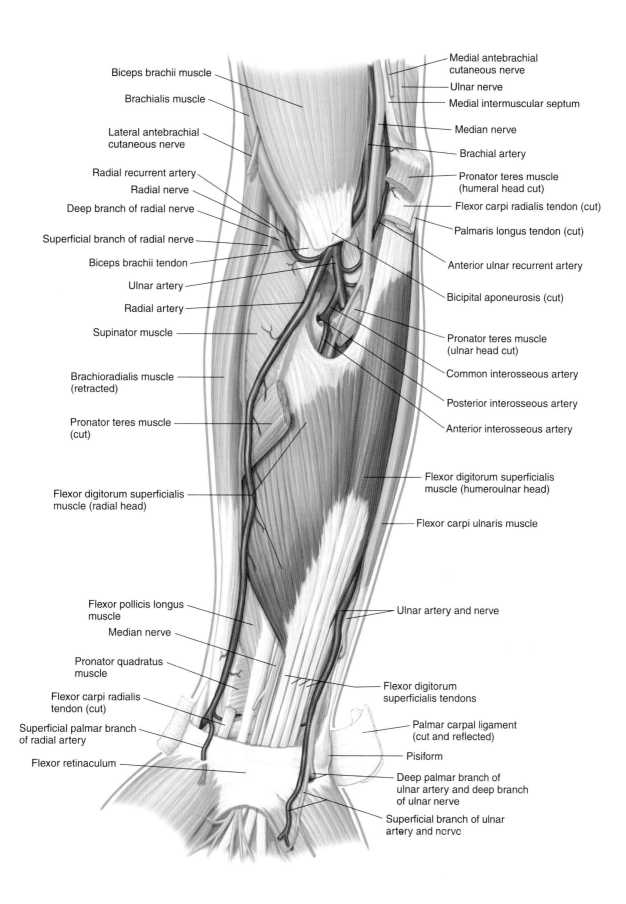

Biceps brachii muscle

Brachialis muscle

Lateral antebrachial cutaneous nerve

Radial recurrent artery

Radial nerve

Deep branch of radial nerve

Superficial branch of radial nerve

Biceps brachii tendon

Ulnar artery

Radial artery

Supinator muscle

Brachioradialis muscle (retracted)

Pronator teres muscle (cut)

Flexor digitorum superficialis muscle (radial head)

Flexor pollicis longus muscle

Median nerve

Pronator quadratus muscle

Flexor carpi radialis tendon (cut)

Superficial palmar branch of radial artery

Flexor retinaculum

Medial antebrachial cutaneous nerve

Ulnar nerve

Medial intermuscular septum

Median nerve

Brachial artery

Pronator teres muscle (humeral head cut)

Flexor carpi radialis tendon (cut)

Palmaris longus tendon (cut)

Anterior ulnar recurrent artery

Bicipital aponeurosis (cut)

Pronator teres muscle (ulnar head cut)

Common interosseous artery

Posterior interosseous artery

Anterior interosseous artery

Flexor digitorum superficialis muscle (humeroulnar head)

Flexor carpi ulnaris muscle

Ulnar artery and nerve

Flexor digitorum superficialis tendons

Palmar carpal ligament (cut and reflected)

Pisiform

Deep palmar branch of ulnar artery and deep branch of ulnar nerve

Superficial branch of ulnar artery and nerve

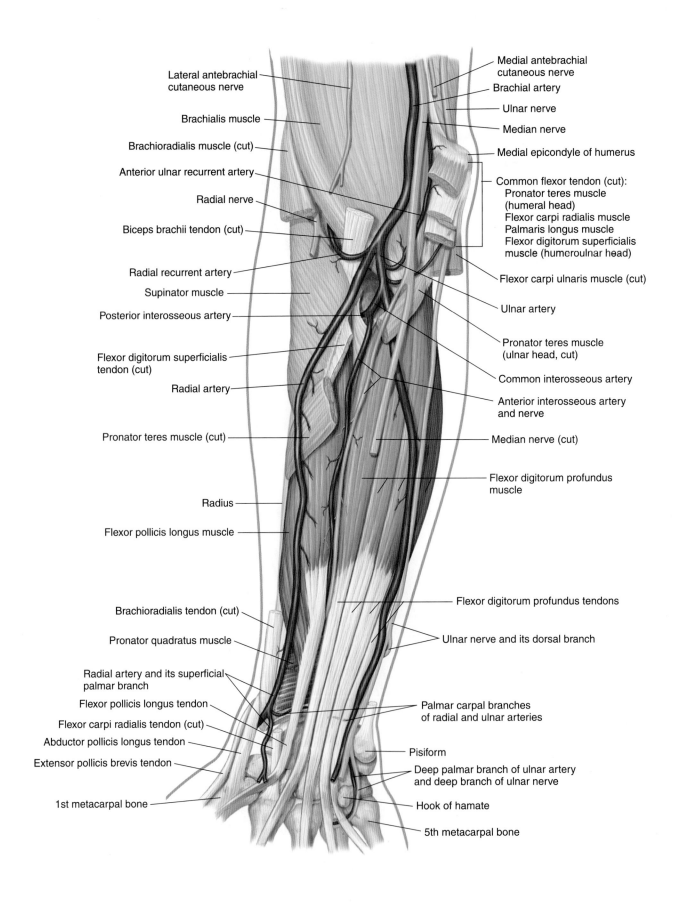

Lateral antebrachial cutaneous nerve

Brachialis muscle

Brachioradialis muscle (cut)

Anterior ulnar recurrent artery

Radial nerve

Biceps brachii tendon (cut)

Radial recurrent artery

Supinator muscle

Posterior interosseous artery

Flexor digitorum superficialis tendon (cut)

Radial artery

Pronator teres muscle (cut)

Radius

Flexor pollicis longus muscle

Brachioradialis tendon (cut)

Pronator quadratus muscle

Radial artery and its superficial palmar branch

Flexor pollicis longus tendon

Flexor carpi radialis tendon (cut)

Abductor pollicis longus tendon

Extensor pollicis brevis tendon

1st metacarpal bone

Medial antebrachial cutaneous nerve

Brachial artery

Ulnar nerve

Median nerve

Medial epicondyle of humerus

Common flexor tendon (cut):
Pronator teres muscle (humeral head)
Flexor carpi radialis muscle
Palmaris longus muscle
Flexor digitorum superficialis muscle (humeroulnar head)

Flexor carpi ulnaris muscle (cut)

Ulnar artery

Pronator teres muscle (ulnar head, cut)

Common interosseous artery

Anterior interosseous artery and nerve

Median nerve (cut)

Flexor digitorum profundus muscle

Flexor digitorum profundus tendons

Ulnar nerve and its dorsal branch

Palmar carpal branches of radial and ulnar arteries

Pisiform

Deep palmar branch of ulnar artery and deep branch of ulnar nerve

Hook of hamate

5th metacarpal bone

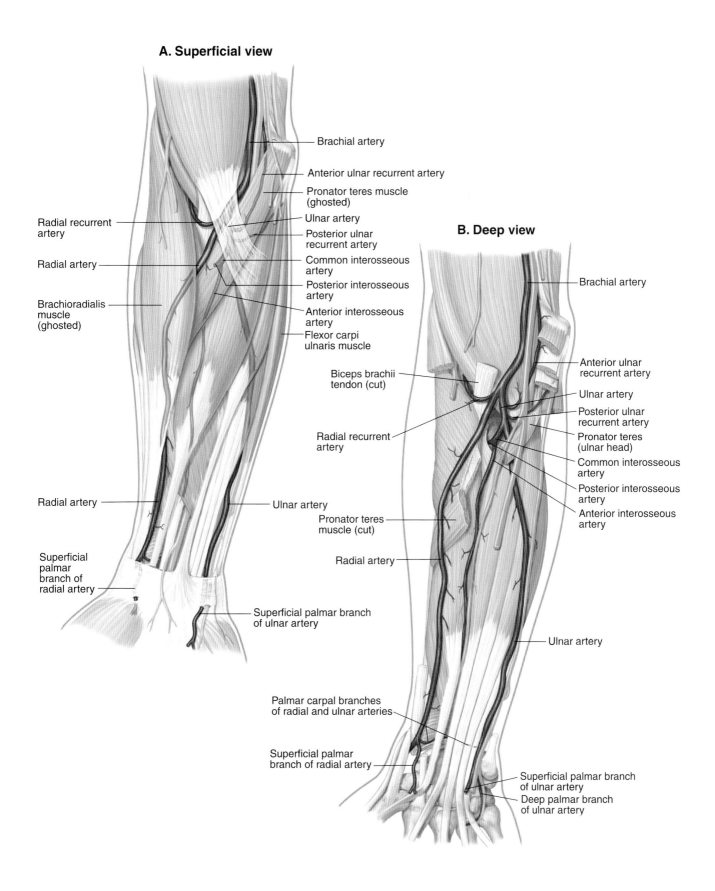

A. Superficial view

Brachial artery

Anterior ulnar recurrent artery

Pronator teres muscle (ghosted)

Ulnar artery

Posterior ulnar recurrent artery

Common interosseous artery

Posterior interosseous artery

Anterior interosseous artery

Flexor carpi ulnaris muscle

Radial recurrent artery

Radial artery

Brachioradialis muscle (ghosted)

Radial artery

Superficial palmar branch of radial artery

Ulnar artery

Superficial palmar branch of ulnar artery

B. Deep view

Brachial artery

Anterior ulnar recurrent artery

Ulnar artery

Posterior ulnar recurrent artery

Pronator teres (ulnar head)

Common interosseous artery

Posterior interosseous artery

Anterior interosseous artery

Biceps brachii tendon (cut)

Radial recurrent artery

Pronator teres muscle (cut)

Radial artery

Ulnar artery

Palmar carpal branches of radial and ulnar arteries

Superficial palmar branch of radial artery

Superficial palmar branch of ulnar artery

Deep palmar branch of ulnar artery

PLATE 2-27   **Nerves of the Anterior Forearm**

A. Superficial view

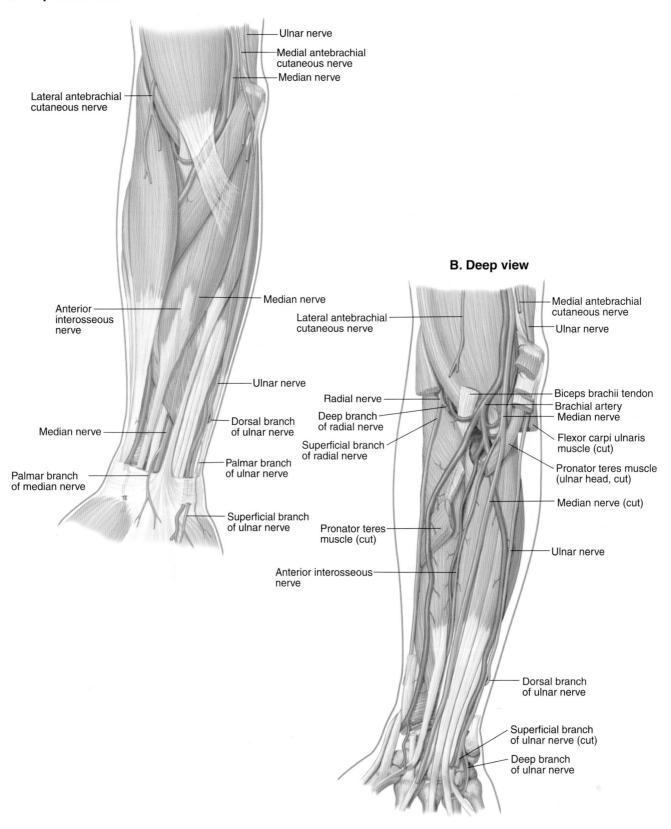

Ulnar nerve

Medial antebrachial
cutaneous nerve

Median nerve

Lateral antebrachial
cutaneous nerve

B. Deep view

Median nerve

Anterior
interosseous
nerve

Lateral antebrachial
cutaneous nerve

Medial antebrachial
cutaneous nerve

Ulnar nerve

Ulnar nerve

Radial nerve

Biceps brachii tendon

Deep branch
of radial nerve

Brachial artery

Median nerve

Superficial branch
of radial nerve

Flexor carpi ulnaris
muscle (cut)

Dorsal branch
of ulnar nerve

Pronator teres muscle
(ulnar head, cut)

Median nerve

Palmar branch
of ulnar nerve

Median nerve (cut)

Pronator teres
muscle (cut)

Palmar branch
of median nerve

Ulnar nerve

Superficial branch
of ulnar nerve

Anterior interosseous
nerve

Dorsal branch
of ulnar nerve

Superficial branch
of ulnar nerve (cut)

Deep branch
of ulnar nerve

A. Orientation

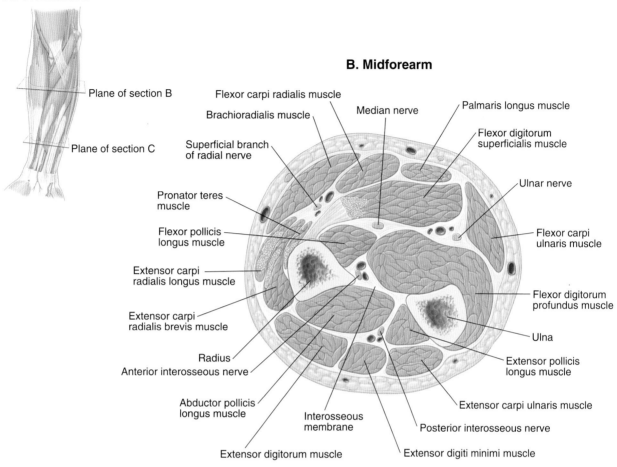

Plane of section B

Plane of section C

B. Midforearm

Flexor carpi radialis muscle

Brachioradialis muscle

Median nerve

Palmaris longus muscle

Superficial branch of radial nerve

Flexor digitorum superficialis muscle

Pronator teres muscle

Ulnar nerve

Flexor pollicis longus muscle

Flexor carpi ulnaris muscle

Extensor carpi radialis longus muscle

Flexor digitorum profundus muscle

Extensor carpi radialis brevis muscle

Ulna

Radius

Extensor pollicis longus muscle

Anterior interosseous nerve

Abductor pollicis longus muscle

Extensor carpi ulnaris muscle

Interosseous membrane

Posterior interosseous nerve

Extensor digitorum muscle

Extensor digiti minimi muscle

C. Distal forearm

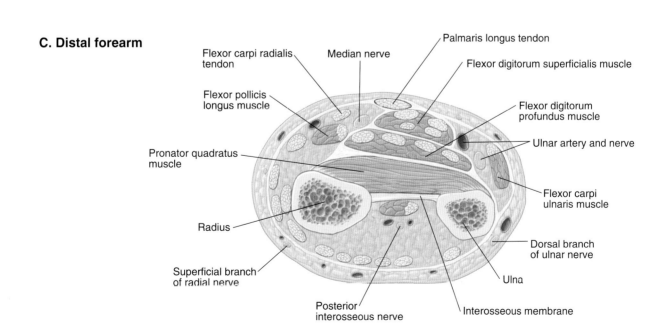

Flexor carpi radialis tendon

Median nerve

Palmaris longus tendon

Flexor pollicis longus muscle

Flexor digitorum superficialis muscle

Pronator quadratus muscle

Flexor digitorum profundus muscle

Ulnar artery and nerve

Radius

Flexor carpi ulnaris muscle

Superficial branch of radial nerve

Dorsal branch of ulnar nerve

Ulna

Posterior interosseous nerve

Interosseous membrane

PLATE 2-29   **Muscles of the Posterior Forearm, Superficial Dissection**

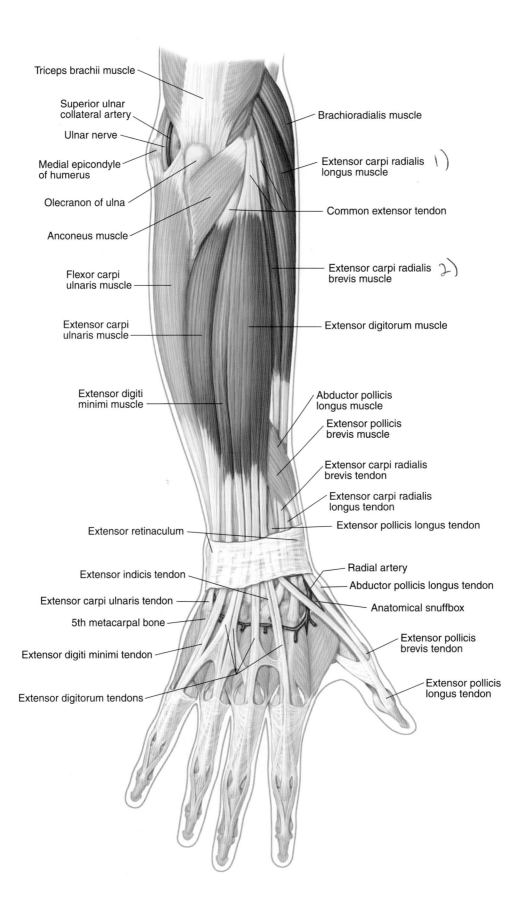

Triceps brachii muscle

Superior ulnar collateral artery

Ulnar nerve

Medial epicondyle of humerus

Olecranon of ulna

Anconeus muscle

Flexor carpi ulnaris muscle

Extensor carpi ulnaris muscle

Extensor digiti minimi muscle

Extensor retinaculum

Extensor indicis tendon

Extensor carpi ulnaris tendon

5th metacarpal bone

Extensor digiti minimi tendon

Extensor digitorum tendons

Brachioradialis muscle

Extensor carpi radialis longus muscle

Common extensor tendon

Extensor carpi radialis brevis muscle

Extensor digitorum muscle

Abductor pollicis longus muscle

Extensor pollicis brevis muscle

Extensor carpi radialis brevis tendon

Extensor carpi radialis longus tendon

Extensor pollicis longus tendon

Radial artery

Abductor pollicis longus tendon

Anatomical snuffbox

Extensor pollicis brevis tendon

Extensor pollicis longus tendon

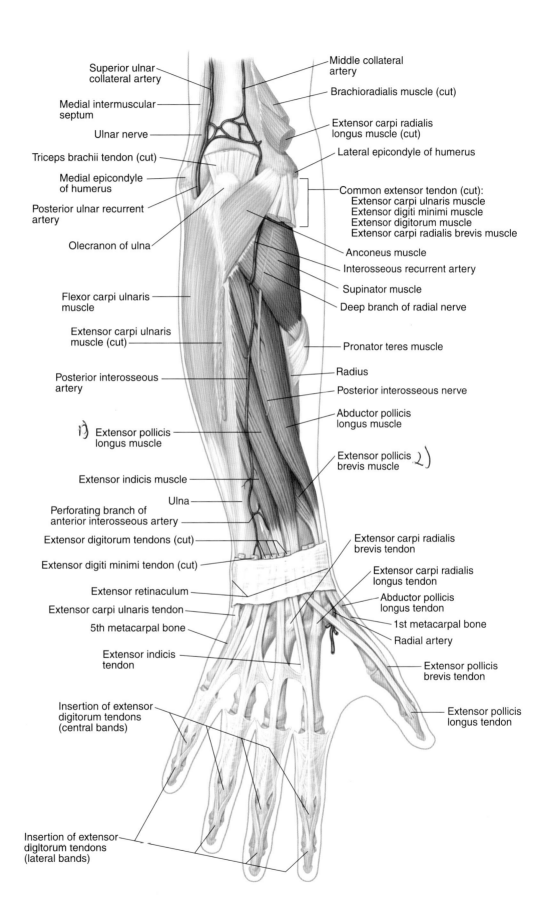

Superior ulnar collateral artery

Medial intermuscular septum

Ulnar nerve

Triceps brachii tendon (cut)

Medial epicondyle of humerus

Posterior ulnar recurrent artery

Olecranon of ulna

Flexor carpi ulnaris muscle

Extensor carpi ulnaris muscle (cut)

Posterior interosseous artery

Extensor pollicis longus muscle

Extensor indicis muscle

Ulna

Perforating branch of anterior interosseous artery

Extensor digitorum tendons (cut)

Extensor digiti minimi tendon (cut)

Extensor retinaculum

Extensor carpi ulnaris tendon

5th metacarpal bone

Extensor indicis tendon

Insertion of extensor digitorum tendons (central bands)

Insertion of extensor digltorum tendons (lateral bands)

Middle collateral artery

Brachioradialis muscle (cut)

Extensor carpi radialis longus muscle (cut)

Lateral epicondyle of humerus

Common extensor tendon (cut):
Extensor carpi ulnaris muscle
Extensor digiti minimi muscle
Extensor digitorum muscle
Extensor carpi radialis brevis muscle

Anconeus muscle

Interosseous recurrent artery

Supinator muscle

Deep branch of radial nerve

Pronator teres muscle

Radius

Posterior interosseous nerve

Abductor pollicis longus muscle

Extensor pollicis brevis muscle

Extensor carpi radialis brevis tendon

Extensor carpi radialis longus tendon

Abductor pollicis longus tendon

1st metacarpal bone

Radial artery

Extensor pollicis brevis tendon

Extensor pollicis longus tendon

A. Bones

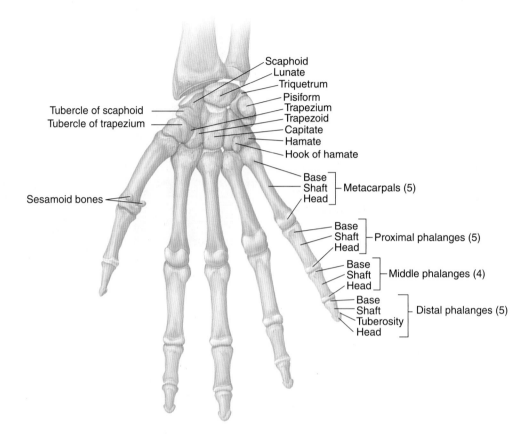

Scaphoid
Lunate
Triquetrum
Pisiform
Trapezium
Trapezoid
Capitate
Hamate
Hook of hamate

Tubercle of scaphoid
Tubercle of trapezium

Sesamoid bones

Base
Shaft ⎦ Metacarpals (5)
Head

Base
Shaft ⎦ Proximal phalanges (5)
Head

Base
Shaft ⎦ Middle phalanges (4)
Head

Base
Shaft
Tuberosity ⎦ Distal phalanges (5)
Head

B. Muscle attachments

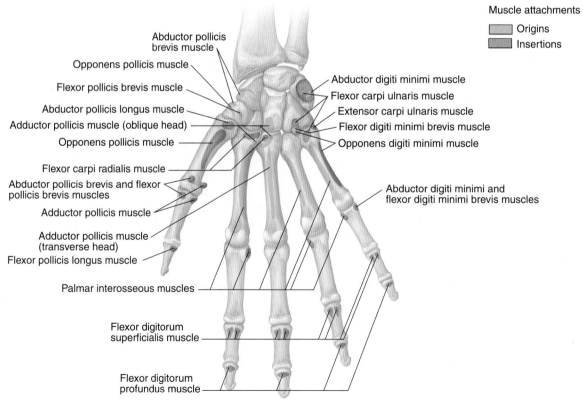

Muscle attachments
Origins
Insertions

Abductor pollicis
brevis muscle

Opponens pollicis muscle

Flexor pollicis brevis muscle

Abductor pollicis longus muscle

Adductor pollicis muscle (oblique head)

Opponens pollicis muscle

Flexor carpi radialis muscle

Abductor pollicis brevis and flexor
pollicis brevis muscles

Adductor pollicis muscle

Adductor pollicis muscle
(transverse head)

Flexor pollicis longus muscle

Palmar interosseous muscles

Flexor digitorum
superficialis muscle

Flexor digitorum
profundus muscle

Abductor digiti minimi muscle
Flexor carpi ulnaris muscle
Extensor carpi ulnaris muscle
Flexor digiti minimi brevis muscle
Opponens digiti minimi muscle

Abductor digiti minimi and
flexor digiti minimi brevis muscles

A. Bones

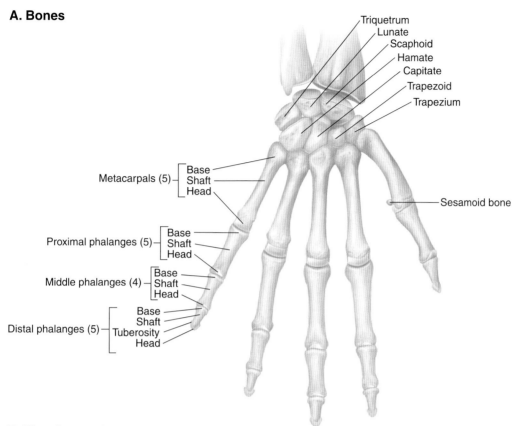

Triquetrum
Lunate
Scaphoid
Hamate
Capitate
Trapezoid
Trapezium

Metacarpals (5) — Base / Shaft / Head

Sesamoid bone

Proximal phalanges (5) — Base / Shaft / Head

Middle phalanges (4) — Base / Shaft / Head

Distal phalanges (5) — Base / Shaft / Tuberosity / Head

B. Muscle attachments

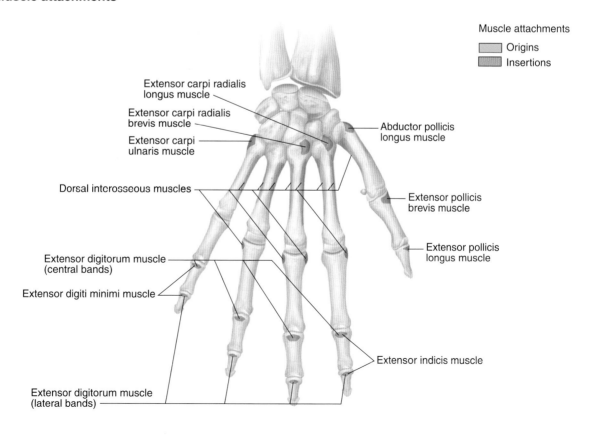

Muscle attachments
▢ Origins
▨ Insertions

Extensor carpi radialis longus muscle

Extensor carpi radialis brevis muscle

Extensor carpi ulnaris muscle

Dorsal interosseous muscles

Extensor digitorum muscle (central bands)

Extensor digiti minimi muscle

Extensor digitorum muscle (lateral bands)

Abductor pollicis longus muscle

Extensor pollicis brevis muscle

Extensor pollicis longus muscle

Extensor indicis muscle

PLATE 2-33   **Cutaneous Nerves of the Hand, Anterior View**

A. Dissection

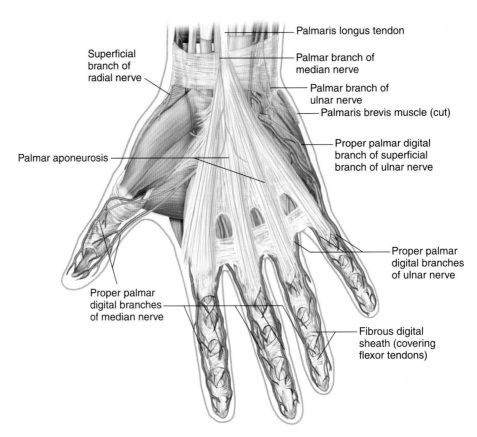

Superficial branch of radial nerve

Palmaris longus tendon

Palmar branch of median nerve

Palmar branch of ulnar nerve

Palmaris brevis muscle (cut)

Proper palmar digital branch of superficial branch of ulnar nerve

Palmar aponeurosis

Proper palmar digital branches of ulnar nerve

Proper palmar digital branches of median nerve

Fibrous digital sheath (covering flexor tendons)

B. Nerve territories

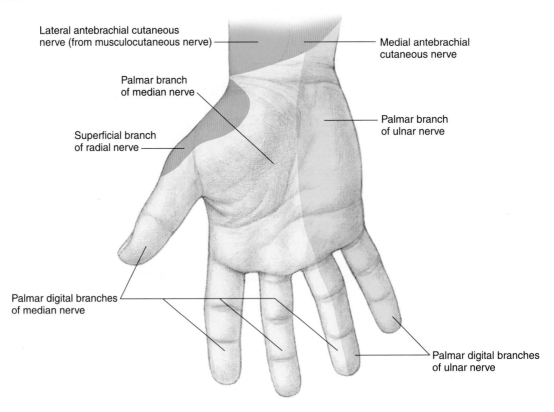

Lateral antebrachial cutaneous nerve (from musculocutaneous nerve)

Medial antebrachial cutaneous nerve

Palmar branch of median nerve

Palmar branch of ulnar nerve

Superficial branch of radial nerve

Palmar digital branches of median nerve

Palmar digital branches of ulnar nerve

A. Superficial dissection

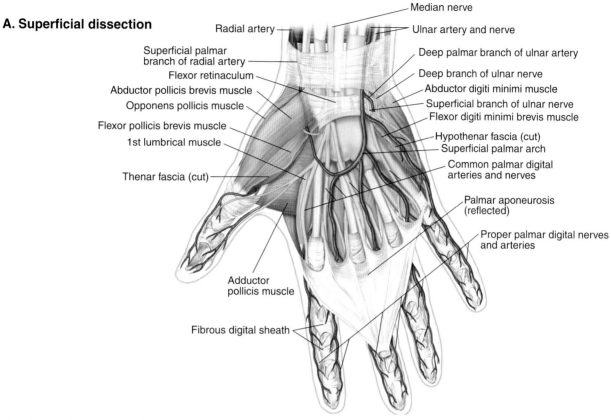

Median nerve

Radial artery

Ulnar artery and nerve

Superficial palmar branch of radial artery

Deep palmar branch of ulnar artery

Flexor retinaculum

Deep branch of ulnar nerve

Abductor pollicis brevis muscle

Abductor digiti minimi muscle

Opponens pollicis muscle

Superficial branch of ulnar nerve

Flexor pollicis brevis muscle

Flexor digiti minimi brevis muscle

1st lumbrical muscle

Hypothenar fascia (cut)

Superficial palmar arch

Common palmar digital arteries and nerves

Thenar fascia (cut)

Palmar aponeurosis (reflected)

Proper palmar digital nerves and arteries

Adductor pollicis muscle

Fibrous digital sheath

B. Intermediate dissection

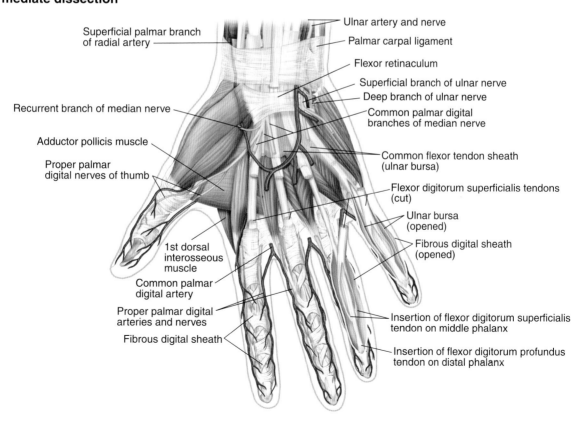

Superficial palmar branch of radial artery

Ulnar artery and nerve

Palmar carpal ligament

Flexor retinaculum

Superficial branch of ulnar nerve

Recurrent branch of median nerve

Deep branch of ulnar nerve

Common palmar digital branches of median nerve

Adductor pollicis muscle

Proper palmar digital nerves of thumb

Common flexor tendon sheath (ulnar bursa)

Flexor digitorum superficialis tendons (cut)

Ulnar bursa (opened)

1st dorsal interosseous muscle

Fibrous digital sheath (opened)

Common palmar digital artery

Proper palmar digital arteries and nerves

Insertion of flexor digitorum superficialis tendon on middle phalanx

Fibrous digital sheath

Insertion of flexor digitorum profundus tendon on distal phalanx

PLATE 2-35   Wrist and Palm of the Hand II

A. Deep dissection

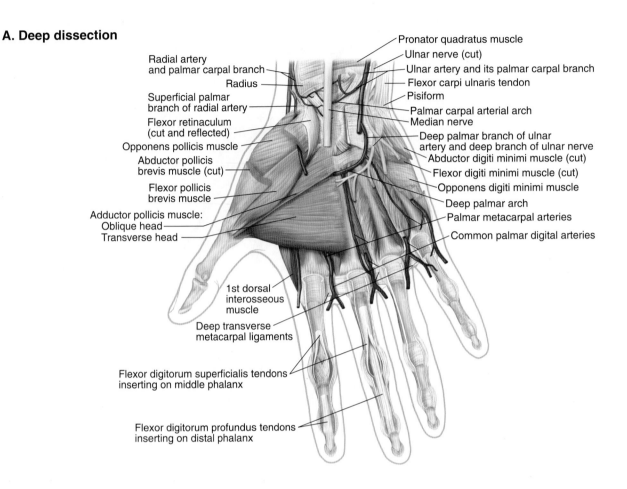

Radial artery and palmar carpal branch
Radius
Superficial palmar branch of radial artery
Flexor retinaculum (cut and reflected)
Opponens pollicis muscle
Abductor pollicis brevis muscle (cut)
Flexor pollicis brevis muscle
Adductor pollicis muscle:
Oblique head
Transverse head

Pronator quadratus muscle
Ulnar nerve (cut)
Ulnar artery and its palmar carpal branch
Flexor carpi ulnaris tendon
Pisiform
Palmar carpal arterial arch
Median nerve
Deep palmar branch of ulnar artery and deep branch of ulnar nerve
Abductor digiti minimi muscle (cut)
Flexor digiti minimi muscle (cut)
Opponens digiti minimi muscle
Deep palmar arch
Palmar metacarpal arteries
Common palmar digital arteries

1st dorsal interosseous muscle
Deep transverse metacarpal ligaments
Flexor digitorum superficialis tendons inserting on middle phalanx
Flexor digitorum profundus tendons inserting on distal phalanx

B. Palmar interosseous muscles   ## C. Dorsal interosseous muscles

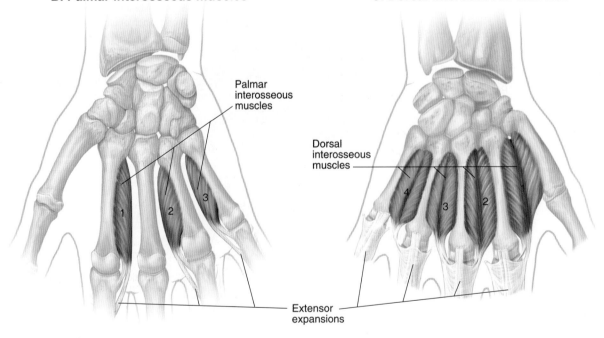

Palmar interosseous muscles

1
2
3

Dorsal interosseous muscles

4
3
2
1

Extensor expansions

A. Orientation

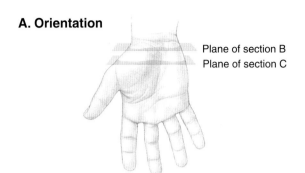

Plane of section B
Plane of section C

B. Wrist

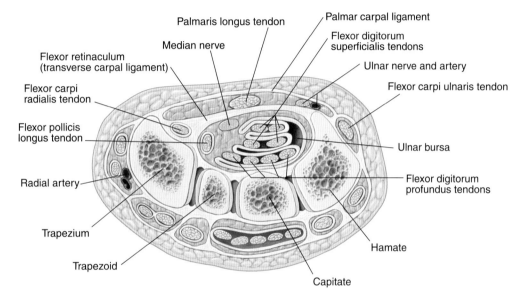

Palmaris longus tendon

Palmar carpal ligament

Median nerve

Flexor digitorum
superficialis tendons

Flexor retinaculum
(transverse carpal ligament)

Ulnar nerve and artery

Flexor carpi
radialis tendon

Flexor carpi ulnaris tendon

Flexor pollicis
longus tendon

Ulnar bursa

Radial artery

Flexor digitorum
profundus tendons

Trapezium

Hamate

Trapezoid

Capitate

C. Palm

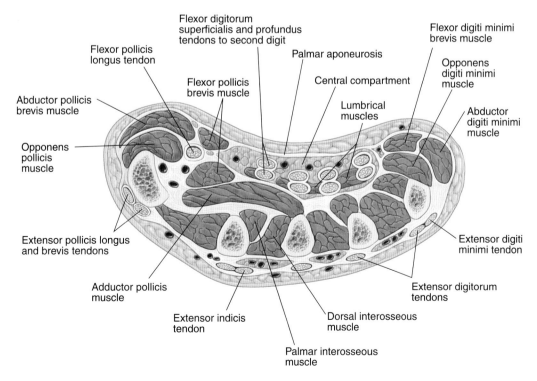

Flexor digitorum
superficialis and profundus
tendons to second digit

Flexor digiti minimi
brevis muscle

Flexor pollicis
longus tendon

Palmar aponeurosis

Opponens
digiti minimi
muscle

Flexor pollicis
brevis muscle

Central compartment

Abductor pollicis
brevis muscle

Lumbrical
muscles

Abductor
digiti minimi
muscle

Opponens
pollicis
muscle

Extensor digiti
minimi tendon

Extensor pollicis longus
and brevis tendons

Extensor digitorum
tendons

Adductor pollicis
muscle

Dorsal interosseous
muscle

Extensor indicis
tendon

Palmar interosseous
muscle

PLATE 2-37   **Arteries of the Hand, Anterior View**

A. Superficial view

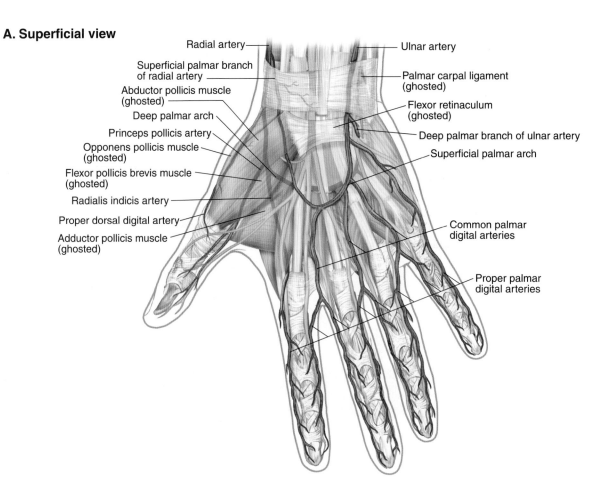

Radial artery

Superficial palmar branch of radial artery

Abductor pollicis muscle (ghosted)

Deep palmar arch

Princeps pollicis artery

Opponens pollicis muscle (ghosted)

Flexor pollicis brevis muscle (ghosted)

Radialis indicis artery

Proper dorsal digital artery

Adductor pollicis muscle (ghosted)

Ulnar artery

Palmar carpal ligament (ghosted)

Flexor retinaculum (ghosted)

Deep palmar branch of ulnar artery

Superficial palmar arch

Common palmar digital arteries

Proper palmar digital arteries

B. Deep view

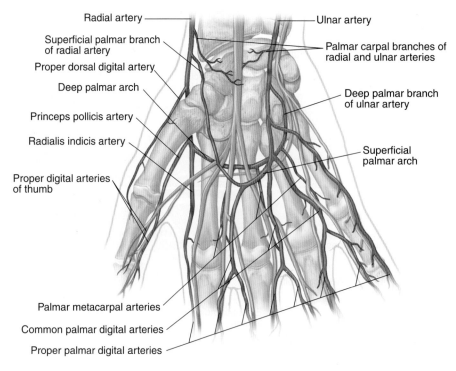

Radial artery

Superficial palmar branch of radial artery

Proper dorsal digital artery

Deep palmar arch

Princeps pollicis artery

Radialis indicis artery

Proper digital arteries of thumb

Ulnar artery

Palmar carpal branches of radial and ulnar arteries

Deep palmar branch of ulnar artery

Superficial palmar arch

Palmar metacarpal arteries

Common palmar digital arteries

Proper palmar digital arteries

A. Anterior view

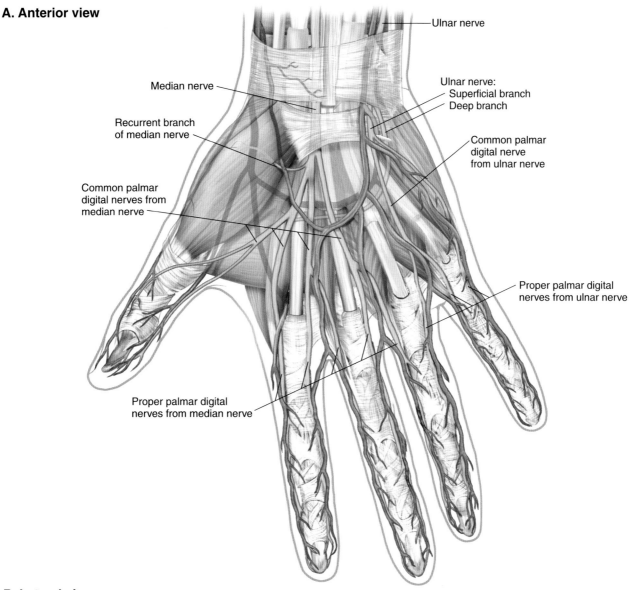

Ulnar nerve

Median nerve

Ulnar nerve:
Superficial branch
Deep branch

Recurrent branch
of median nerve

Common palmar
digital nerve
from ulnar nerve

Common palmar
digital nerves from
median nerve

Proper palmar digital
nerves from ulnar nerve

Proper palmar digital
nerves from median nerve

B. Lateral view

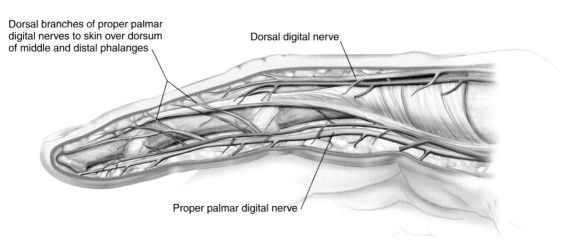

Dorsal branches of proper palmar
digital nerves to skin over dorsum
of middle and distal phalanges

Dorsal digital nerve

Proper palmar digital nerve

A. Dissection

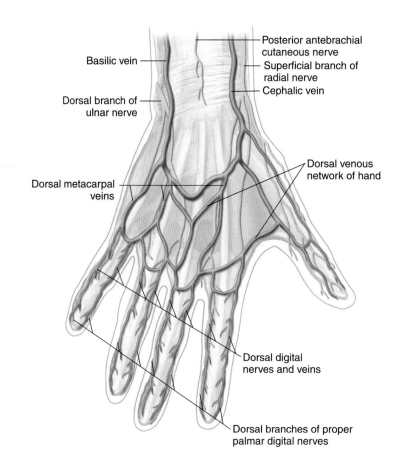

Basilic vein

Posterior antebrachial cutaneous nerve

Superficial branch of radial nerve

Cephalic vein

Dorsal branch of ulnar nerve

Dorsal venous network of hand

Dorsal metacarpal veins

Dorsal digital nerves and veins

Dorsal branches of proper palmar digital nerves

B. Nerve territories

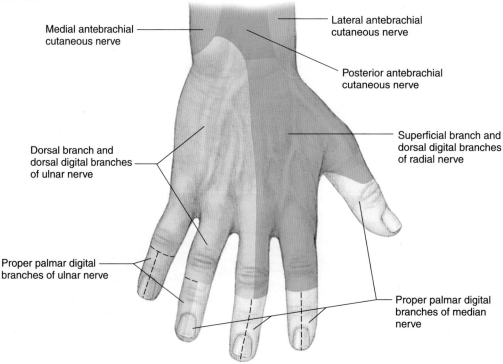

Medial antebrachial cutaneous nerve

Lateral antebrachial cutaneous nerve

Posterior antebrachial cutaneous nerve

Dorsal branch and dorsal digital branches of ulnar nerve

Superficial branch and dorsal digital branches of radial nerve

Proper palmar digital branches of ulnar nerve

Proper palmar digital branches of median nerve

A. Dissection

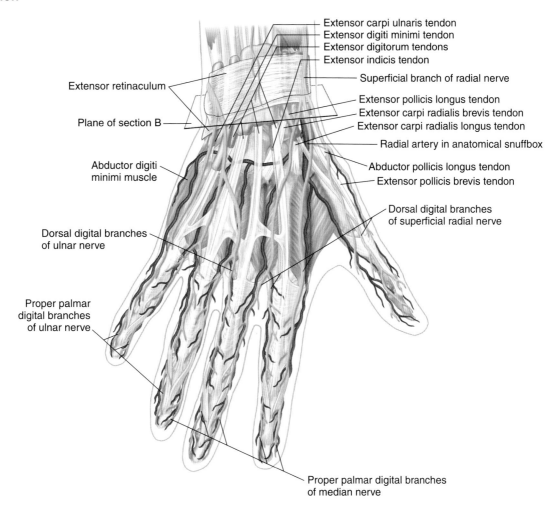

Extensor carpi ulnaris tendon
Extensor digiti minimi tendon
Extensor digitorum tendons
Extensor indicis tendon
Superficial branch of radial nerve
Extensor pollicis longus tendon
Extensor carpi radialis brevis tendon
Extensor carpi radialis longus tendon
Radial artery in anatomical snuffbox
Abductor pollicis longus tendon
Extensor pollicis brevis tendon
Dorsal digital branches of superficial radial nerve

Extensor retinaculum
Plane of section B
Abductor digiti minimi muscle
Dorsal digital branches of ulnar nerve
Proper palmar digital branches of ulnar nerve
Proper palmar digital branches of median nerve

B. Cross section through the wrist

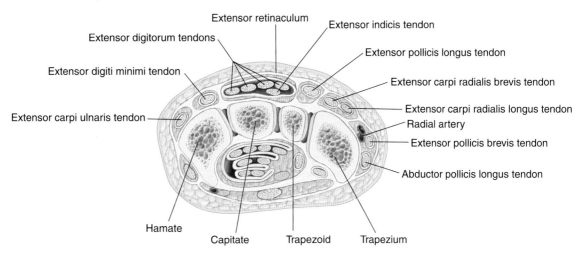

Extensor retinaculum
Extensor indicis tendon
Extensor digitorum tendons
Extensor pollicis longus tendon
Extensor digiti minimi tendon
Extensor carpi radialis brevis tendon
Extensor carpi ulnaris tendon
Extensor carpi radialis longus tendon
Radial artery
Extensor pollicis brevis tendon
Abductor pollicis longus tendon
Hamate
Capitate
Trapezoid
Trapezium

A. Dissection

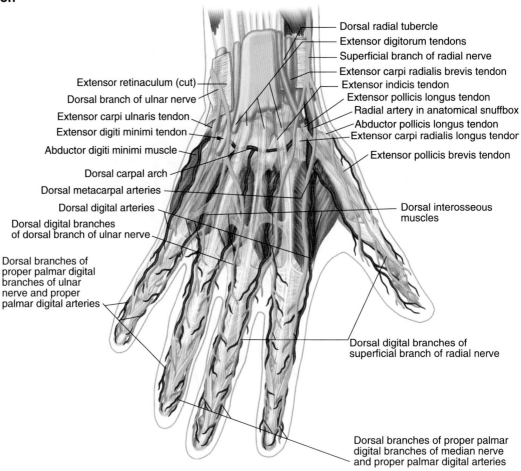

Dorsal radial tubercle
Extensor digitorum tendons
Superficial branch of radial nerve
Extensor carpi radialis brevis tendon
Extensor indicis tendon
Extensor pollicis longus tendon
Radial artery in anatomical snuffbox
Abductor pollicis longus tendon
Extensor carpi radialis longus tendon
Extensor pollicis brevis tendon

Extensor retinaculum (cut)
Dorsal branch of ulnar nerve
Extensor carpi ulnaris tendon
Extensor digiti minimi tendon
Abductor digiti minimi muscle
Dorsal carpal arch
Dorsal metacarpal arteries
Dorsal digital arteries
Dorsal digital branches
of dorsal branch of ulnar nerve

Dorsal interosseous
muscles

Dorsal branches of
proper palmar digital
branches of ulnar
nerve and proper
palmar digital arteries

Dorsal digital branches of
superficial branch of radial nerve

Dorsal branches of proper palmar
digital branches of median nerve
and proper palmar digital arteries

B. Extensor expansion, right index finger

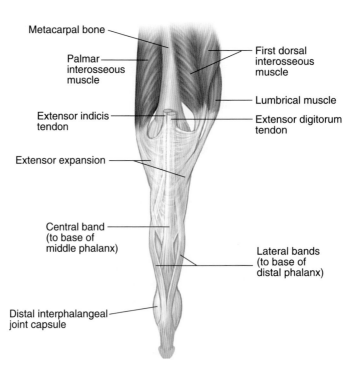

Metacarpal bone
Palmar interosseous muscle
Extensor indicis tendon
Extensor expansion
Central band (to base of middle phalanx)
Distal interphalangeal joint capsule

First dorsal interosseous muscle
Lumbrical muscle
Extensor digitorum tendon
Lateral bands (to base of distal phalanx)

A. Dissection

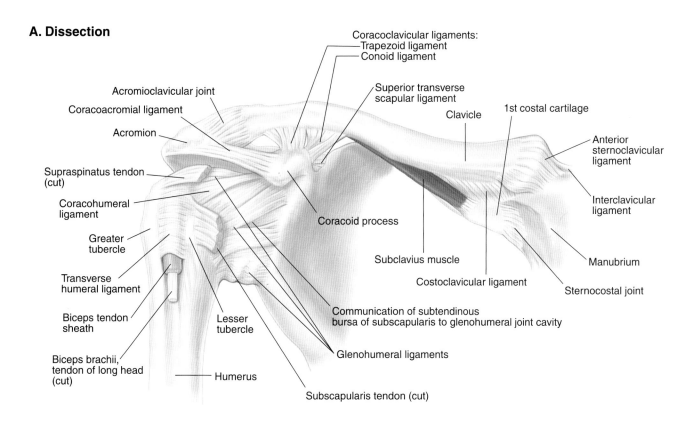

Coracoclavicular ligaments:
Trapezoid ligament
Conoid ligament

Acromioclavicular joint

Coracoacromial ligament

Superior transverse
scapular ligament

Clavicle

1st costal cartilage

Acromion

Anterior
sternoclavicular
ligament

Supraspinatus tendon
(cut)

Coracohumeral
ligament

Interclavicular
ligament

Greater
tubercle

Coracoid process

Transverse
humeral ligament

Subclavius muscle

Manubrium

Biceps tendon
sheath

Costoclavicular ligament

Sternocostal joint

Lesser
tubercle

Communication of subtendinous
bursa of subscapularis to glenohumeral joint cavity

Biceps brachii,
tendon of long head
(cut)

Humerus

Glenohumeral ligaments

Subscapularis tendon (cut)

B. Shoulder joint, coronal section

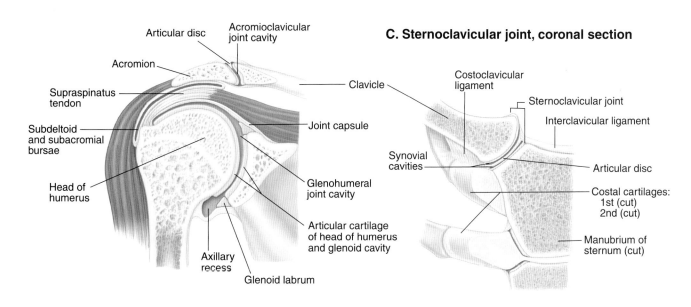

Articular disc

Acromioclavicular
joint cavity

C. Sternoclavicular joint, coronal section

Acromion

Clavicle

Costoclavicular
ligament

Supraspinatus
tendon

Sternoclavicular joint

Subdeltoid
and subacromial
bursae

Joint capsule

Interclavicular ligament

Synovial
cavities

Head of
humerus

Glenohumeral
joint cavity

Articular disc

Articular cartilage
of head of humerus
and glenoid cavity

Costal cartilages:
1st (cut)
2nd (cut)

Axillary
recess

Glenoid labrum

Manubrium of
sternum (cut)

PLATE 2-43   Elbow Joint

A. Anterior view

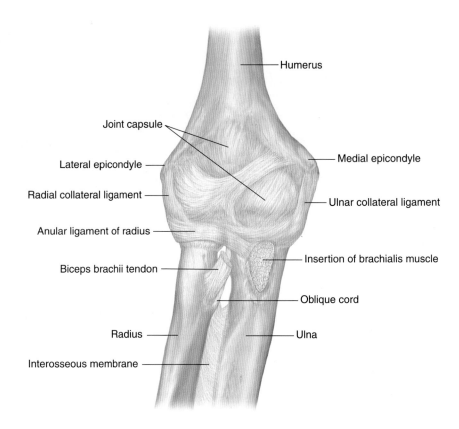

Humerus

Joint capsule

Lateral epicondyle

Medial epicondyle

Radial collateral ligament

Ulnar collateral ligament

Anular ligament of radius

Biceps brachii tendon

Insertion of brachialis muscle

Oblique cord

Radius

Ulna

Interosseous membrane

B. Lateral view

C. Medial view

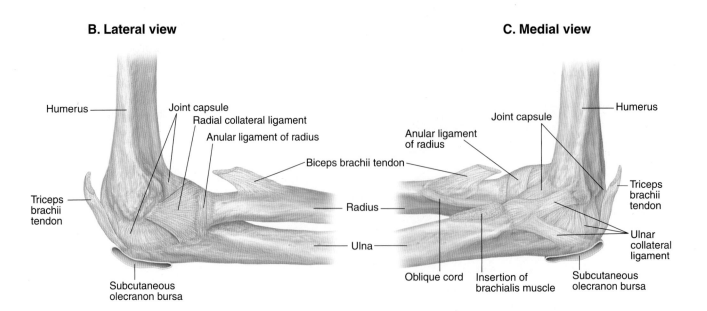

Humerus

Joint capsule

Radial collateral ligament

Anular ligament of radius

Biceps brachii tendon

Triceps brachii tendon

Subcutaneous olecranon bursa

Anular ligament of radius

Joint capsule

Humerus

Biceps brachii tendon

Radius

Triceps brachii tendon

Ulna

Ulnar collateral ligament

Oblique cord

Insertion of brachialis muscle

Subcutaneous olecranon bursa

A. Anterior view

Radius

Ulna

Interosseous membrane

Palmar radioulnar ligament

Lunate

Palmar radiocarpal ligament

Ulnar collateral ligament

Radial collateral ligament

Flexor carpi ulnaris tendon (cut)

Tubercle of scaphoid

Pisiform

Tubercle of trapezium

Pisohamate ligament

Attachment of flexor retinaculum (cut)

Attachment of flexor retinaculum (cut)

Articular capsule of carpometacarpal joint of thumb

Hook of hamate

Capitate

Palmar metacarpal ligaments

Palmar carpometacarpal ligaments

1

2

3

4

5

Metacarpal bones

B. Posterior view

Ulna

Radius

Interosseous membrane

Dorsal radiocarpal ligament

Dorsal radioulnar ligament

Lunate (covered by ligament)

Dorsal ulnocarpal ligament

Scaphoid

Ulnar collateral ligament

Radial collateral ligament

Dorsal intercarpal ligament

Trapezium

Triquetrum

Trapezoid

Hamate

Capitate

Dorsal carpometacarpal ligaments

1st metacarpal

Dorsal metacarpal ligaments

C. Coronal section, posterior view

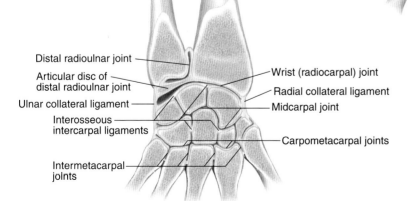

Distal radioulnar joint

Wrist (radiocarpal) joint

Articular disc of distal radioulnar joint

Radial collateral ligament

Ulnar collateral ligament

Midcarpal joint

Interosseous intercarpal ligaments

Carpometacarpal joints

Intermetacarpal joints

PLATE 2-45   Joints of the Hand and Digits

A. Anterior view

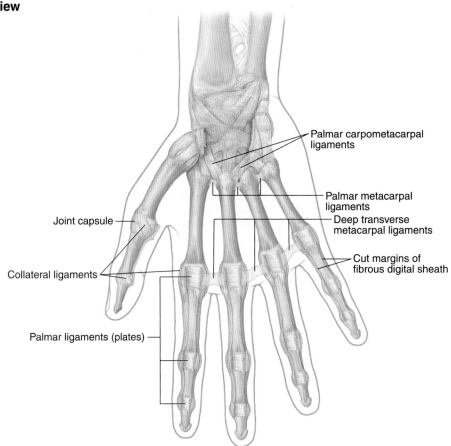

Palmar carpometacarpal ligaments

Palmar metacarpal ligaments

Deep transverse metacarpal ligaments

Cut margins of fibrous digital sheath

Joint capsule

Collateral ligaments

Palmar ligaments (plates)

B. Joints of the digits

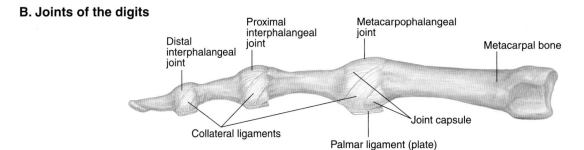

Distal interphalangeal joint

Proximal interphalangeal joint

Metacarpophalangeal joint

Metacarpal bone

Collateral ligaments

Palmar ligament (plate)

Joint capsule

C. Extensor expansion

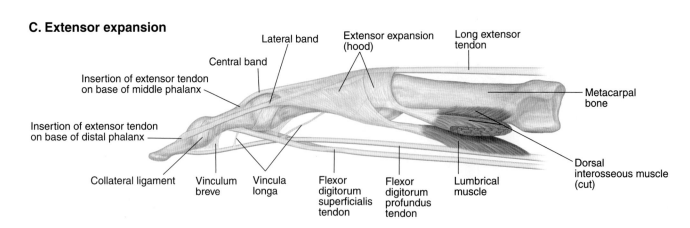

Lateral band

Central band

Extensor expansion (hood)

Long extensor tendon

Insertion of extensor tendon on base of middle phalanx

Metacarpal bone

Insertion of extensor tendon on base of distal phalanx

Collateral ligament

Vinculum breve

Vincula longa

Flexor digitorum superficialis tendon

Flexor digitorum profundus tendon

Lumbrical muscle

Dorsal interosseous muscle (cut)

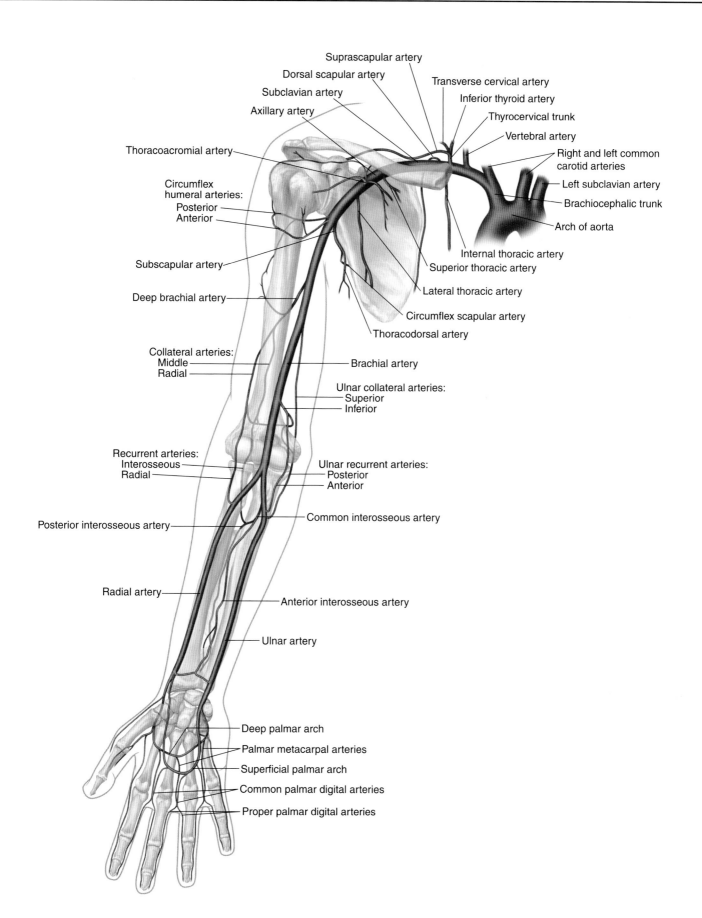

Suprascapular artery
Dorsal scapular artery
Subclavian artery
Axillary artery
Transverse cervical artery
Inferior thyroid artery
Thyrocervical trunk
Vertebral artery
Thoracoacromial artery
Right and left common carotid arteries
Circumflex humeral arteries:
Posterior
Anterior
Left subclavian artery
Brachiocephalic trunk
Arch of aorta
Subscapular artery
Internal thoracic artery
Superior thoracic artery
Deep brachial artery
Lateral thoracic artery
Circumflex scapular artery
Thoracodorsal artery
Collateral arteries:
Middle
Radial
Brachial artery
Ulnar collateral arteries:
Superior
Inferior
Recurrent arteries:
Interosseous
Radial
Ulnar recurrent arteries:
Posterior
Anterior
Posterior interosseous artery
Common interosseous artery
Radial artery
Anterior interosseous artery
Ulnar artery
Deep palmar arch
Palmar metacarpal arteries
Superficial palmar arch
Common palmar digital arteries
Proper palmar digital arteries

PLATE 2-47   Musculocutaneous Nerve

A. Anterior view

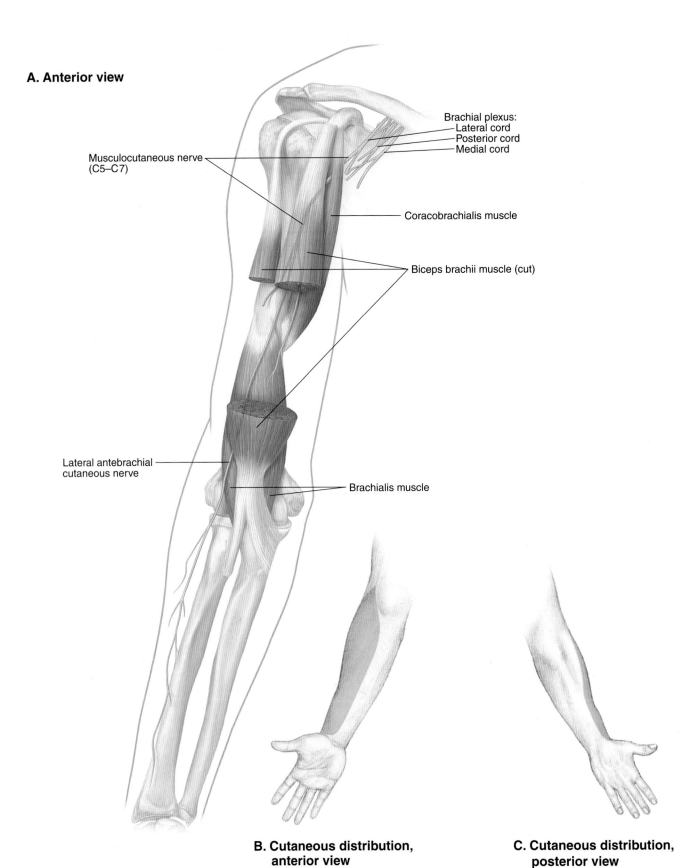

Brachial plexus:
Lateral cord
Posterior cord
Medial cord

Musculocutaneous nerve
(C5–C7)

Coracobrachialis muscle

Biceps brachii muscle (cut)

Lateral antebrachial
cutaneous nerve

Brachialis muscle

B. Cutaneous distribution,
anterior view

C. Cutaneous distribution,
posterior view

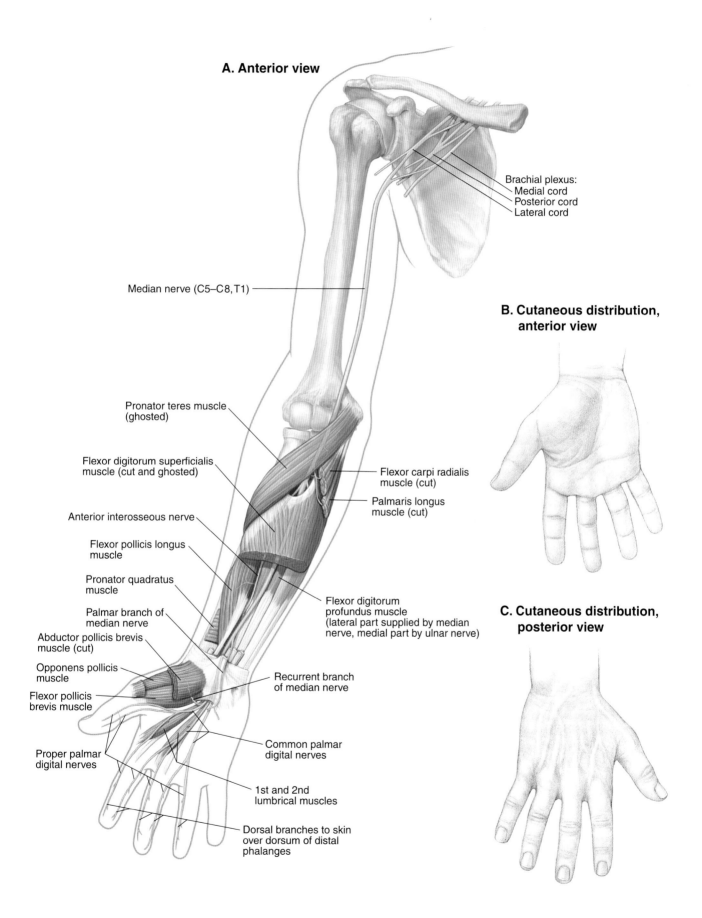

A. Anterior view

Brachial plexus:
Medial cord
Posterior cord
Lateral cord

Median nerve (C5–C8, T1)

B. Cutaneous distribution, anterior view

Pronator teres muscle (ghosted)

Flexor digitorum superficialis muscle (cut and ghosted)

Flexor carpi radialis muscle (cut)

Palmaris longus muscle (cut)

Anterior interosseous nerve

Flexor pollicis longus muscle

Pronator quadratus muscle

Palmar branch of median nerve

Flexor digitorum profundus muscle (lateral part supplied by median nerve, medial part by ulnar nerve)

Abductor pollicis brevis muscle (cut)

C. Cutaneous distribution, posterior view

Opponens pollicis muscle

Recurrent branch of median nerve

Flexor pollicis brevis muscle

Proper palmar digital nerves

Common palmar digital nerves

1st and 2nd lumbrical muscles

Dorsal branches to skin over dorsum of distal phalanges

PLATE 2-49   Ulnar Nerve

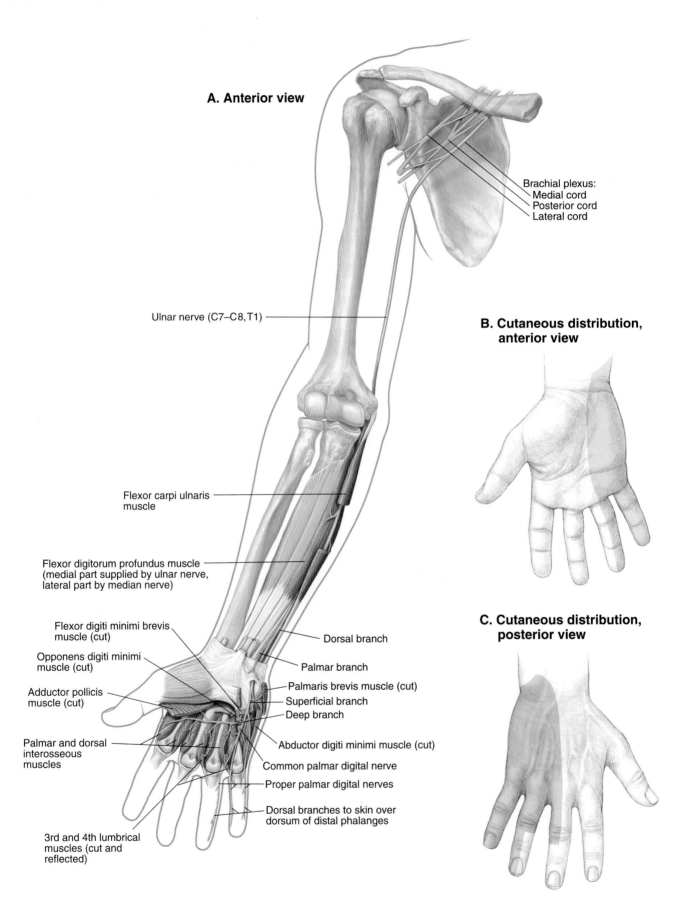

A. Anterior view

Brachial plexus:
Medial cord
Posterior cord
Lateral cord

Ulnar nerve (C7–C8, T1)

B. Cutaneous distribution, anterior view

Flexor carpi ulnaris muscle

Flexor digitorum profundus muscle (medial part supplied by ulnar nerve, lateral part by median nerve)

C. Cutaneous distribution, posterior view

Flexor digiti minimi brevis muscle (cut)

Dorsal branch

Opponens digiti minimi muscle (cut)

Palmar branch

Palmaris brevis muscle (cut)

Adductor pollicis muscle (cut)

Superficial branch

Deep branch

Abductor digiti minimi muscle (cut)

Palmar and dorsal interosseous muscles

Common palmar digital nerve

Proper palmar digital nerves

Dorsal branches to skin over dorsum of distal phalanges

3rd and 4th lumbrical muscles (cut and reflected)

A. Posterior view

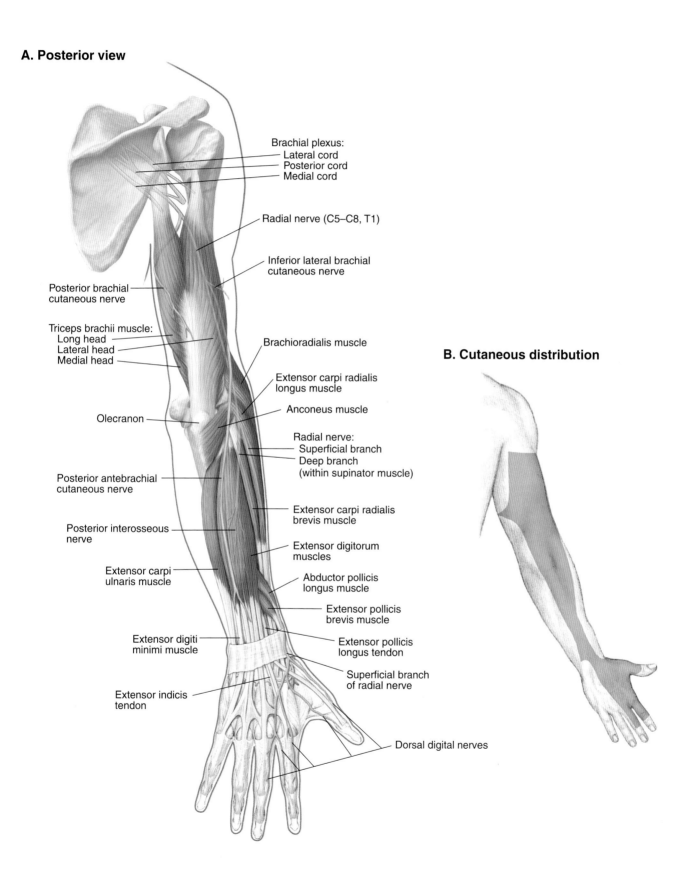

Brachial plexus:
Lateral cord
Posterior cord
Medial cord

Radial nerve (C5–C8, T1)

Inferior lateral brachial
cutaneous nerve

Posterior brachial
cutaneous nerve

Triceps brachii muscle:
Long head
Lateral head
Medial head

Brachioradialis muscle

Extensor carpi radialis
longus muscle

Anconeus muscle

B. Cutaneous distribution

Olecranon

Radial nerve:
Superficial branch
Deep branch
(within supinator muscle)

Posterior antebrachial
cutaneous nerve

Extensor carpi radialis
brevis muscle

Posterior interosseous
nerve

Extensor digitorum
muscles

Extensor carpi
ulnaris muscle

Abductor pollicis
longus muscle

Extensor pollicis
brevis muscle

Extensor digiti
minimi muscle

Extensor pollicis
longus tendon

Superficial branch
of radial nerve

Extensor indicis
tendon

Dorsal digital nerves

PLATE 2-51   **Cutaneous Innervation of the Upper Limb, Summary**

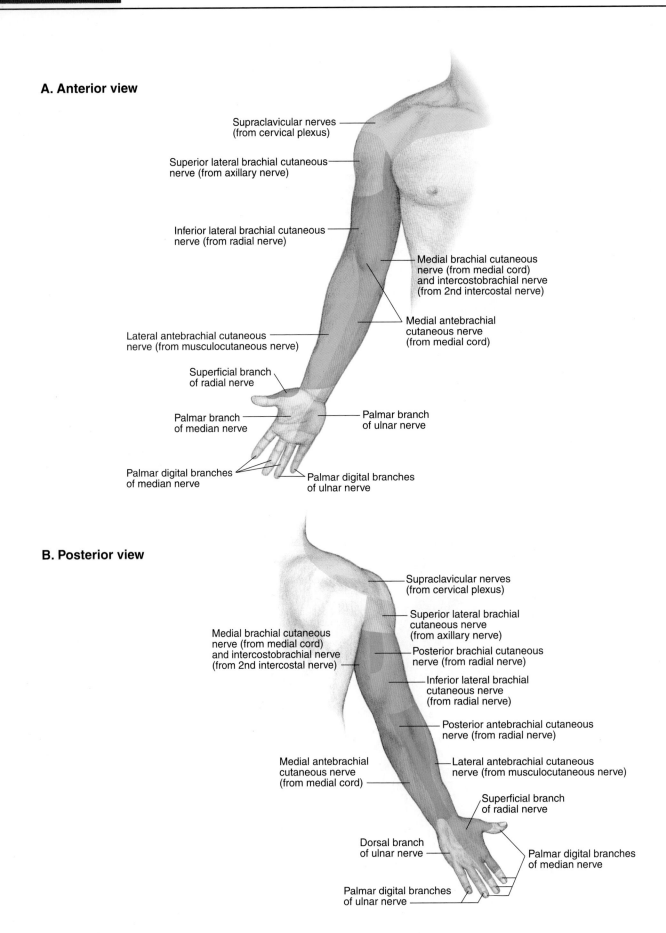

A. Anterior view

Supraclavicular nerves
(from cervical plexus)

Superior lateral brachial cutaneous
nerve (from axillary nerve)

Inferior lateral brachial cutaneous
nerve (from radial nerve)

Medial brachial cutaneous
nerve (from medial cord)
and intercostobrachial nerve
(from 2nd intercostal nerve)

Medial antebrachial
cutaneous nerve
(from medial cord)

Lateral antebrachial cutaneous
nerve (from musculocutaneous nerve)

Superficial branch
of radial nerve

Palmar branch
of median nerve

Palmar branch
of ulnar nerve

Palmar digital branches
of median nerve

Palmar digital branches
of ulnar nerve

B. Posterior view

Supraclavicular nerves
(from cervical plexus)

Superior lateral brachial
cutaneous nerve
(from axillary nerve)

Medial brachial cutaneous
nerve (from medial cord)
and intercostobrachial nerve
(from 2nd intercostal nerve)

Posterior brachial cutaneous
nerve (from radial nerve)

Inferior lateral brachial
cutaneous nerve
(from radial nerve)

Posterior antebrachial cutaneous
nerve (from radial nerve)

Medial antebrachial
cutaneous nerve
(from medial cord)

Lateral antebrachial cutaneous
nerve (from musculocutaneous nerve)

Superficial branch
of radial nerve

Dorsal branch
of ulnar nerve

Palmar digital branches
of median nerve

Palmar digital branches
of ulnar nerve

A. Posterior view

B. Anterior view

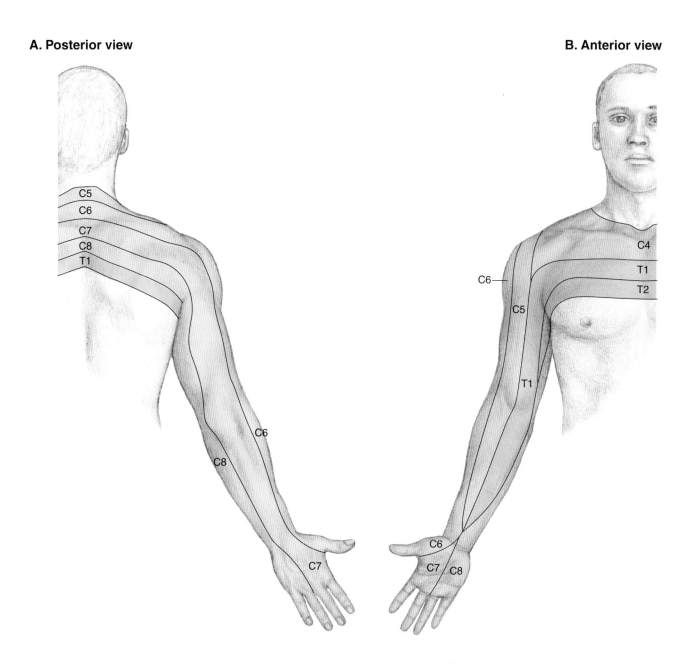

C5
C6
C7
C8
T1

C6

C8

C7

C4
T1
T2

C6

C5

T1

C6

C7　C8

PLATE 2-53 **Lymphatics of the Upper Limb**

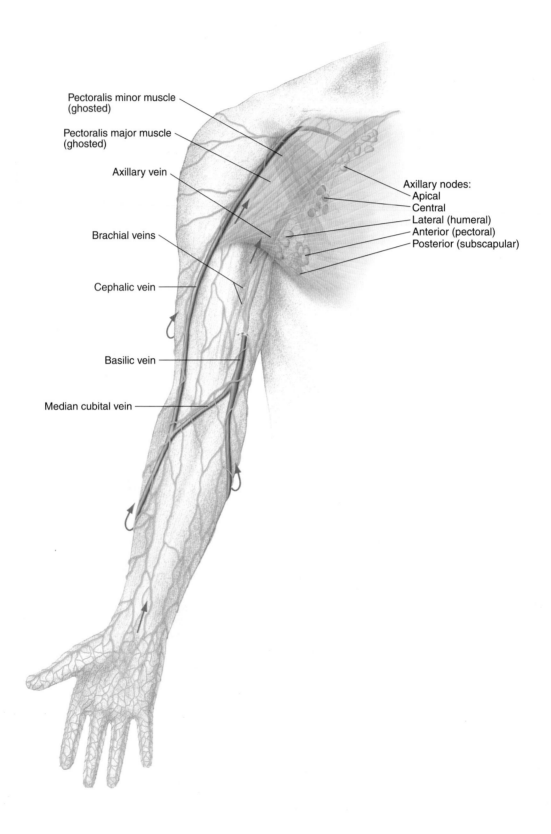

Pectoralis minor muscle (ghosted)

Pectoralis major muscle (ghosted)

Axillary vein

Brachial veins

Cephalic vein

Basilic vein

Median cubital vein

Axillary nodes:
Apical
Central
Lateral (humeral)
Anterior (pectoral)
Posterior (subscapular)

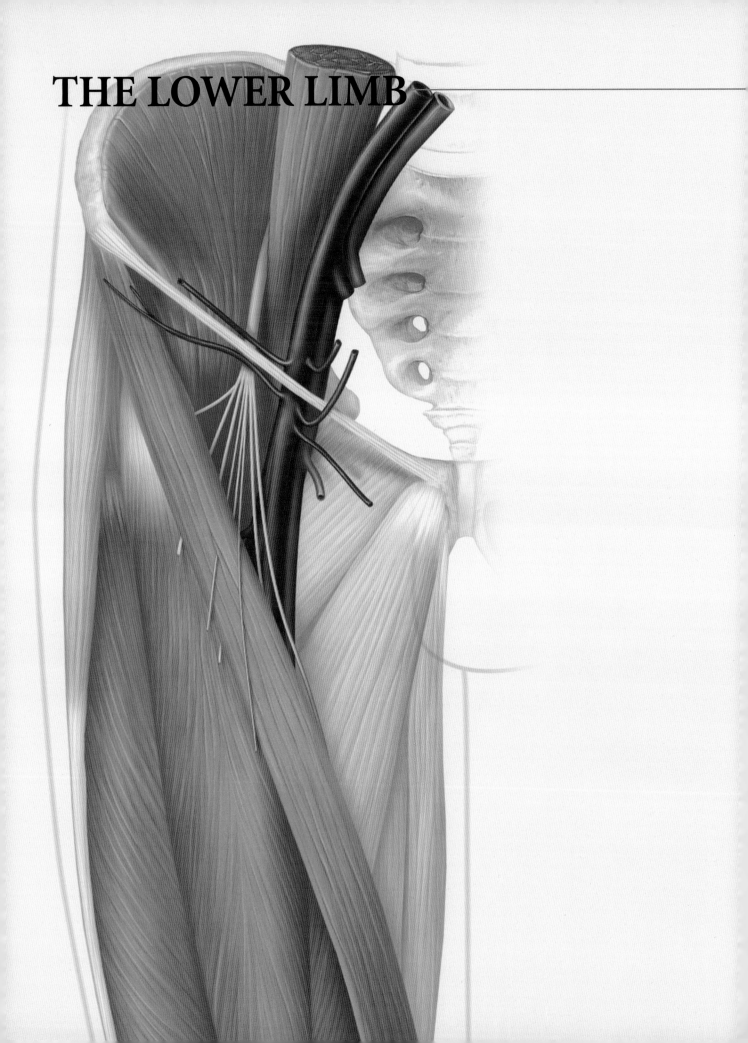

THE LOWER LIMB

Palpable bony structures

A. Anterior view   **B. Posterior view**

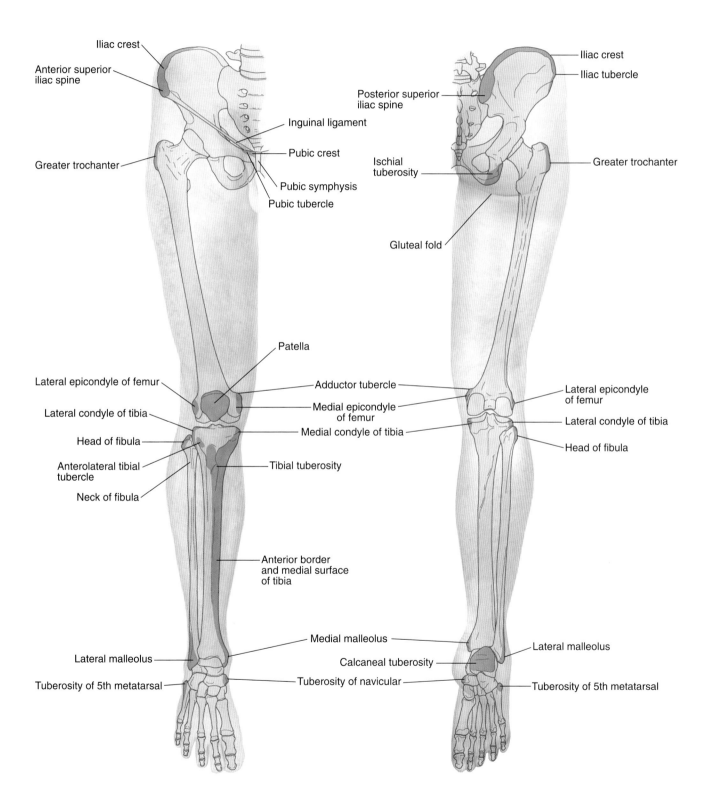

Iliac crest

Anterior superior
iliac spine

Greater trochanter

Inguinal ligament

Pubic crest

Pubic symphysis
Pubic tubercle

Iliac crest

Iliac tubercle

Posterior superior
iliac spine

Ischial
tuberosity

Greater trochanter

Gluteal fold

Patella

Lateral epicondyle of femur

Lateral condyle of tibia

Head of fibula

Anterolateral tibial
tubercle

Neck of fibula

Adductor tubercle

Medial epicondyle
of femur

Medial condyle of tibia

Tibial tuberosity

Lateral epicondyle
of femur

Lateral condyle of tibia

Head of fibula

Anterior border
and medial surface
of tibia

Medial malleolus

Lateral malleolus

Calcaneal tuberosity

Lateral malleolus

Tuberosity of 5th metatarsal

Tuberosity of navicular

Tuberosity of 5th metatarsal

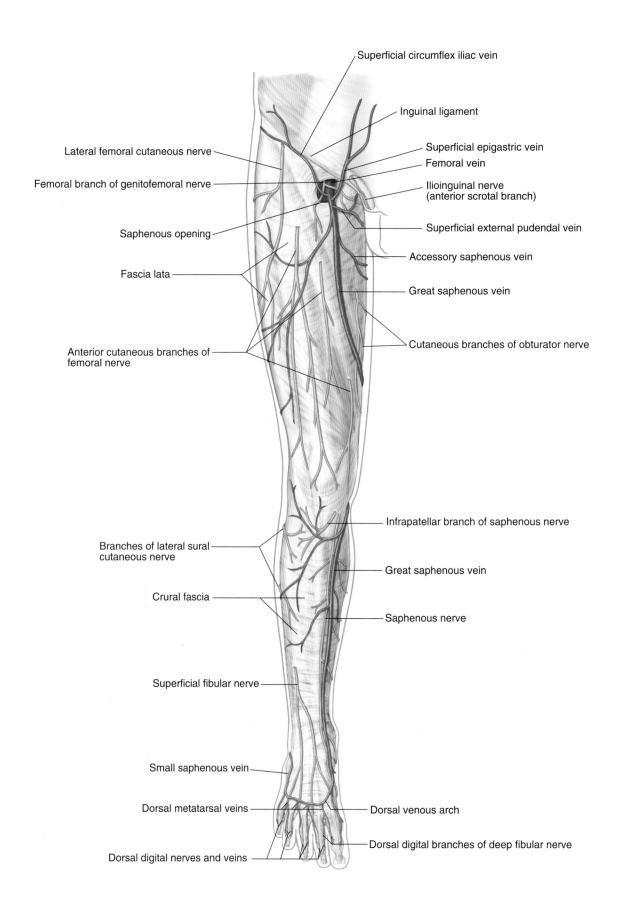

Superficial circumflex iliac vein

Inguinal ligament

Lateral femoral cutaneous nerve

Superficial epigastric vein

Femoral vein

Femoral branch of genitofemoral nerve

Ilioinguinal nerve
(anterior scrotal branch)

Saphenous opening

Superficial external pudendal vein

Accessory saphenous vein

Fascia lata

Great saphenous vein

Anterior cutaneous branches of
femoral nerve

Cutaneous branches of obturator nerve

Infrapatellar branch of saphenous nerve

Branches of lateral sural
cutaneous nerve

Great saphenous vein

Crural fascia

Saphenous nerve

Superficial fibular nerve

Small saphenous vein

Dorsal metatarsal veins

Dorsal venous arch

Dorsal digital branches of deep fibular nerve

Dorsal digital nerves and veins

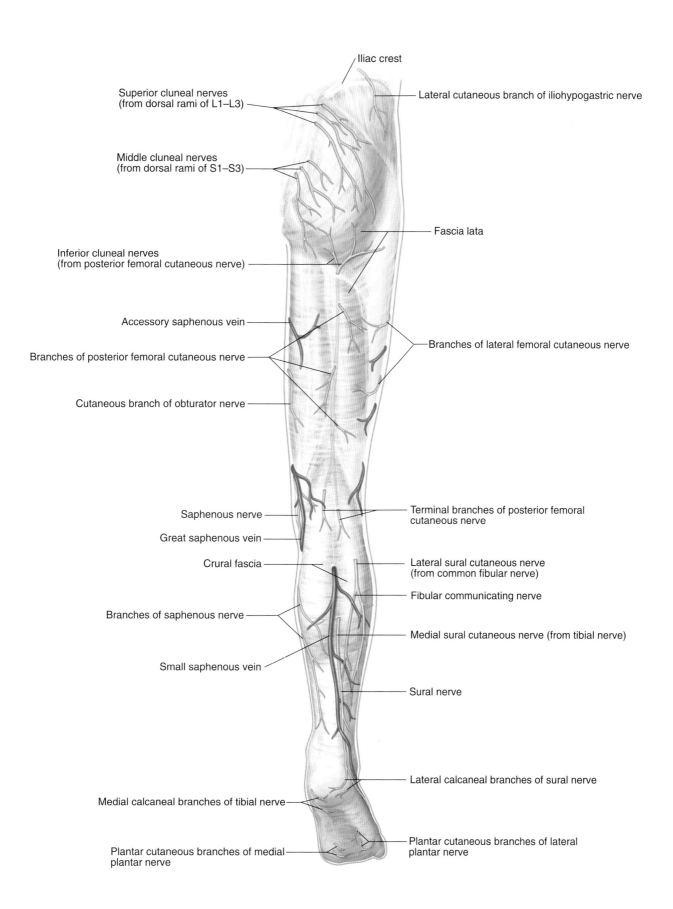

Iliac crest

Superior cluneal nerves
(from dorsal rami of L1–L3)

Lateral cutaneous branch of iliohypogastric nerve

Middle cluneal nerves
(from dorsal rami of S1–S3)

Fascia lata

Inferior cluneal nerves
(from posterior femoral cutaneous nerve)

Accessory saphenous vein

Branches of lateral femoral cutaneous nerve

Branches of posterior femoral cutaneous nerve

Cutaneous branch of obturator nerve

Saphenous nerve

Terminal branches of posterior femoral cutaneous nerve

Great saphenous vein

Crural fascia

Lateral sural cutaneous nerve
(from common fibular nerve)

Fibular communicating nerve

Branches of saphenous nerve

Medial sural cutaneous nerve (from tibial nerve)

Small saphenous vein

Sural nerve

Lateral calcaneal branches of sural nerve

Medial calcaneal branches of tibial nerve

Plantar cutaneous branches of lateral plantar nerve

Plantar cutaneous branches of medial plantar nerve

A. Bony features

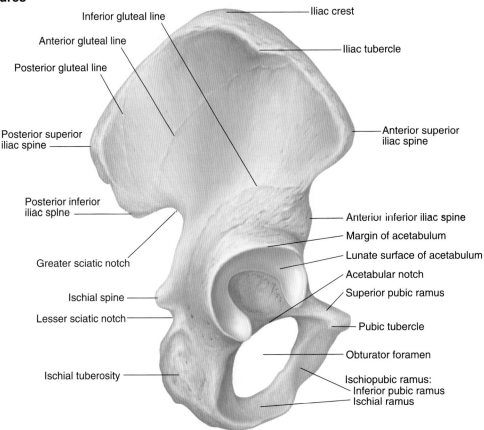

Inferior gluteal line

Anterior gluteal line

Posterior gluteal line

Posterior superior iliac spine

Posterior inferior iliac splne

Greater sciatic notch

Ischial spine

Lesser sciatic notch

Ischial tuberosity

Iliac crest

Iliac tubercle

Anterior superior iliac spine

Anterior inferior iliac spine

Margin of acetabulum

Lunate surface of acetabulum

Acetabular notch

Superior pubic ramus

Pubic tubercle

Obturator foramen

Ischiopubic ramus:
Inferior pubic ramus
Ischial ramus

B. Parts of os coxae

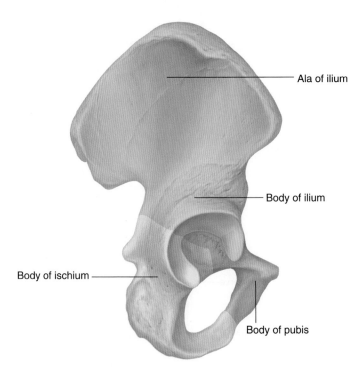

Ala of ilium

Body of ilium

Body of ischium

Body of pubis

A. Bony features

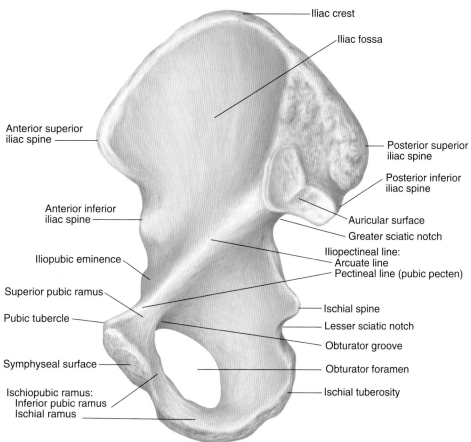

Iliac crest

Iliac fossa

Anterior superior iliac spine

Posterior superior iliac spine

Posterior inferior iliac spine

Anterior inferior iliac spine

Auricular surface

Greater sciatic notch

Iliopubic eminence

Iliopectineal line:
Arcuate line
Pectineal line (pubic pecten)

Superior pubic ramus

Pubic tubercle

Ischial spine

Lesser sciatic notch

Obturator groove

Symphyseal surface

Obturator foramen

Ischiopubic ramus:
Inferior pubic ramus
Ischial ramus

Ischial tuberosity

B. Parts of os coxae

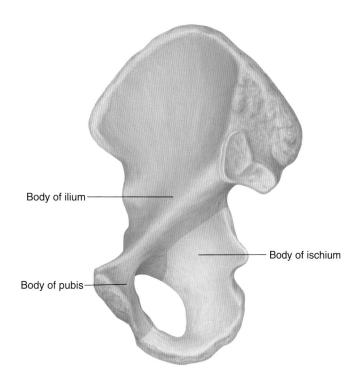

Body of ilium

Body of ischium

Body of pubis

PLATE 3-06   **Skeleton of the Proximal Lower Limb, Anterior View**

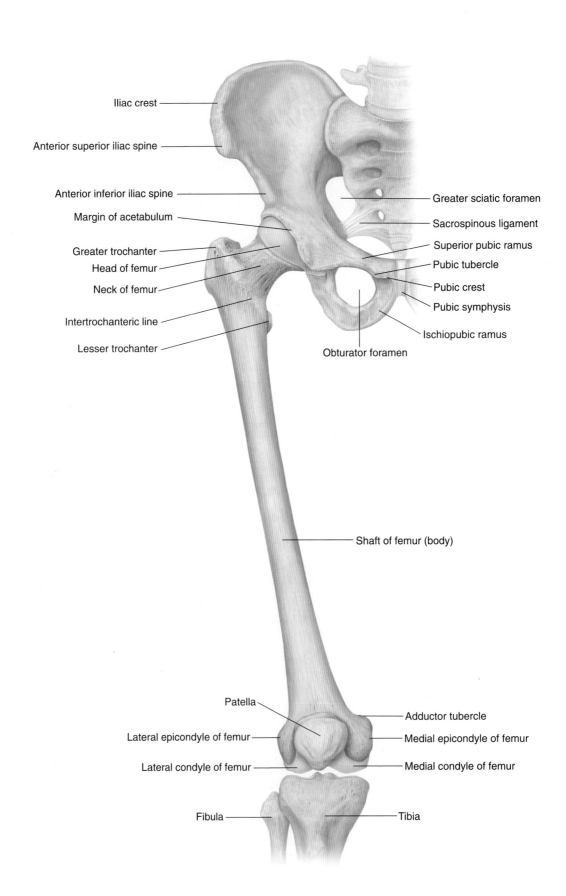

Iliac crest

Anterior superior iliac spine

Anterior inferior iliac spine

Margin of acetabulum

Greater trochanter

Head of femur

Neck of femur

Intertrochanteric line

Lesser trochanter

Greater sciatic foramen

Sacrospinous ligament

Superior pubic ramus

Pubic tubercle

Pubic crest

Pubic symphysis

Ischiopubic ramus

Obturator foramen

Shaft of femur (body)

Patella

Lateral epicondyle of femur

Lateral condyle of femur

Adductor tubercle

Medial epicondyle of femur

Medial condyle of femur

Fibula

Tibia

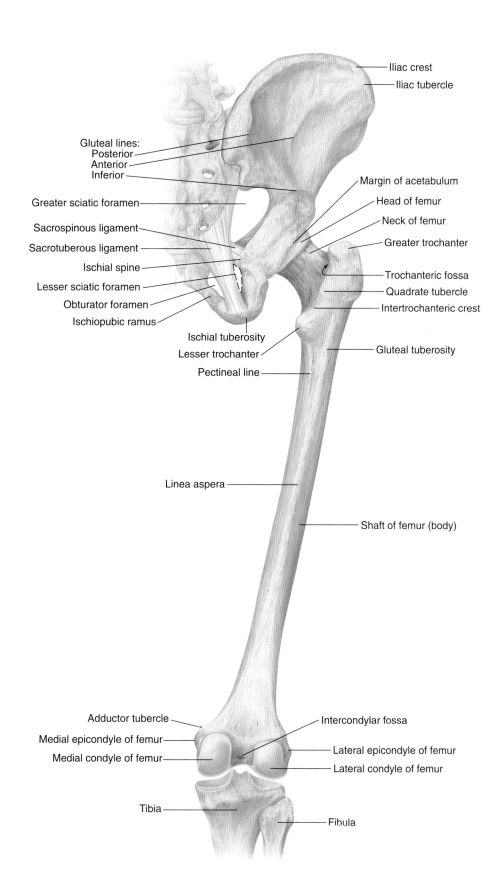

Iliac crest

Iliac tubercle

Gluteal lines:
Posterior
Anterior
Inferior

Greater sciatic foramen

Sacrospinous ligament

Sacrotuberous ligament

Ischial spine

Lesser sciatic foramen

Obturator foramen

Ischiopubic ramus

Ischial tuberosity

Lesser trochanter

Pectineal line

Margin of acetabulum

Head of femur

Neck of femur

Greater trochanter

Trochanteric fossa

Quadrate tubercle

Intertrochanteric crest

Gluteal tuberosity

Linea aspera

Shaft of femur (body)

Adductor tubercle

Medial epicondyle of femur

Medial condyle of femur

Intercondylar fossa

Lateral epicondyle of femur

Lateral condyle of femur

Tibia

Fibula

PLATE 3-08   **Skeleton of the Distal Lower Limb, Anterior View**

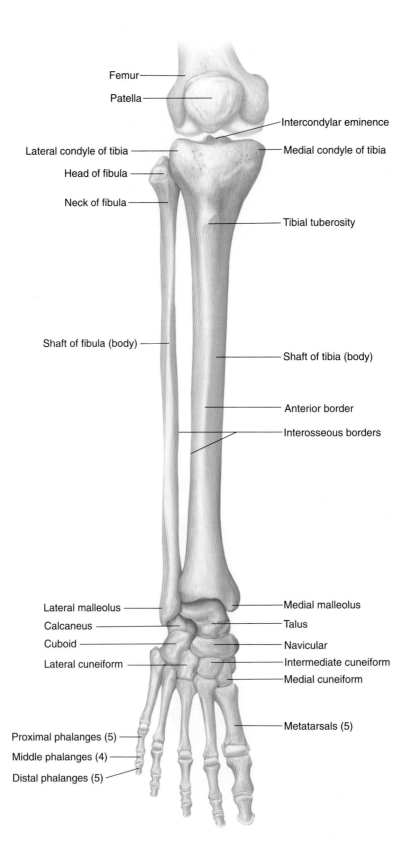

Femur

Patella

Intercondylar eminence

Lateral condyle of tibia

Medial condyle of tibia

Head of fibula

Neck of fibula

Tibial tuberosity

Shaft of fibula (body)

Shaft of tibia (body)

Anterior border

Interosseous borders

Lateral malleolus

Medial malleolus

Calcaneus

Talus

Cuboid

Navicular

Lateral cuneiform

Intermediate cuneiform

Medial cuneiform

Metatarsals (5)

Proximal phalanges (5)

Middle phalanges (4)

Distal phalanges (5)

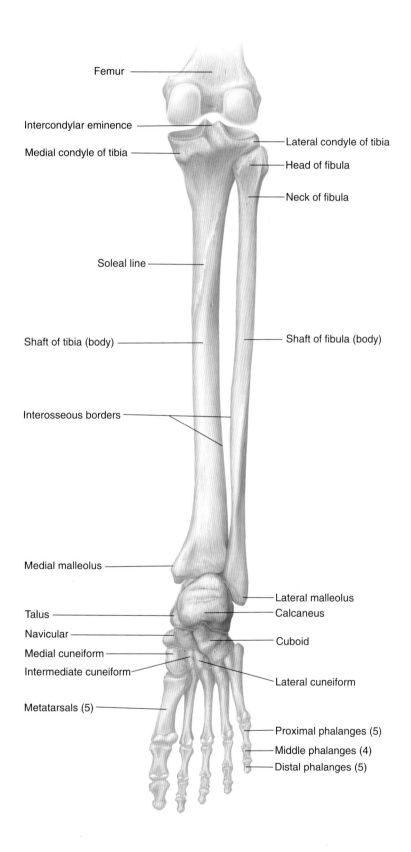

Femur

Intercondylar eminence

Medial condyle of tibia

Lateral condyle of tibia

Head of fibula

Neck of fibula

Soleal line

Shaft of tibia (body)

Shaft of fibula (body)

Interosseous borders

Medial malleolus

Lateral malleolus

Talus

Calcaneus

Navicular

Cuboid

Medial cuneiform

Intermediate cuneiform

Lateral cuneiform

Metatarsals (5)

Proximal phalanges (5)

Middle phalanges (4)

Distal phalanges (5)

PLATE 3-10   **Radiographs of the Lower Limb**

A. Hip joint, anterior view

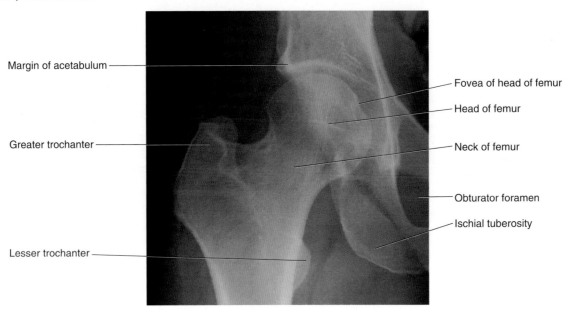

Margin of acetabulum

Greater trochanter

Lesser trochanter

Fovea of head of femur

Head of femur

Neck of femur

Obturator foramen

Ischial tuberosity

B. Knee joint, anterior view

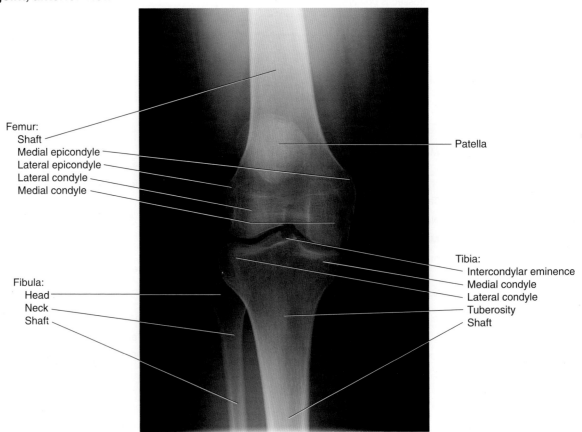

Femur:
    Shaft
    Medial epicondyle
    Lateral epicondyle
    Lateral condyle
    Medial condyle

Fibula:
    Head
    Neck
    Shaft

Patella

Tibia:
    Intercondylar eminence
    Medial condyle
    Lateral condyle
    Tuberosity
    Shaft

A. Anterior view

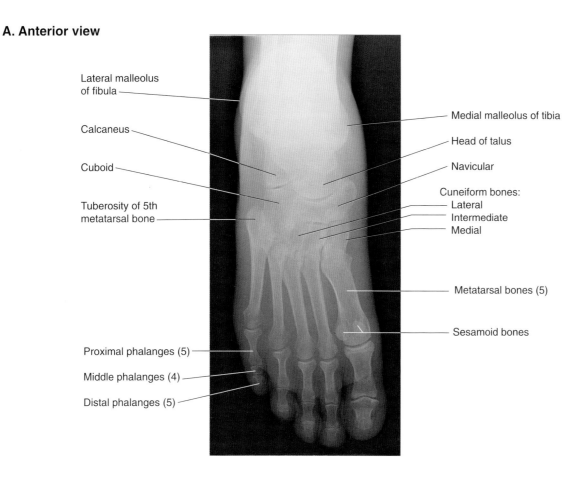

Lateral malleolus of fibula

Calcaneus

Cuboid

Tuberosity of 5th metatarsal bone

Medial malleolus of tibia

Head of talus

Navicular

Cuneiform bones:
Lateral
Intermediate
Medial

Metatarsal bones (5)

Sesamoid bones

Proximal phalanges (5)

Middle phalanges (4)

Distal phalanges (5)

B. Lateral view

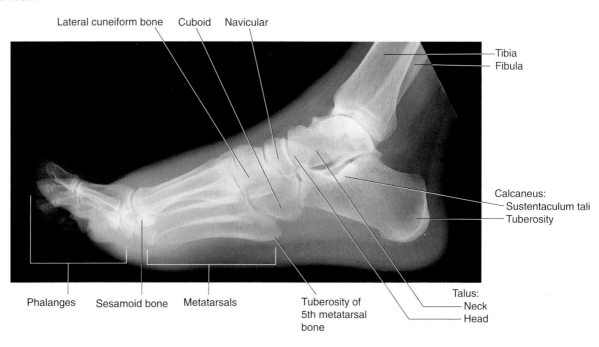

Lateral cuneiform bone   Cuboid   Navicular

Tibia

Fibula

Calcaneus:
Sustentaculum tali
Tuberosity

Phalanges   Sesamoid bone   Metatarsals

Tuberosity of 5th metatarsal bone

Talus:
Neck
Head

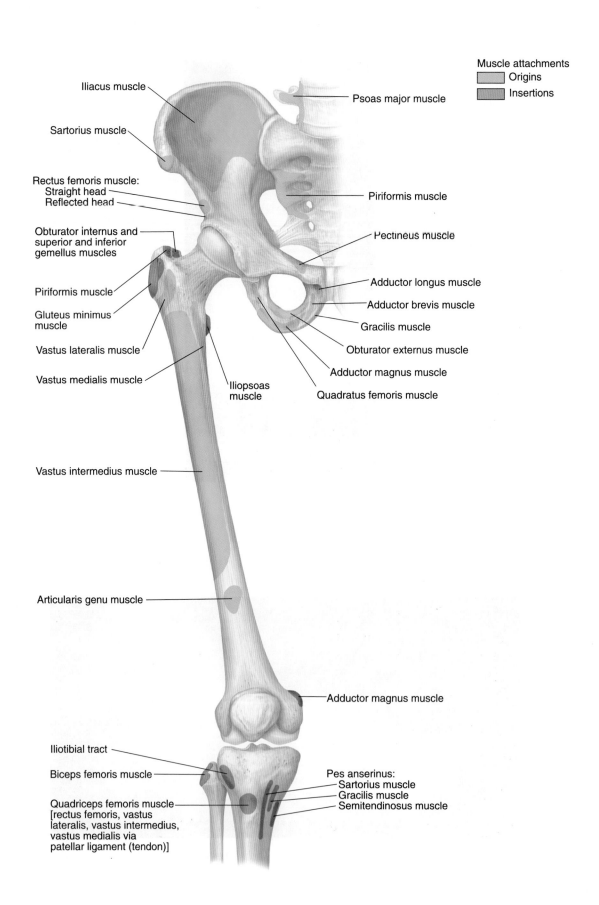

Muscle attachments
Origins
Insertions

Iliacus muscle

Psoas major muscle

Sartorius muscle

Rectus femoris muscle:
  Straight head
  Reflected head

Piriformis muscle

Obturator internus and
superior and inferior
gemellus muscles

Pectineus muscle

Piriformis muscle

Adductor longus muscle

Gluteus minimus
muscle

Adductor brevis muscle

Gracilis muscle

Vastus lateralis muscle

Obturator externus muscle

Vastus medialis muscle

Adductor magnus muscle

Iliopsoas
muscle

Quadratus femoris muscle

Vastus intermedius muscle

Articularis genu muscle

Adductor magnus muscle

Iliotibial tract

Biceps femoris muscle

Pes anserinus:
  Sartorius muscle
  Gracilis muscle
  Semitendinosus muscle

Quadriceps femoris muscle
[rectus femoris, vastus
lateralis, vastus intermedius,
vastus medialis via
patellar ligament (tendon)]

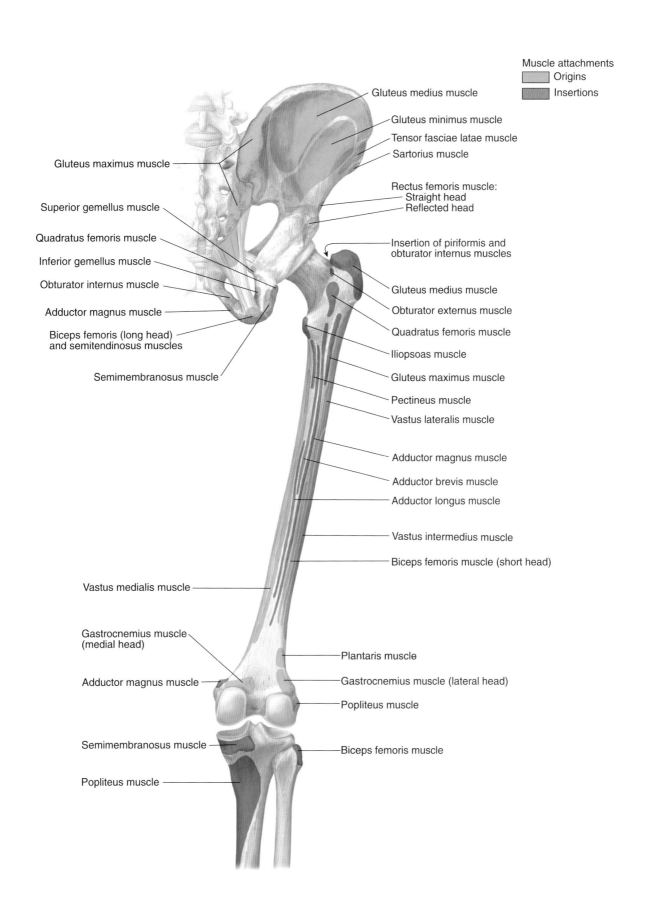

Muscle attachments
- Origins
- Insertions

Gluteus medius muscle

Gluteus minimus muscle

Tensor fasciae latae muscle

Sartorius muscle

Rectus femoris muscle:
Straight head
Reflected head

Insertion of piriformis and obturator internus muscles

Gluteus medius muscle

Obturator externus muscle

Quadratus femoris muscle

Iliopsoas muscle

Gluteus maximus muscle

Pectineus muscle

Vastus lateralis muscle

Adductor magnus muscle

Adductor brevis muscle

Adductor longus muscle

Vastus intermedius muscle

Biceps femoris muscle (short head)

Plantaris muscle

Gastrocnemius muscle (lateral head)

Popliteus muscle

Biceps femoris muscle

Gluteus maximus muscle

Superior gemellus muscle

Quadratus femoris muscle

Inferior gemellus muscle

Obturator internus muscle

Adductor magnus muscle

Biceps femoris (long head) and semitendinosus muscles

Semimembranosus muscle

Vastus medialis muscle

Gastrocnemius muscle (medial head)

Adductor magnus muscle

Semimembranosus muscle

Popliteus muscle

PLATE 3-14   Lumbar Plexus

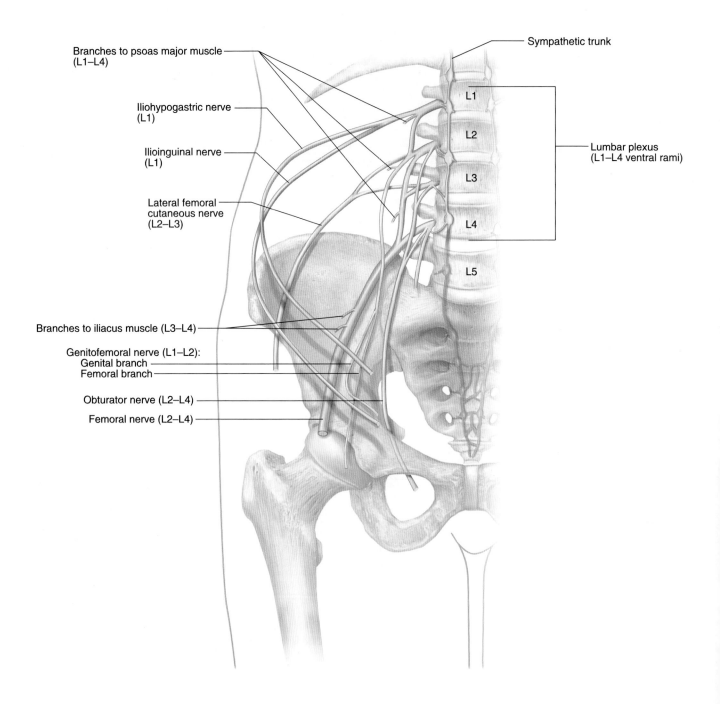

Branches to psoas major muscle
(L1–L4)

Iliohypogastric nerve
(L1)

Ilioinguinal nerve
(L1)

Lateral femoral
cutaneous nerve
(L2–L3)

Branches to iliacus muscle (L3–L4)

Genitofemoral nerve (L1–L2):
Genital branch
Femoral branch

Obturator nerve (L2–L4)

Femoral nerve (L2–L4)

Sympathetic trunk

L1

L2

L3

L4

L5

Lumbar plexus
(L1–L4 ventral rami)

A. Orientation

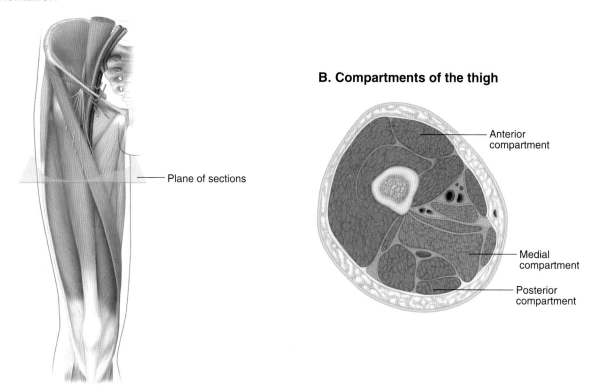

Plane of sections

B. Compartments of the thigh

Anterior compartment

Medial compartment

Posterior compartment

C. Cross section

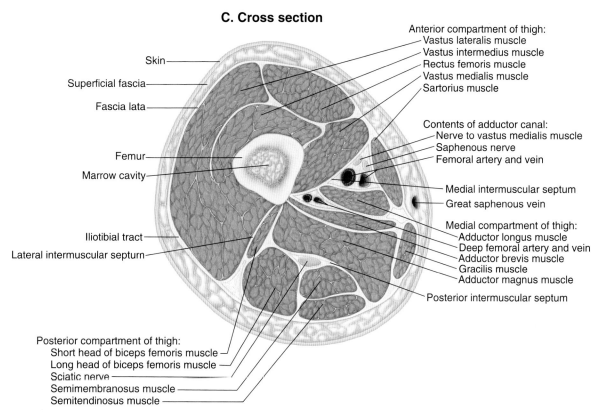

Skin

Superficial fascia

Fascia lata

Femur

Marrow cavity

Iliotibial tract

Lateral intermuscular septurn

Anterior compartment of thigh:
Vastus lateralis muscle
Vastus intermedius muscle
Rectus femoris muscle
Vastus medialis muscle
Sartorius muscle

Contents of adductor canal:
Nerve to vastus medialis muscle
Saphenous nerve
Femoral artery and vein

Medial intermuscular septum
Great saphenous vein

Medial compartment of thigh:
Adductor longus muscle
Deep femoral artery and vein
Adductor brevis muscle
Gracilis muscle
Adductor magnus muscle

Posterior intermuscular septum

Posterior compartment of thigh:
Short head of biceps femoris muscle
Long head of biceps femoris muscle
Sciatic nerve
Semimembranosus muscle
Semitendinosus muscle

PLATE 3-16   **Muscles of the Anterior Thigh, Superficial Dissection**

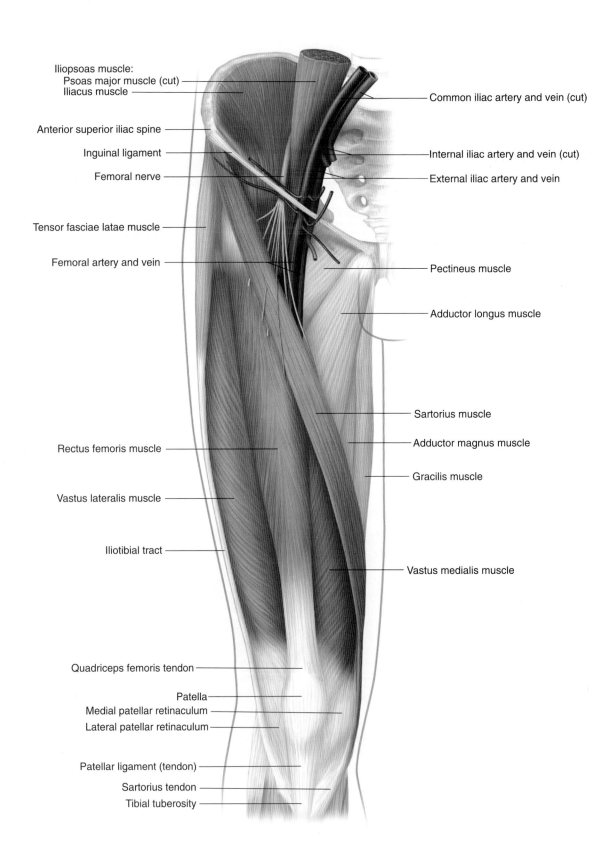

Iliopsoas muscle:
Psoas major muscle (cut)
Iliacus muscle

Anterior superior iliac spine

Inguinal ligament

Femoral nerve

Tensor fasciae latae muscle

Femoral artery and vein

Rectus femoris muscle

Vastus lateralis muscle

Iliotibial tract

Quadriceps femoris tendon

Patella
Medial patellar retinaculum
Lateral patellar retinaculum

Patellar ligament (tendon)
Sartorius tendon
Tibial tuberosity

Common iliac artery and vein (cut)

Internal iliac artery and vein (cut)

External iliac artery and vein

Pectineus muscle

Adductor longus muscle

Sartorius muscle

Adductor magnus muscle

Gracilis muscle

Vastus medialis muscle

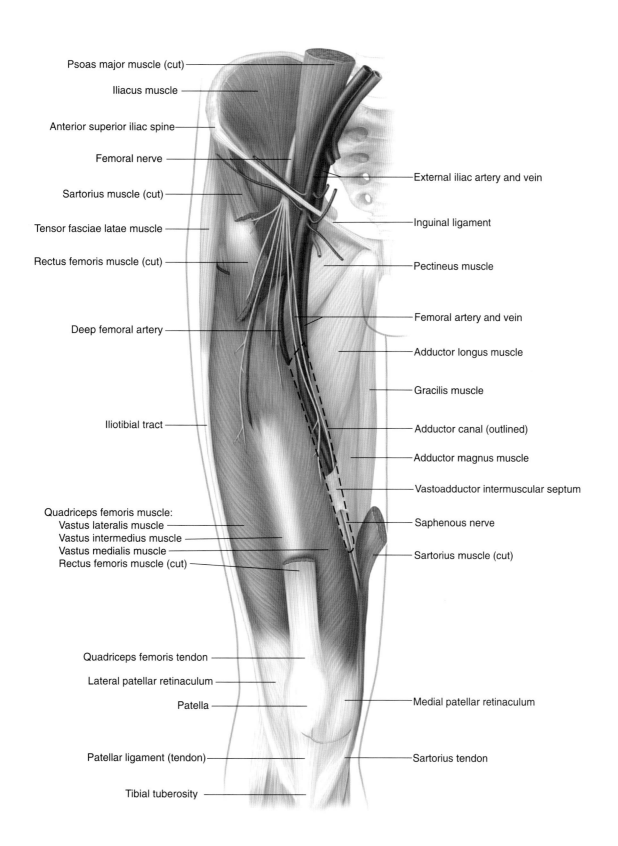

Psoas major muscle (cut)

Iliacus muscle

Anterior superior iliac spine

Femoral nerve

Sartorius muscle (cut)

Tensor fasciae latae muscle

Rectus femoris muscle (cut)

Deep femoral artery

Iliotibial tract

Quadriceps femoris muscle:
Vastus lateralis muscle
Vastus intermedius muscle
Vastus medialis muscle
Rectus femoris muscle (cut)

Quadriceps femoris tendon

Lateral patellar retinaculum

Patella

Patellar ligament (tendon)

Tibial tuberosity

External iliac artery and vein

Inguinal ligament

Pectineus muscle

Femoral artery and vein

Adductor longus muscle

Gracilis muscle

Adductor canal (outlined)

Adductor magnus muscle

Vastoadductor intermuscular septum

Saphenous nerve

Sartorius muscle (cut)

Medial patellar retinaculum

Sartorius tendon

PLATE 3-18   Femoral Triangle

A. Anterior view

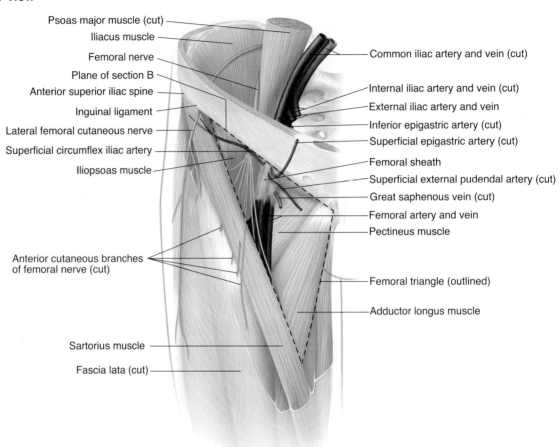

Psoas major muscle (cut)

Iliacus muscle

Femoral nerve

Plane of section B

Anterior superior iliac spine

Inguinal ligament

Lateral femoral cutaneous nerve

Superficial circumflex iliac artery

Iliopsoas muscle

Anterior cutaneous branches
of femoral nerve (cut)

Sartorius muscle

Fascia lata (cut)

Common iliac artery and vein (cut)

Internal iliac artery and vein (cut)

External iliac artery and vein

Inferior epigastric artery (cut)

Superficial epigastric artery (cut)

Femoral sheath

Superficial external pudendal artery (cut)

Great saphenous vein (cut)

Femoral artery and vein

Pectineus muscle

Femoral triangle (outlined)

Adductor longus muscle

B. Section through the femoral sheath

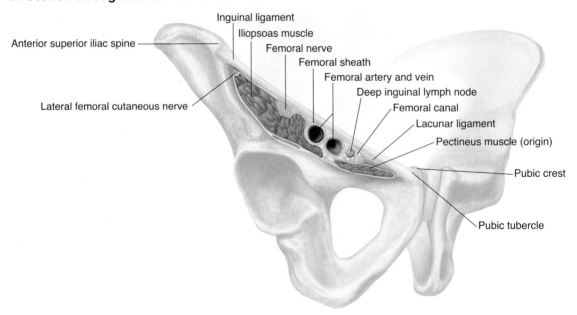

Inguinal ligament

Iliopsoas muscle

Femoral nerve

Femoral sheath

Femoral artery and vein

Deep inguinal lymph node

Femoral canal

Lacunar ligament

Pectineus muscle (origin)

Pubic crest

Pubic tubercle

Anterior superior iliac spine

Lateral femoral cutaneous nerve

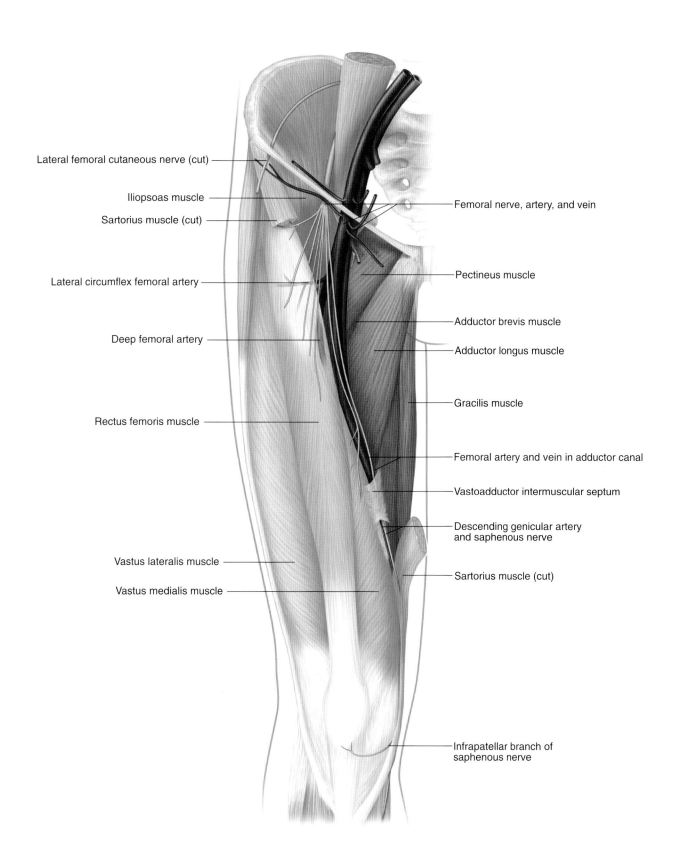

Lateral femoral cutaneous nerve (cut)

Iliopsoas muscle

Sartorius muscle (cut)

Lateral circumflex femoral artery

Deep femoral artery

Rectus femoris muscle

Vastus lateralis muscle

Vastus medialis muscle

Femoral nerve, artery, and vein

Pectineus muscle

Adductor brevis muscle

Adductor longus muscle

Gracilis muscle

Femoral artery and vein in adductor canal

Vastoadductor intermuscular septum

Descending genicular artery and saphenous nerve

Sartorius muscle (cut)

Infrapatellar branch of saphenous nerve

PLATE 3-20   **Muscles of the Medial Thigh, Intermediate Dissection**

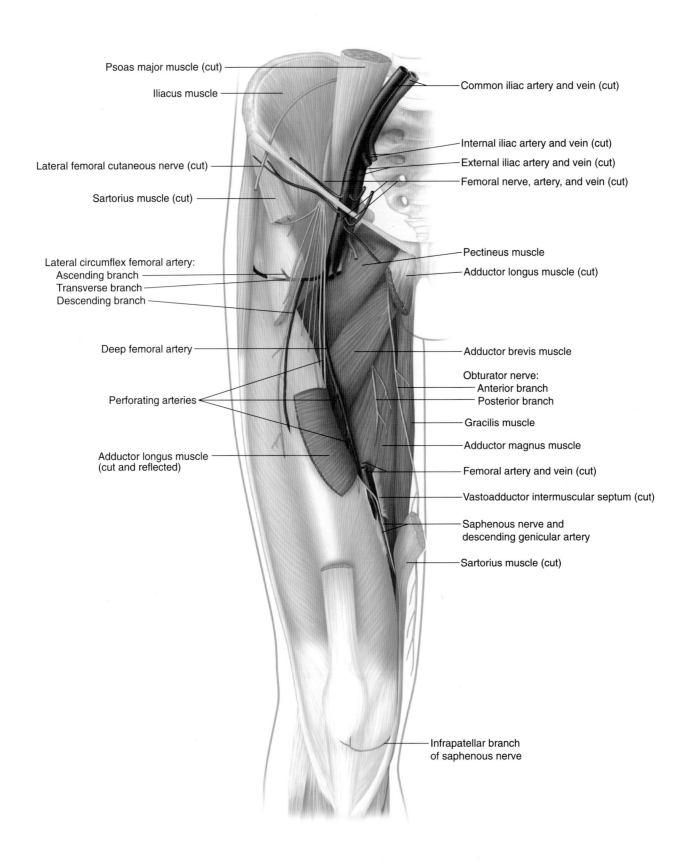

Psoas major muscle (cut)

Iliacus muscle

Common iliac artery and vein (cut)

Internal iliac artery and vein (cut)

External iliac artery and vein (cut)

Femoral nerve, artery, and vein (cut)

Lateral femoral cutaneous nerve (cut)

Sartorius muscle (cut)

Pectineus muscle

Adductor longus muscle (cut)

Lateral circumflex femoral artery:
  Ascending branch
  Transverse branch
  Descending branch

Deep femoral artery

Adductor brevis muscle

Obturator nerve:
  Anterior branch
  Posterior branch

Gracilis muscle

Perforating arteries

Adductor magnus muscle

Adductor longus muscle
(cut and reflected)

Femoral artery and vein (cut)

Vastoadductor intermuscular septum (cut)

Saphenous nerve and
descending genicular artery

Sartorius muscle (cut)

Infrapatellar branch
of saphenous nerve

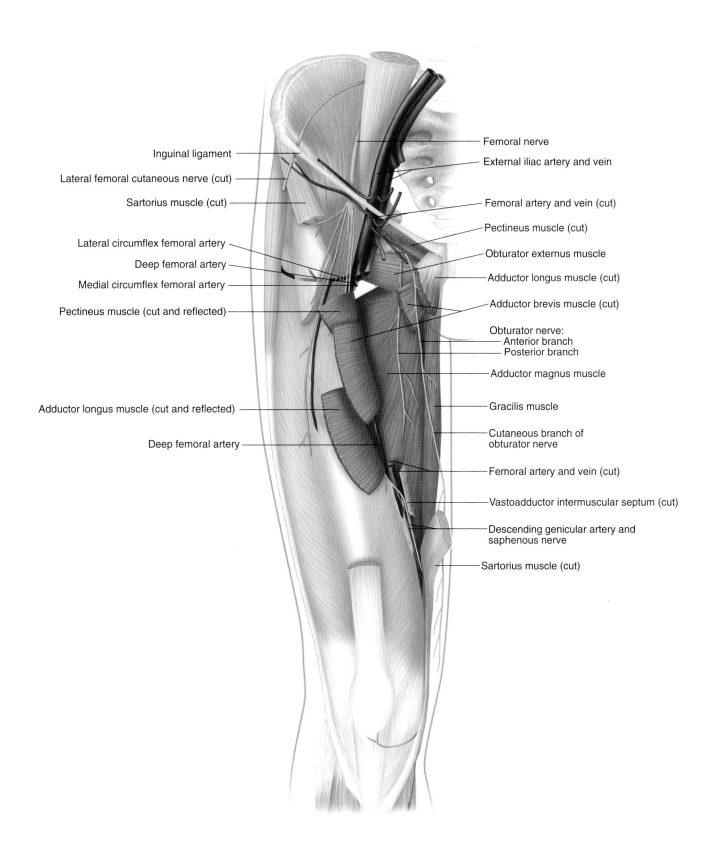

Inguinal ligament

Lateral femoral cutaneous nerve (cut)

Sartorius muscle (cut)

Lateral circumflex femoral artery

Deep femoral artery

Medial circumflex femoral artery

Pectineus muscle (cut and reflected)

Adductor longus muscle (cut and reflected)

Deep femoral artery

Femoral nerve

External iliac artery and vein

Femoral artery and vein (cut)

Pectineus muscle (cut)

Obturator externus muscle

Adductor longus muscle (cut)

Adductor brevis muscle (cut)

Obturator nerve:
Anterior branch
Posterior branch

Adductor magnus muscle

Gracilis muscle

Cutaneous branch of
obturator nerve

Femoral artery and vein (cut)

Vastoadductor intermuscular septum (cut)

Descending genicular artery and
saphenous nerve

Sartorius muscle (cut)

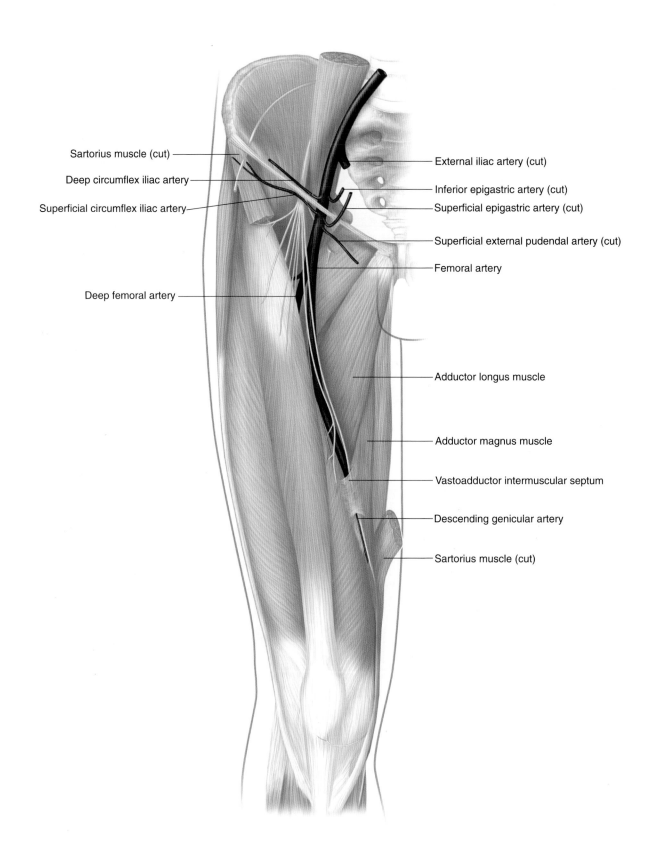

Sartorius muscle (cut)

Deep circumflex iliac artery

Superficial circumflex iliac artery

Deep femoral artery

External iliac artery (cut)

Inferior epigastric artery (cut)

Superficial epigastric artery (cut)

Superficial external pudendal artery (cut)

Femoral artery

Adductor longus muscle

Adductor magnus muscle

Vastoadductor intermuscular septum

Descending genicular artery

Sartorius muscle (cut)

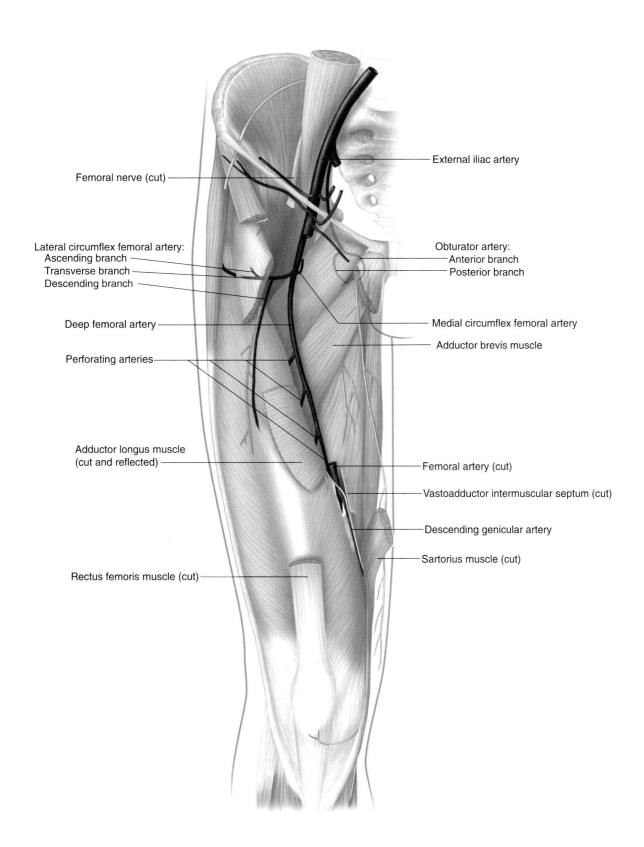

Femoral nerve (cut)

External iliac artery

Lateral circumflex femoral artery:
Ascending branch
Transverse branch
Descending branch

Obturator artery:
Anterior branch
Posterior branch

Deep femoral artery

Medial circumflex femoral artery

Perforating arteries

Adductor brevis muscle

Adductor longus muscle
(cut and reflected)

Femoral artery (cut)

Vastoadductor intermuscular septum (cut)

Descending genicular artery

Sartorius muscle (cut)

Rectus femoris muscle (cut)

PLATE 3-24   **Nerves of the Anterior and Medial Thigh**

A. Superficial dissection

B. Deep dissection

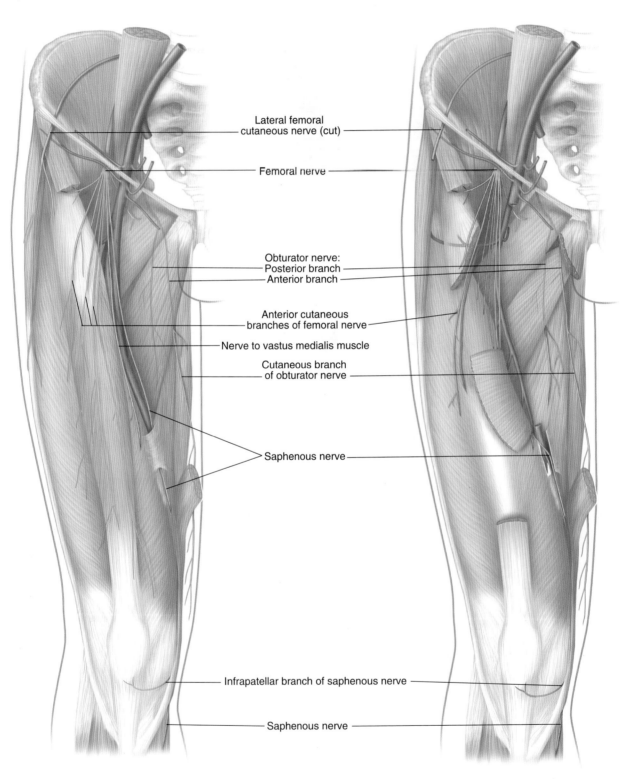

Lateral femoral cutaneous nerve (cut)

Femoral nerve

Obturator nerve:
Posterior branch
Anterior branch

Anterior cutaneous branches of femoral nerve

Nerve to vastus medialis muscle

Cutaneous branch of obturator nerve

Saphenous nerve

Infrapatellar branch of saphenous nerve

Saphenous nerve

A. Anterior view

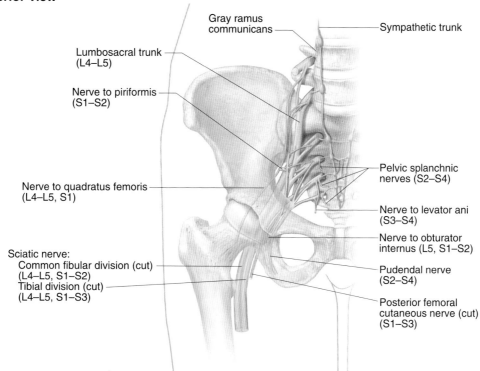

Gray ramus communicans

Sympathetic trunk

Lumbosacral trunk (L4–L5)

Nerve to piriformis (S1–S2)

Nerve to quadratus femoris (L4–L5, S1)

Pelvic splanchnic nerves (S2–S4)

Nerve to levator ani (S3–S4)

Nerve to obturator internus (L5, S1–S2)

Sciatic nerve:
Common fibular division (cut) (L4–L5, S1–S2)
Tibial division (cut) (L4–L5, S1–S3)

Pudendal nerve (S2–S4)

Posterior femoral cutaneous nerve (cut) (S1–S3)

B. Posterior view

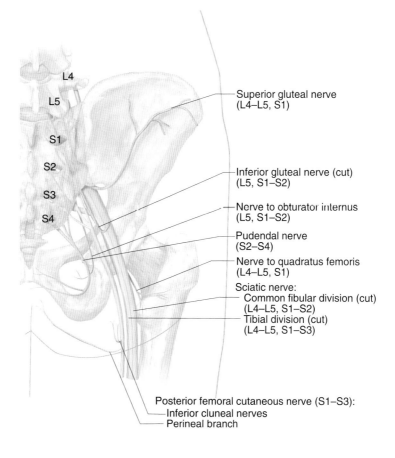

L4

L5

S1

S2

S3

S4

Superior gluteal nerve (L4–L5, S1)

Inferior gluteal nerve (cut) (L5, S1–S2)

Nerve to obturator internus (L5, S1–S2)

Pudendal nerve (S2–S4)

Nerve to quadratus femoris (L4–L5, S1)

Sciatic nerve:
Common fibular division (cut) (L4–L5, S1–S2)
Tibial division (cut) (L4–L5, S1–S3)

Posterior femoral cutaneous nerve (S1–S3):
Inferior cluneal nerves
Perineal branch

PLATE 3-26   Muscles of the Gluteal Region

A. Superficial dissection

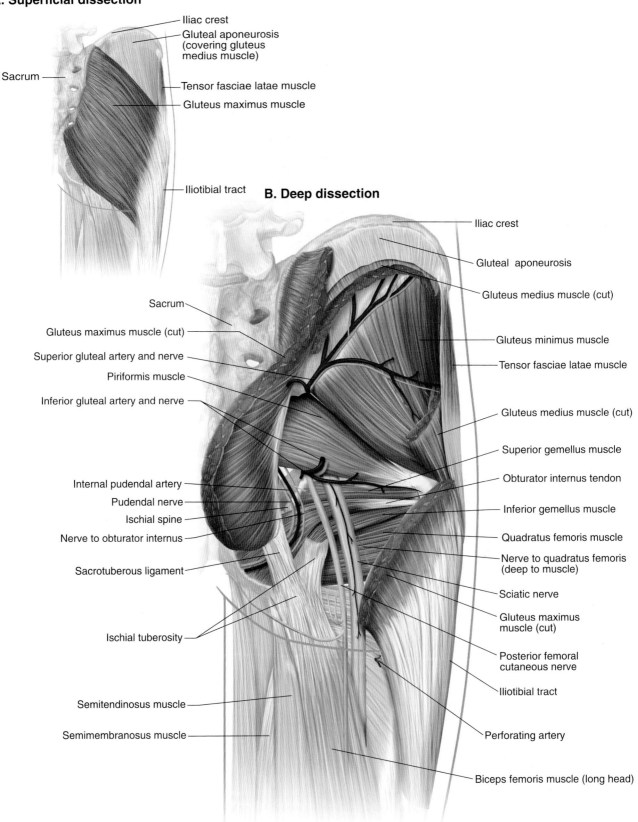

Iliac crest

Gluteal aponeurosis (covering gluteus medius muscle)

Sacrum

Tensor fasciae latae muscle

Gluteus maximus muscle

Iliotibial tract

B. Deep dissection

Iliac crest

Gluteal aponeurosis

Gluteus medius muscle (cut)

Sacrum

Gluteus maximus muscle (cut)

Superior gluteal artery and nerve

Piriformis muscle

Inferior gluteal artery and nerve

Gluteus minimus muscle

Tensor fasciae latae muscle

Gluteus medius muscle (cut)

Superior gemellus muscle

Obturator internus tendon

Internal pudendal artery

Pudendal nerve

Ischial spine

Nerve to obturator internus

Sacrotuberous ligament

Inferior gemellus muscle

Quadratus femoris muscle

Nerve to quadratus femoris (deep to muscle)

Sciatic nerve

Gluteus maximus muscle (cut)

Ischial tuberosity

Posterior femoral cutaneous nerve

Iliotibial tract

Semitendinosus muscle

Semimembranosus muscle

Perforating artery

Biceps femoris muscle (long head)

A. Arteries

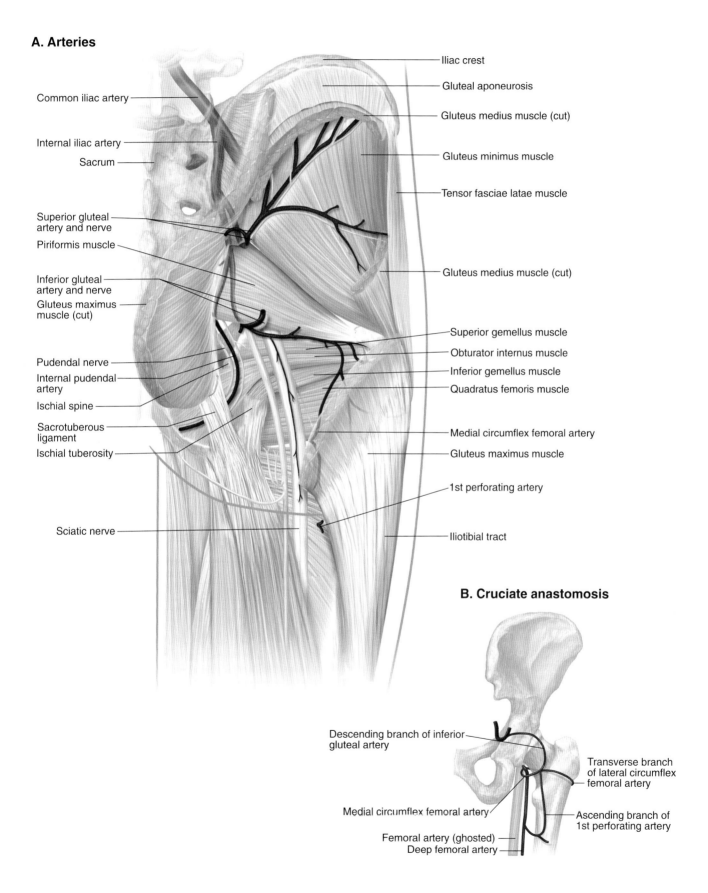

Common iliac artery

Internal iliac artery

Sacrum

Superior gluteal artery and nerve

Piriformis muscle

Inferior gluteal artery and nerve

Gluteus maximus muscle (cut)

Pudendal nerve

Internal pudendal artery

Ischial spine

Sacrotuberous ligament

Ischial tuberosity

Sciatic nerve

Iliac crest

Gluteal aponeurosis

Gluteus medius muscle (cut)

Gluteus minimus muscle

Tensor fasciae latae muscle

Gluteus medius muscle (cut)

Superior gemellus muscle

Obturator internus muscle

Inferior gemellus muscle

Quadratus femoris muscle

Medial circumflex femoral artery

Gluteus maximus muscle

1st perforating artery

Iliotibial tract

B. Cruciate anastomosis

Descending branch of inferior gluteal artery

Transverse branch of lateral circumflex femoral artery

Medial circumflex femoral artery

Ascending branch of 1st perforating artery

Femoral artery (ghosted)

Deep femoral artery

PLATE 3-28   **Nerves of the Gluteal Region**

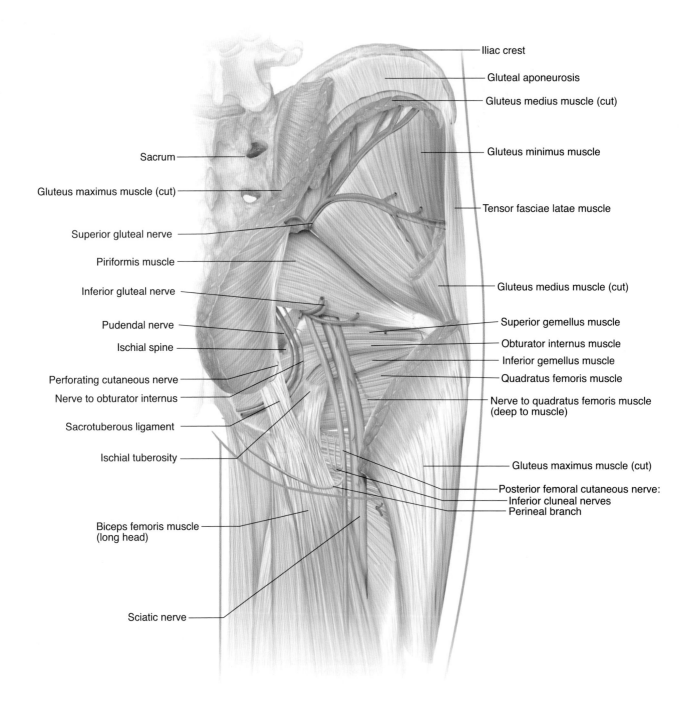

Iliac crest

Gluteal aponeurosis

Gluteus medius muscle (cut)

Gluteus minimus muscle

Sacrum

Tensor fasciae latae muscle

Gluteus maximus muscle (cut)

Superior gluteal nerve

Piriformis muscle

Gluteus medius muscle (cut)

Inferior gluteal nerve

Superior gemellus muscle

Pudendal nerve

Obturator internus muscle

Ischial spine

Inferior gemellus muscle

Quadratus femoris muscle

Perforating cutaneous nerve

Nerve to obturator internus

Nerve to quadratus femoris muscle
(deep to muscle)

Sacrotuberous ligament

Ischial tuberosity

Gluteus maximus muscle (cut)

Posterior femoral cutaneous nerve:
Inferior cluneal nerves
Perineal branch

Biceps femoris muscle
(long head)

Sciatic nerve

A. Superficial dissection

B. Deep dissection

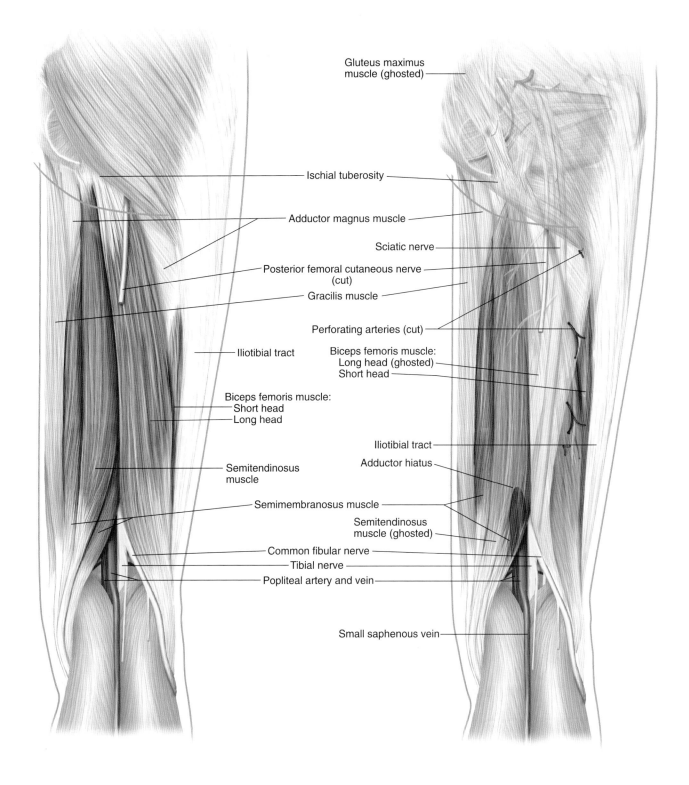

Gluteus maximus
muscle (ghosted)

Ischial tuberosity

Adductor magnus muscle

Sciatic nerve

Posterior femoral cutaneous nerve
(cut)

Gracilis muscle

Perforating arteries (cut)

Iliotibial tract

Biceps femoris muscle:
Long head (ghosted)
Short head

Biceps femoris muscle:
Short head
Long head

Iliotibial tract

Adductor hiatus

Semitendinosus
muscle

Semimembranosus muscle

Semitendinosus
muscle (ghosted)

Common fibular nerve

Tibial nerve

Popliteal artery and vein

Small saphenous vein

PLATE 3-30   **Muscle Attachments of the Distal Lower Limb**

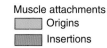

Muscle attachments
☐ Origins
▨ Insertions

A. Anterior view

B. Posterior view

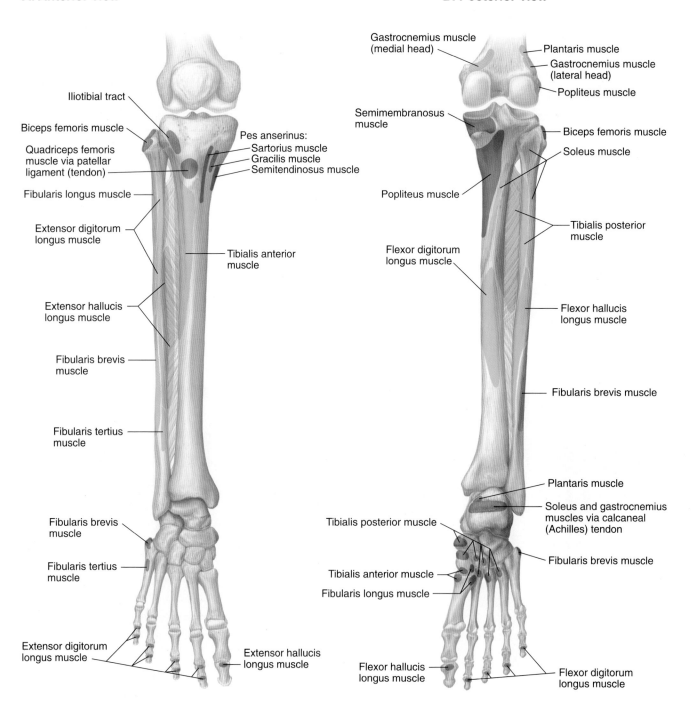

Iliotibial tract

Biceps femoris muscle

Quadriceps femoris muscle via patellar ligament (tendon)

Fibularis longus muscle

Extensor digitorum longus muscle

Extensor hallucis longus muscle

Fibularis brevis muscle

Fibularis tertius muscle

Fibularis brevis muscle

Fibularis tertius muscle

Extensor digitorum longus muscle

Pes anserinus:
Sartorius muscle
Gracilis muscle
Semitendinosus muscle

Tibialis anterior muscle

Extensor hallucis longus muscle

Gastrocnemius muscle (medial head)

Semimembranosus muscle

Popliteus muscle

Flexor digitorum longus muscle

Tibialis posterior muscle

Tibialis anterior muscle

Fibularis longus muscle

Flexor hallucis longus muscle

Plantaris muscle

Gastrocnemius muscle (lateral head)

Popliteus muscle

Biceps femoris muscle

Soleus muscle

Tibialis posterior muscle

Flexor hallucis longus muscle

Fibularis brevis muscle

Plantaris muscle

Soleus and gastrocnemius muscles via calcaneal (Achilles) tendon

Fibularis brevis muscle

Flexor digitorum longus muscle

Note: Attachments of intrinsic muscles of foot not shown

A. Superficial dissection

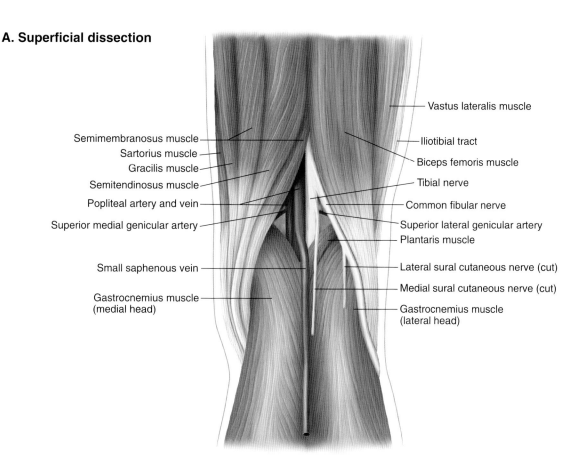

Semimembranosus muscle
Sartorius muscle
Gracilis muscle
Semitendinosus muscle
Popliteal artery and vein
Superior medial genicular artery

Small saphenous vein

Gastrocnemius muscle
(medial head)

Vastus lateralis muscle
Iliotibial tract
Biceps femoris muscle
Tibial nerve
Common fibular nerve
Superior lateral genicular artery
Plantaris muscle
Lateral sural cutaneous nerve (cut)
Medial sural cutaneous nerve (cut)
Gastrocnemius muscle
(lateral head)

B. Deep dissection

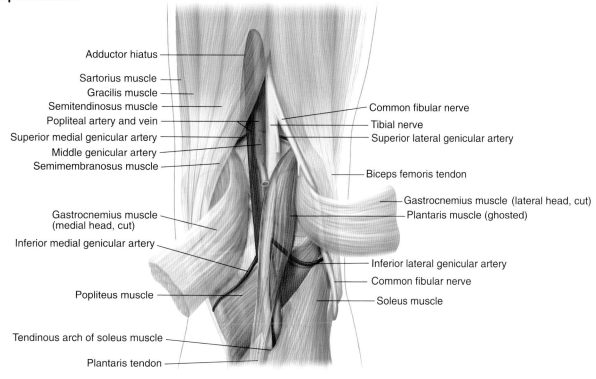

Adductor hiatus
Sartorius muscle
Gracilis muscle
Semitendinosus muscle
Popliteal artery and vein
Superior medial genicular artery
Middle genicular artery
Semimembranosus muscle

Gastrocnemius muscle
(medial head, cut)
Inferior medial genicular artery

Popliteus muscle

Tendinous arch of soleus muscle
Plantaris tendon

Common fibular nerve
Tibial nerve
Superior lateral genicular artery

Biceps femoris tendon
Gastrocnemius muscle (lateral head, cut)
Plantaris muscle (ghosted)

Inferior lateral genicular artery
Common fibular nerve
Soleus muscle

PLATE 3-32   **Compartmental Organization of the Leg**

A. Orientation

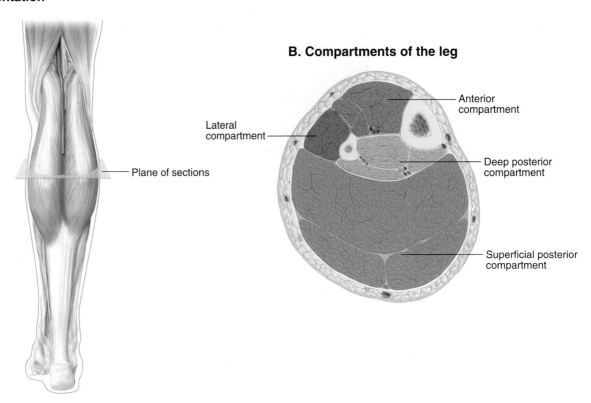

Plane of sections

B. Compartments of the leg

Anterior compartment

Lateral compartment

Deep posterior compartment

Superficial posterior compartment

C. Cross section

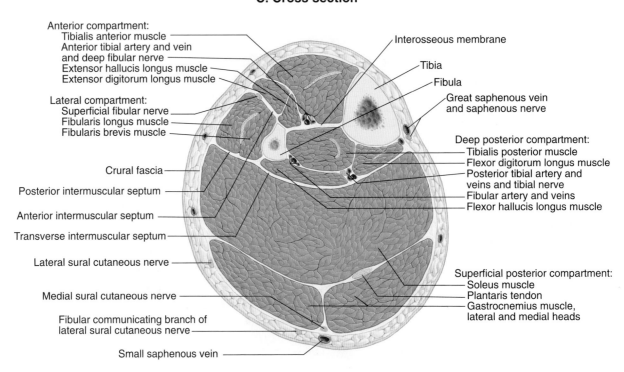

Anterior compartment:
Tibialis anterior muscle
Anterior tibial artery and vein
and deep fibular nerve
Extensor hallucis longus muscle
Extensor digitorum longus muscle

Interosseous membrane

Tibia

Fibula

Great saphenous vein
and saphenous nerve

Lateral compartment:
Superficial fibular nerve
Fibularis longus muscle
Fibularis brevis muscle

Deep posterior compartment:
Tibialis posterior muscle
Flexor digitorum longus muscle
Posterior tibial artery and
veins and tibial nerve
Fibular artery and veins
Flexor hallucis longus muscle

Crural fascia

Posterior intermuscular septum

Anterior intermuscular septum

Transverse intermuscular septum

Lateral sural cutaneous nerve

Superficial posterior compartment:
Soleus muscle
Plantaris tendon
Gastrocnemius muscle,
lateral and medial heads

Medial sural cutaneous nerve

Fibular communicating branch of
lateral sural cutaneous nerve

Small saphenous vein

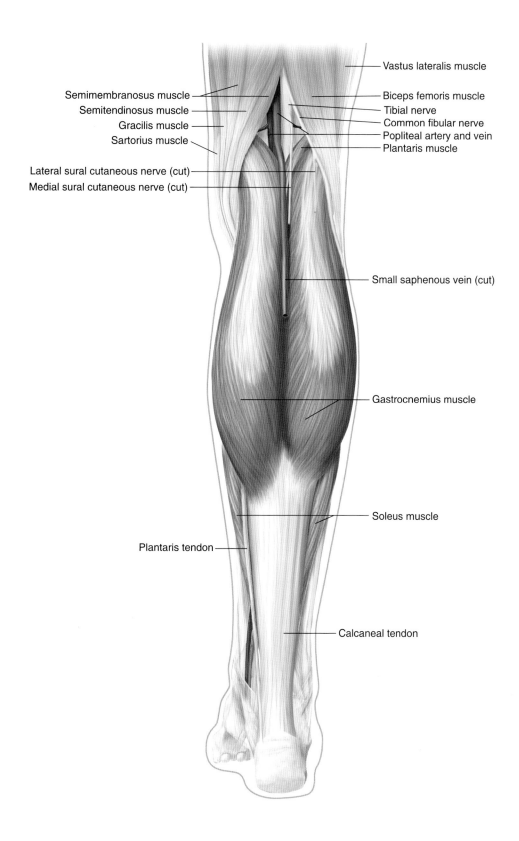

Semimembranosus muscle

Semitendinosus muscle

Gracilis muscle

Sartorius muscle

Lateral sural cutaneous nerve (cut)

Medial sural cutaneous nerve (cut)

Vastus lateralis muscle

Biceps femoris muscle

Tibial nerve

Common fibular nerve

Popliteal artery and vein

Plantaris muscle

Small saphenous vein (cut)

Gastrocnemius muscle

Soleus muscle

Plantaris tendon

Calcaneal tendon

PLATE 3-34   **Muscles of the Posterior Leg, Intermediate Dissection**

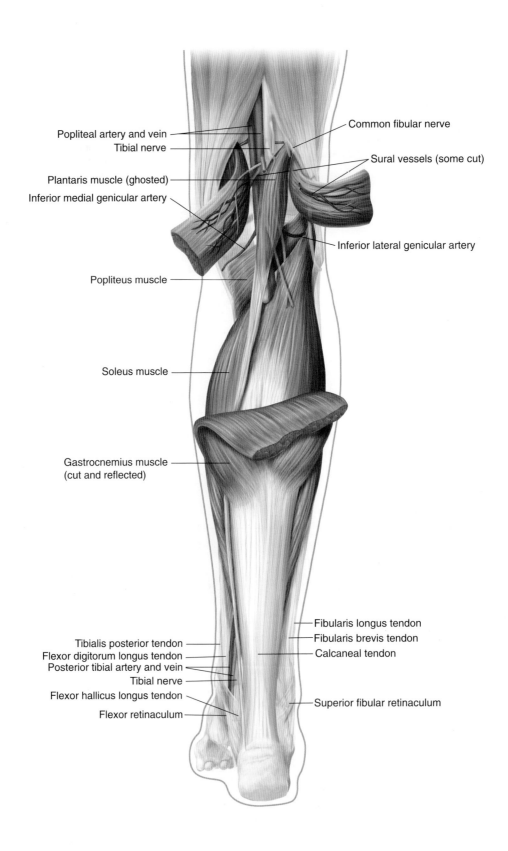

Popliteal artery and vein

Tibial nerve

Plantaris muscle (ghosted)

Inferior medial genicular artery

Popliteus muscle

Soleus muscle

Gastrocnemius muscle
(cut and reflected)

Tibialis posterior tendon

Flexor digitorum longus tendon

Posterior tibial artery and vein

Tibial nerve

Flexor hallicus longus tendon

Flexor retinaculum

Common fibular nerve

Sural vessels (some cut)

Inferior lateral genicular artery

Fibularis longus tendon

Fibularis brevis tendon

Calcaneal tendon

Superior fibular retinaculum

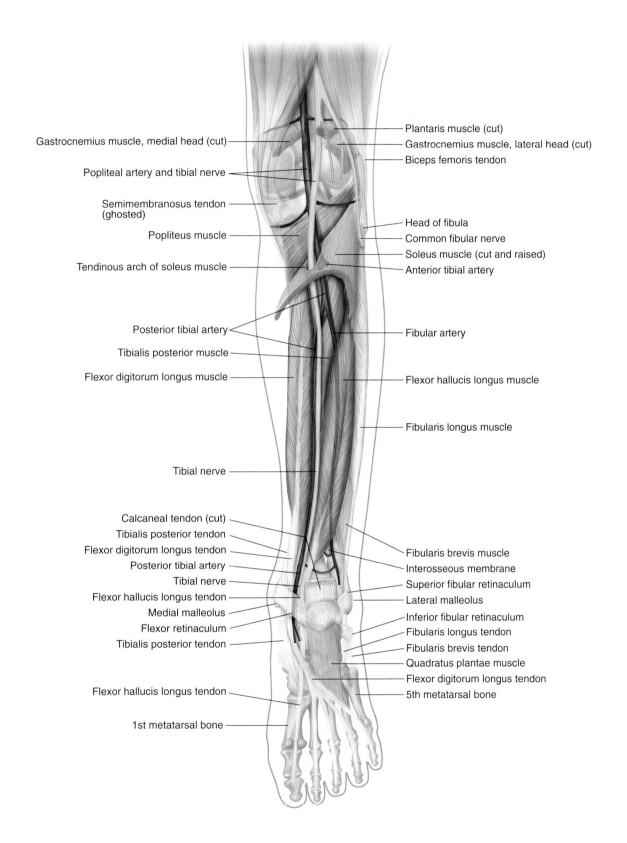

Gastrocnemius muscle, medial head (cut)

Popliteal artery and tibial nerve

Semimembranosus tendon
(ghosted)

Popliteus muscle

Tendinous arch of soleus muscle

Posterior tibial artery

Tibialis posterior muscle

Flexor digitorum longus muscle

Tibial nerve

Calcaneal tendon (cut)
Tibialis posterior tendon
Flexor digitorum longus tendon
Posterior tibial artery
Tibial nerve
Flexor hallucis longus tendon
Medial malleolus
Flexor retinaculum
Tibialis posterior tendon

Flexor hallucis longus tendon

1st metatarsal bone

Plantaris muscle (cut)
Gastrocnemius muscle, lateral head (cut)
Biceps femoris tendon

Head of fibula
Common fibular nerve
Soleus muscle (cut and raised)
Anterior tibial artery

Fibular artery

Flexor hallucis longus muscle

Fibularis longus muscle

Fibularis brevis muscle
Interosseous membrane
Superior fibular retinaculum
Lateral malleolus
Inferior fibular retinaculum
Fibularis longus tendon
Fibularis brevis tendon
Quadratus plantae muscle
Flexor digitorum longus tendon
5th metatarsal bone

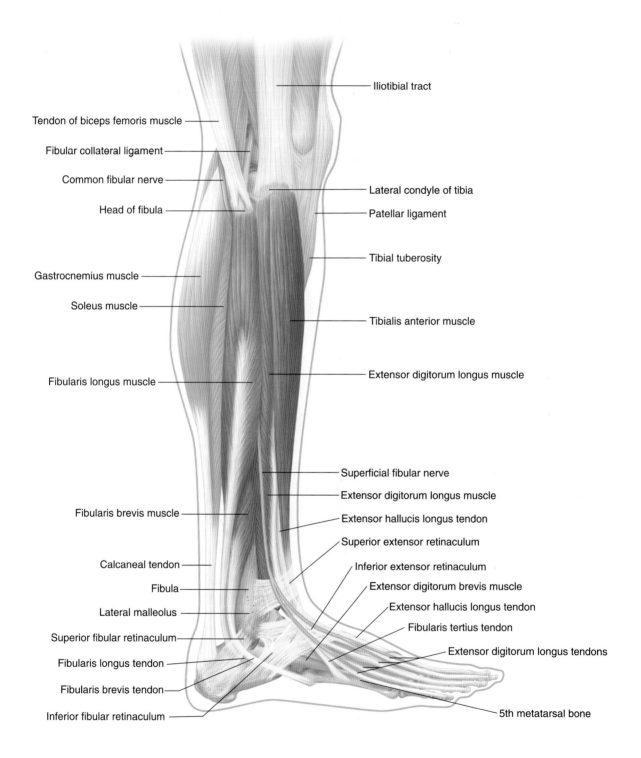

Iliotibial tract

Tendon of biceps femoris muscle

Fibular collateral ligament

Common fibular nerve

Head of fibula

Lateral condyle of tibia

Patellar ligament

Tibial tuberosity

Gastrocnemius muscle

Soleus muscle

Tibialis anterior muscle

Extensor digitorum longus muscle

Fibularis longus muscle

Superficial fibular nerve

Extensor digitorum longus muscle

Extensor hallucis longus tendon

Fibularis brevis muscle

Superior extensor retinaculum

Inferior extensor retinaculum

Extensor digitorum brevis muscle

Calcaneal tendon

Fibula

Extensor hallucis longus tendon

Lateral malleolus

Fibularis tertius tendon

Superior fibular retinaculum

Extensor digitorum longus tendons

Fibularis longus tendon

Fibularis brevis tendon

Inferior fibular retinaculum

5th metatarsal bone

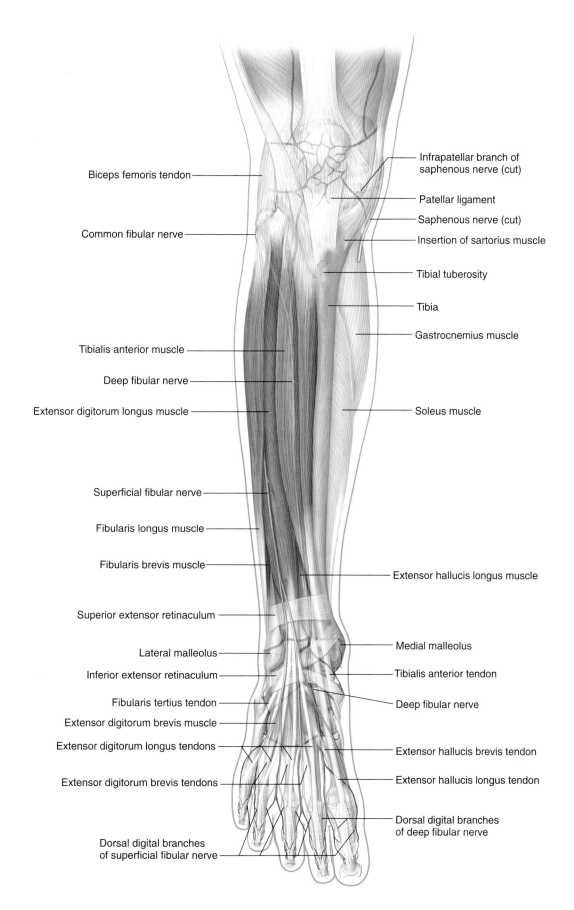

Biceps femoris tendon

Common fibular nerve

Tibialis anterior muscle

Deep fibular nerve

Extensor digitorum longus muscle

Superficial fibular nerve

Fibularis longus muscle

Fibularis brevis muscle

Superior extensor retinaculum

Lateral malleolus

Inferior extensor retinaculum

Fibularis tertius tendon

Extensor digitorum brevis muscle

Extensor digitorum longus tendons

Extensor digitorum brevis tendons

Dorsal digital branches
of superficial fibular nerve

Infrapatellar branch of
saphenous nerve (cut)

Patellar ligament

Saphenous nerve (cut)

Insertion of sartorius muscle

Tibial tuberosity

Tibia

Gastrocnemius muscle

Soleus muscle

Extensor hallucis longus muscle

Medial malleolus

Tibialis anterior tendon

Deep fibular nerve

Extensor hallucis brevis tendon

Extensor hallucis longus tendon

Dorsal digital branches
of deep fibular nerve

PLATE 3-38   **Arteries of the Leg**

A. Posterior view

B. Anterior view

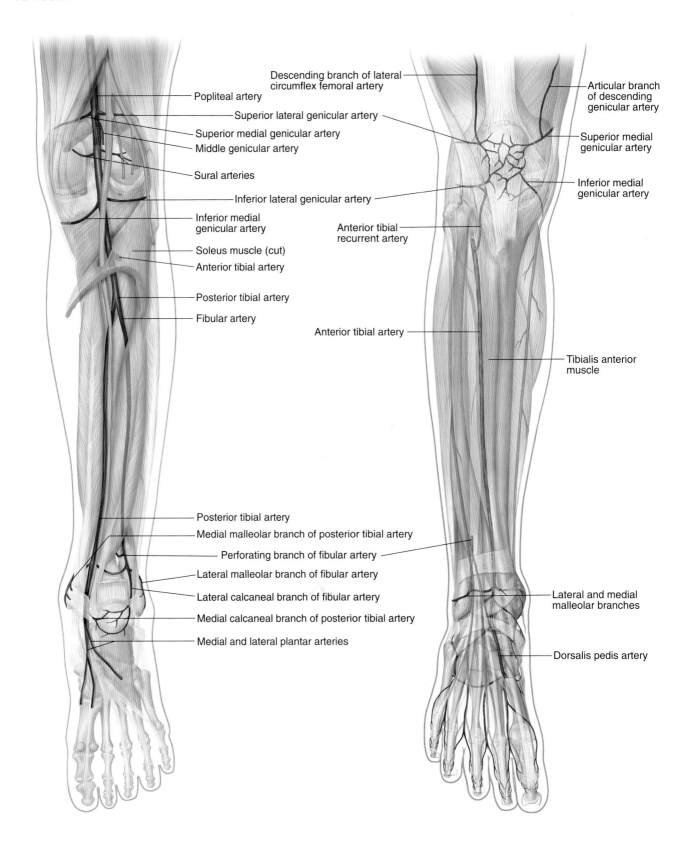

Descending branch of lateral circumflex femoral artery

Popliteal artery

Superior lateral genicular artery

Superior medial genicular artery

Middle genicular artery

Sural arteries

Inferior lateral genicular artery

Inferior medial genicular artery

Soleus muscle (cut)

Anterior tibial artery

Posterior tibial artery

Fibular artery

Articular branch of descending genicular artery

Superior medial genicular artery

Inferior medial genicular artery

Anterior tibial recurrent artery

Anterior tibial artery

Tibialis anterior muscle

Posterior tibial artery

Medial malleolar branch of posterior tibial artery

Perforating branch of fibular artery

Lateral malleolar branch of fibular artery

Lateral calcaneal branch of fibular artery

Medial calcaneal branch of posterior tibial artery

Medial and lateral plantar arteries

Lateral and medial malleolar branches

Dorsalis pedis artery

A. Posterior view

B. Anterior view

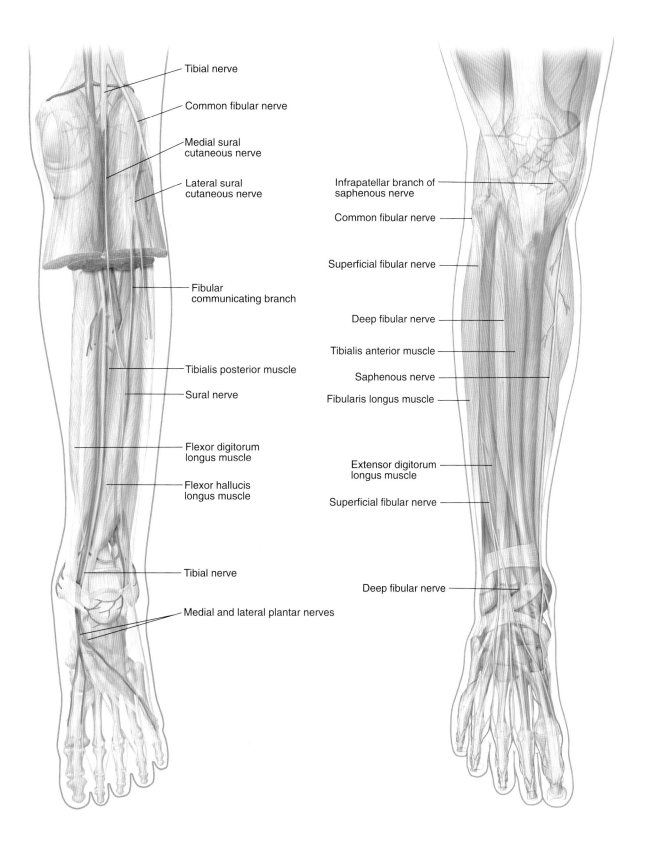

Tibial nerve

Common fibular nerve

Medial sural cutaneous nerve

Lateral sural cutaneous nerve

Fibular communicating branch

Tibialis posterior muscle

Sural nerve

Flexor digitorum longus muscle

Flexor hallucis longus muscle

Tibial nerve

Medial and lateral plantar nerves

Infrapatellar branch of saphenous nerve

Common fibular nerve

Superficial fibular nerve

Deep fibular nerve

Tibialis anterior muscle

Saphenous nerve

Fibularis longus muscle

Extensor digitorum longus muscle

Superficial fibular nerve

Deep fibular nerve

PLATE 3-40   Skeleton of the Foot

A. Dorsal view

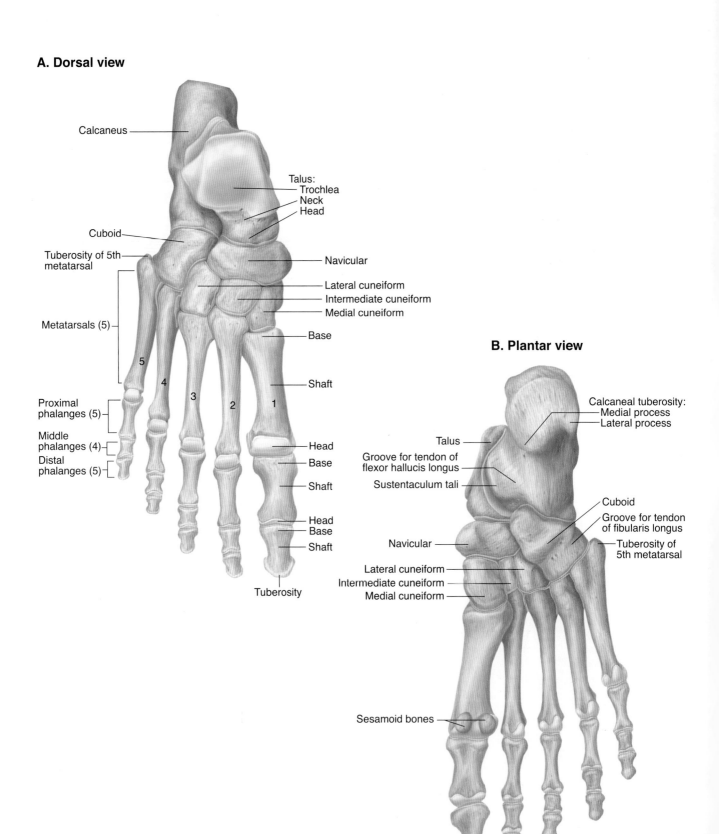

Calcaneus

Talus:
Trochlea
Neck
Head

Cuboid

Tuberosity of 5th metatarsal

Navicular

Lateral cuneiform
Intermediate cuneiform
Medial cuneiform

Metatarsals (5)

Base

5

4

Shaft

3

2

1

Proximal phalanges (5)

Middle phalanges (4)

Distal phalanges (5)

Head

Base

Shaft

Head
Base

Shaft

Tuberosity

B. Plantar view

Calcaneal tuberosity:
Medial process
Lateral process

Talus

Groove for tendon of flexor hallucis longus

Sustentaculum tali

Cuboid

Groove for tendon of fibularis longus

Tuberosity of 5th metatarsal

Navicular

Lateral cuneiform
Intermediate cuneiform
Medial cuneiform

Sesamoid bones

A. Medial view

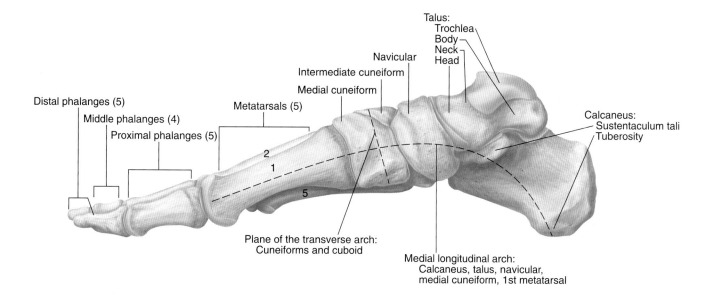

Distal phalanges (5)
Middle phalanges (4)
Proximal phalanges (5)
Metatarsals (5)
Medial cuneiform
Intermediate cuneiform
Navicular
Talus:
Trochlea
Body
Neck
Head
Calcaneus:
Sustentaculum tali
Tuberosity

2
1
5

Plane of the transverse arch:
Cuneiforms and cuboid

Medial longitudinal arch:
Calcaneus, talus, navicular,
medial cuneiform, 1st metatarsal

B. Lateral view

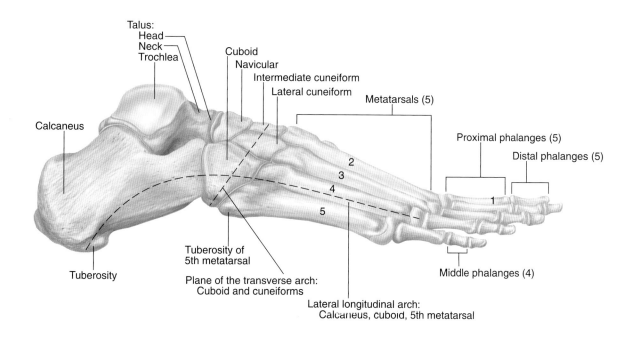

Talus:
Head
Neck
Trochlea
Cuboid
Navicular
Intermediate cuneiform
Lateral cuneiform
Metatarsals (5)
Proximal phalanges (5)
Distal phalanges (5)

Calcaneus

2
3
4
5
1

Tuberosity

Tuberosity of
5th metatarsal

Plane of the transverse arch:
Cuboid and cuneiforms

Lateral longitudinal arch:
Calcaneus, cuboid, 5th metatarsal

Middle phalanges (4)

PLATE 3-42   **Muscle Attachments of the Foot, Dorsal Surface**

Muscle attachments
Origins
Insertions

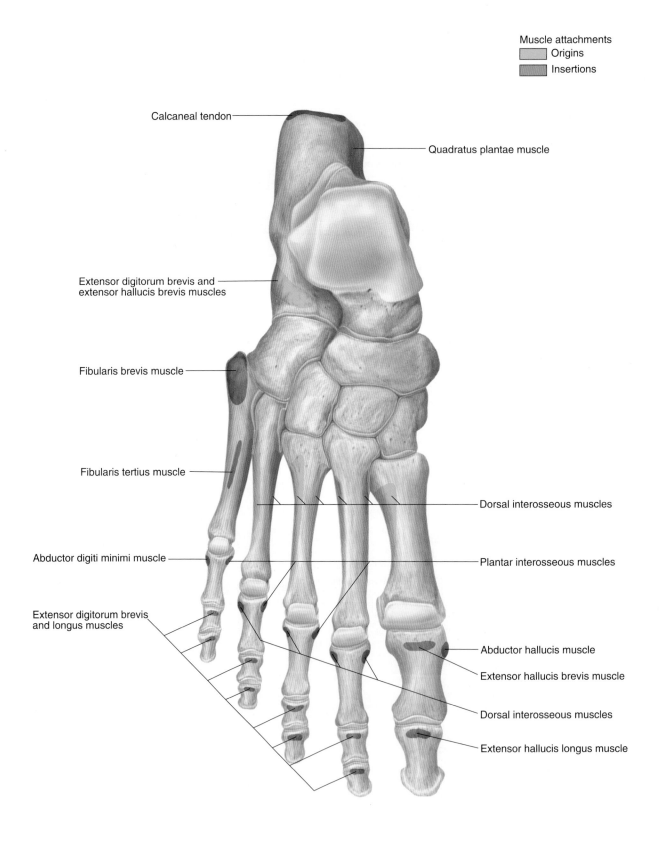

Calcaneal tendon

Quadratus plantae muscle

Extensor digitorum brevis and
extensor hallucis brevis muscles

Fibularis brevis muscle

Fibularis tertius muscle

Dorsal interosseous muscles

Abductor digiti minimi muscle

Plantar interosseous muscles

Extensor digitorum brevis
and longus muscles

Abductor hallucis muscle

Extensor hallucis brevis muscle

Dorsal interosseous muscles

Extensor hallucis longus muscle

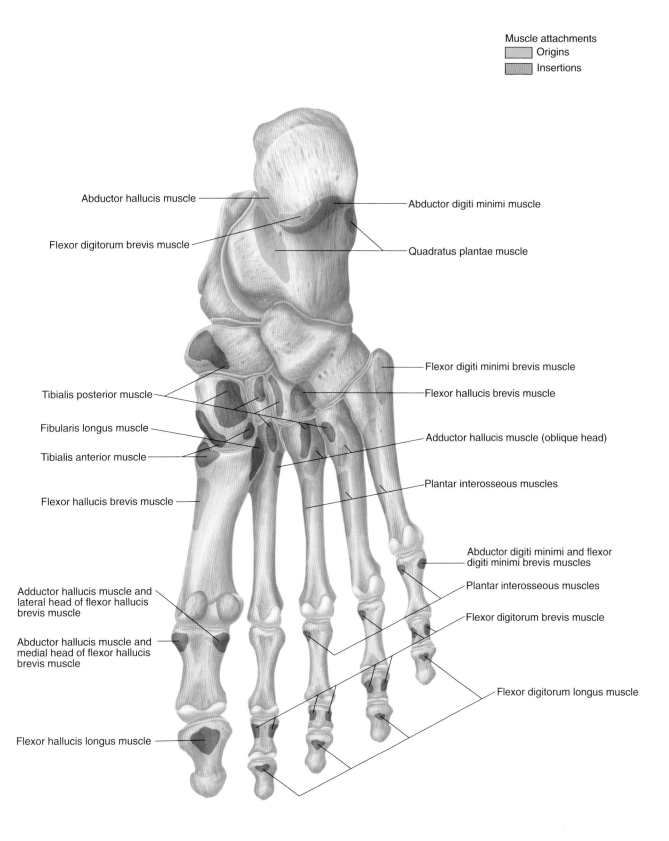

Muscle attachments
Origins
Insertions

Abductor hallucis muscle

Flexor digitorum brevis muscle

Abductor digiti minimi muscle

Quadratus plantae muscle

Tibialis posterior muscle

Fibularis longus muscle

Tibialis anterior muscle

Flexor hallucis brevis muscle

Flexor digiti minimi brevis muscle

Flexor hallucis brevis muscle

Adductor hallucis muscle (oblique head)

Plantar interosseous muscles

Adductor hallucis muscle and
lateral head of flexor hallucis
brevis muscle

Abductor hallucis muscle and
medial head of flexor hallucis
brevis muscle

Flexor hallucis longus muscle

Abductor digiti minimi and flexor
digiti minimi brevis muscles

Plantar interosseous muscles

Flexor digitorum brevis muscle

Flexor digitorum longus muscle

A. Dissection

B. Cutaneous distribution

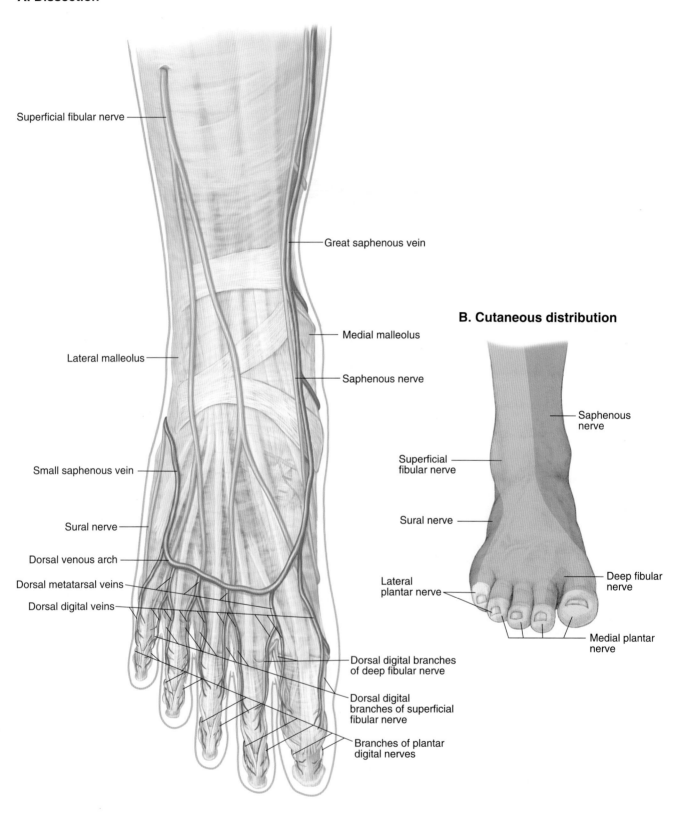

Superficial fibular nerve

Great saphenous vein

Medial malleolus

Saphenous nerve

Lateral malleolus

Small saphenous vein

Sural nerve

Dorsal venous arch

Dorsal metatarsal veins

Dorsal digital veins

Dorsal digital branches
of deep fibular nerve

Dorsal digital
branches of superficial
fibular nerve

Branches of plantar
digital nerves

Saphenous
nerve

Superficial
fibular nerve

Sural nerve

Lateral
plantar nerve

Deep fibular
nerve

Medial plantar
nerve

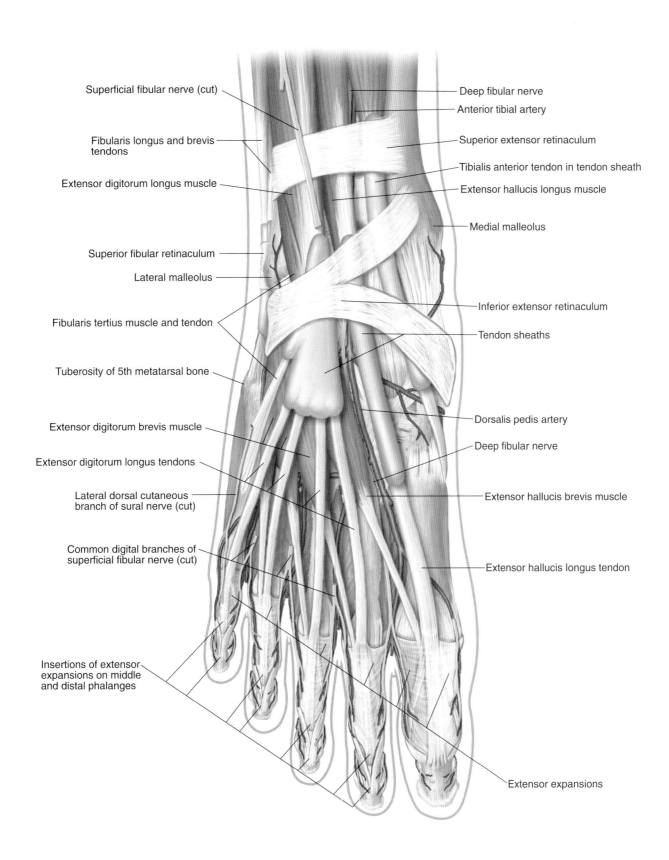

Superficial fibular nerve (cut)

Fibularis longus and brevis tendons

Extensor digitorum longus muscle

Superior fibular retinaculum

Lateral malleolus

Fibularis tertius muscle and tendon

Tuberosity of 5th metatarsal bone

Extensor digitorum brevis muscle

Extensor digitorum longus tendons

Lateral dorsal cutaneous branch of sural nerve (cut)

Common digital branches of superficial fibular nerve (cut)

Insertions of extensor expansions on middle and distal phalanges

Deep fibular nerve

Anterior tibial artery

Superior extensor retinaculum

Tibialis anterior tendon in tendon sheath

Extensor hallucis longus muscle

Medial malleolus

Inferior extensor retinaculum

Tendon sheaths

Dorsalis pedis artery

Deep fibular nerve

Extensor hallucis brevis muscle

Extensor hallucis longus tendon

Extensor expansions

PLATE 3-46 **Dorsum of the Foot, Deep Dissection**

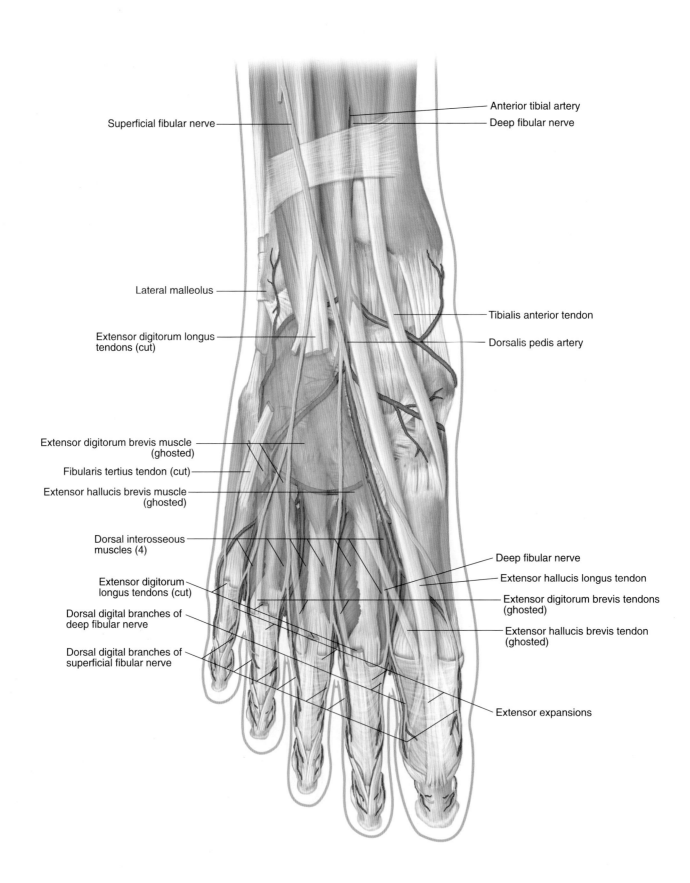

Superficial fibular nerve

Lateral malleolus

Extensor digitorum longus
tendons (cut)

Extensor digitorum brevis muscle
(ghosted)

Fibularis tertius tendon (cut)

Extensor hallucis brevis muscle
(ghosted)

Dorsal interosseous
muscles (4)

Extensor digitorum
longus tendons (cut)

Dorsal digital branches of
deep fibular nerve

Dorsal digital branches of
superficial fibular nerve

Anterior tibial artery

Deep fibular nerve

Tibialis anterior tendon

Dorsalis pedis artery

Deep fibular nerve

Extensor hallucis longus tendon

Extensor digitorum brevis tendons
(ghosted)

Extensor hallucis brevis tendon
(ghosted)

Extensor expansions

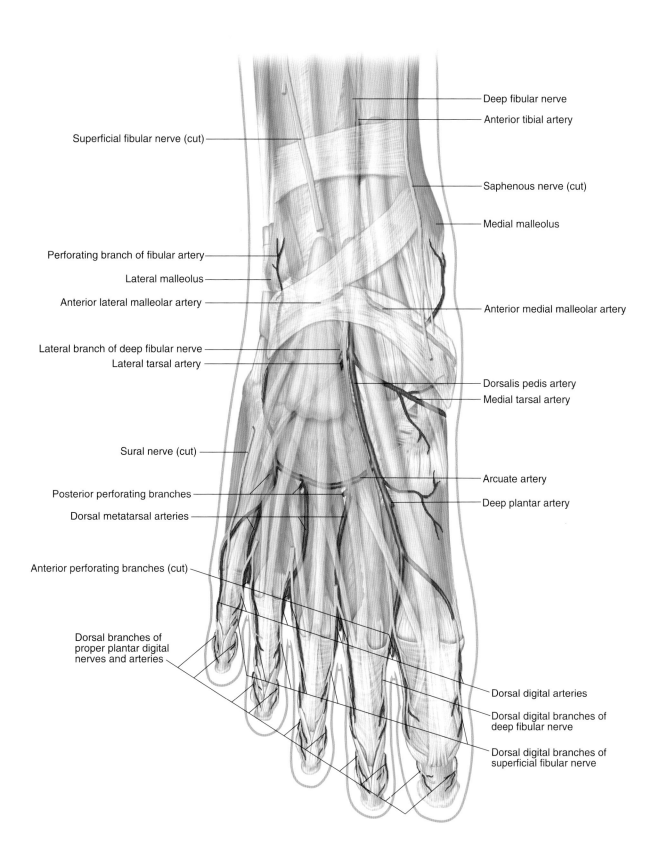

Deep fibular nerve

Anterior tibial artery

Superficial fibular nerve (cut)

Saphenous nerve (cut)

Medial malleolus

Perforating branch of fibular artery

Lateral malleolus

Anterior lateral malleolar artery

Anterior medial malleolar artery

Lateral branch of deep fibular nerve

Lateral tarsal artery

Dorsalis pedis artery

Medial tarsal artery

Sural nerve (cut)

Arcuate artery

Posterior perforating branches

Dorsal metatarsal arteries

Deep plantar artery

Anterior perforating branches (cut)

Dorsal branches of
proper plantar digital
nerves and arteries

Dorsal digital arteries

Dorsal digital branches of
deep fibular nerve

Dorsal digital branches of
superficial fibular nerve

PLATE 3-48 **Cutaneous Nerves of the Sole of the Foot**

A. Dissection

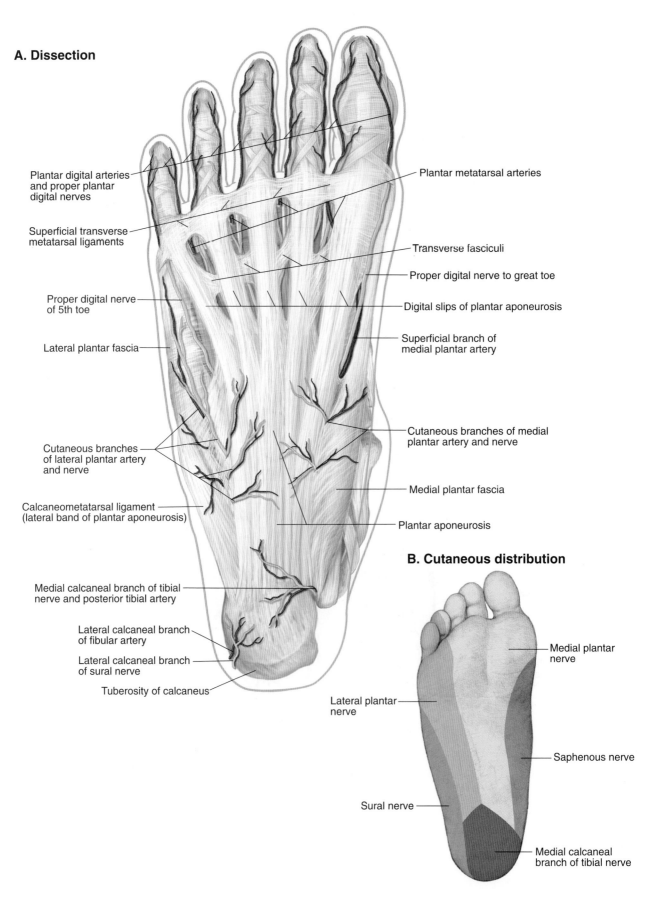

Plantar digital arteries
and proper plantar
digital nerves

Plantar metatarsal arteries

Superficial transverse
metatarsal ligaments

Transverse fasciculi

Proper digital nerve to great toe

Proper digital nerve
of 5th toe

Digital slips of plantar aponeurosis

Lateral plantar fascia

Superficial branch of
medial plantar artery

Cutaneous branches
of lateral plantar artery
and nerve

Cutaneous branches of medial
plantar artery and nerve

Medial plantar fascia

Calcaneometatarsal ligament
(lateral band of plantar aponeurosis)

Plantar aponeurosis

Medial calcaneal branch of tibial
nerve and posterior tibial artery

B. Cutaneous distribution

Lateral calcaneal branch
of fibular artery

Lateral calcaneal branch
of sural nerve

Tuberosity of calcaneus

Medial plantar
nerve

Lateral plantar
nerve

Saphenous nerve

Sural nerve

Medial calcaneal
branch of tibial nerve

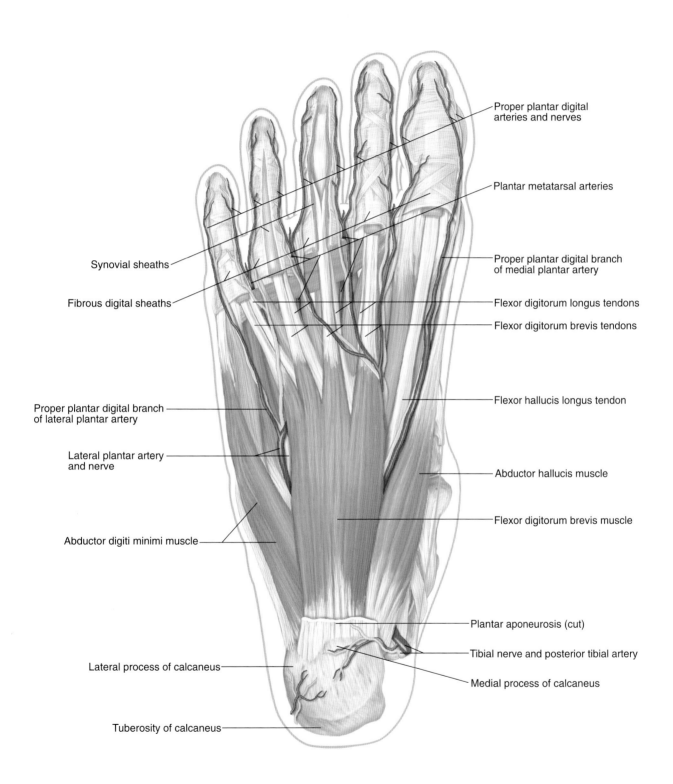

Proper plantar digital
arteries and nerves

Plantar metatarsal arteries

Proper plantar digital branch
of medial plantar artery

Flexor digitorum longus tendons

Flexor digitorum brevis tendons

Flexor hallucis longus tendon

Abductor hallucis muscle

Flexor digitorum brevis muscle

Plantar aponeurosis (cut)

Tibial nerve and posterior tibial artery

Medial process of calcaneus

Synovial sheaths

Fibrous digital sheaths

Proper plantar digital branch
of lateral plantar artery

Lateral plantar artery
and nerve

Abductor digiti minimi muscle

Lateral process of calcaneus

Tuberosity of calcaneus

PLATE 3-50 **Muscles of the Sole of the Foot, Second Layer**

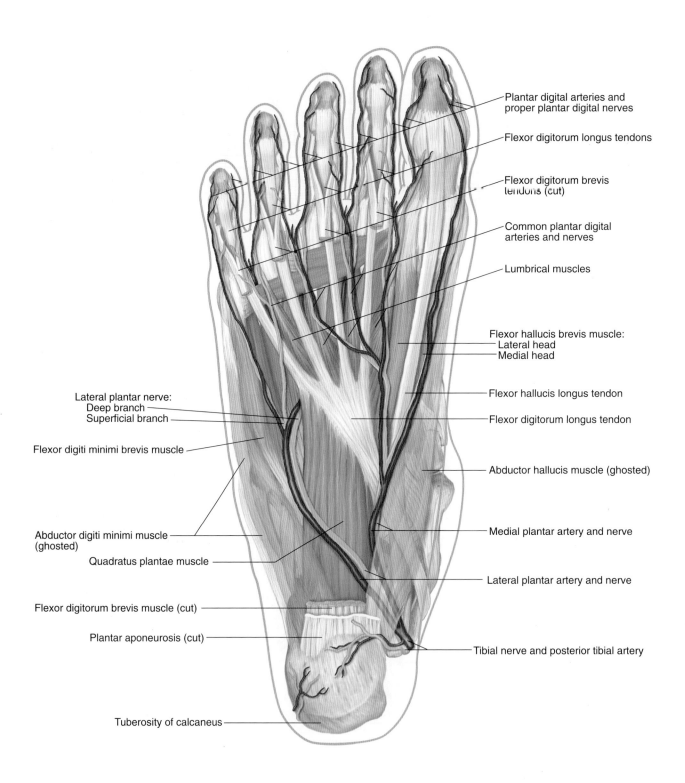

Plantar digital arteries and proper plantar digital nerves

Flexor digitorum longus tendons

Flexor digitorum brevis tendons (cut)

Common plantar digital arteries and nerves

Lumbrical muscles

Flexor hallucis brevis muscle:
Lateral head
Medial head

Flexor hallucis longus tendon

Flexor digitorum longus tendon

Abductor hallucis muscle (ghosted)

Medial plantar artery and nerve

Lateral plantar artery and nerve

Tibial nerve and posterior tibial artery

Lateral plantar nerve:
Deep branch
Superficial branch

Flexor digiti minimi brevis muscle

Abductor digiti minimi muscle (ghosted)

Quadratus plantae muscle

Flexor digitorum brevis muscle (cut)

Plantar aponeurosis (cut)

Tuberosity of calcaneus

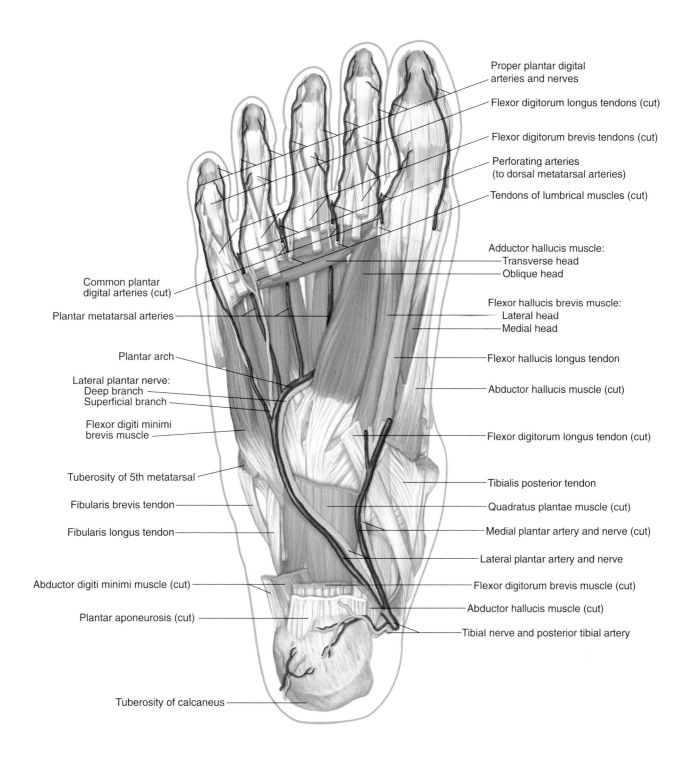

Proper plantar digital
arteries and nerves

Flexor digitorum longus tendons (cut)

Flexor digitorum brevis tendons (cut)

Perforating arteries
(to dorsal metatarsal arteries)

Tendons of lumbrical muscles (cut)

Adductor hallucis muscle:
Transverse head
Oblique head

Flexor hallucis brevis muscle:
Lateral head
Medial head

Flexor hallucis longus tendon

Abductor hallucis muscle (cut)

Flexor digitorum longus tendon (cut)

Tibialis posterior tendon

Quadratus plantae muscle (cut)

Medial plantar artery and nerve (cut)

Lateral plantar artery and nerve

Flexor digitorum brevis muscle (cut)

Abductor hallucis muscle (cut)

Tibial nerve and posterior tibial artery

Common plantar
digital arteries (cut)

Plantar metatarsal arteries

Plantar arch

Lateral plantar nerve:
Deep branch
Superficial branch

Flexor digiti minimi
brevis muscle

Tuberosity of 5th metatarsal

Fibularis brevis tendon

Fibularis longus tendon

Abductor digiti minimi muscle (cut)

Plantar aponeurosis (cut)

Tuberosity of calcaneus

PLATE 3-52 **Muscles of the Sole of the Foot, Fourth Layer**

A. Plantar view

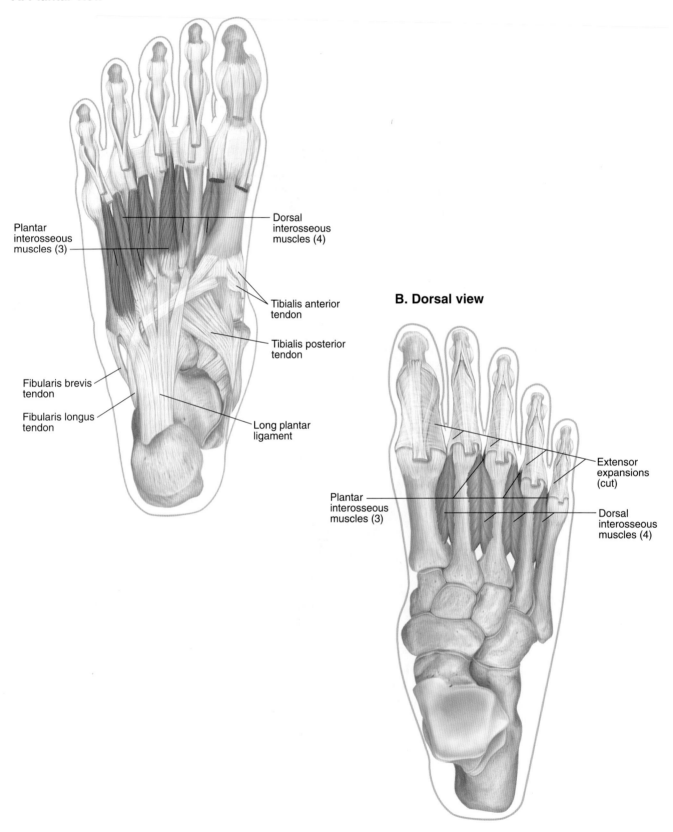

Plantar
interosseous
muscles (3)

Dorsal
interosseous
muscles (4)

Tibialis anterior
tendon

B. Dorsal view

Tibialis posterior
tendon

Fibularis brevis
tendon

Fibularis longus
tendon

Long plantar
ligament

Extensor
expansions
(cut)

Plantar
interosseous
muscles (3)

Dorsal
interosseous
muscles (4)

A. Arteries

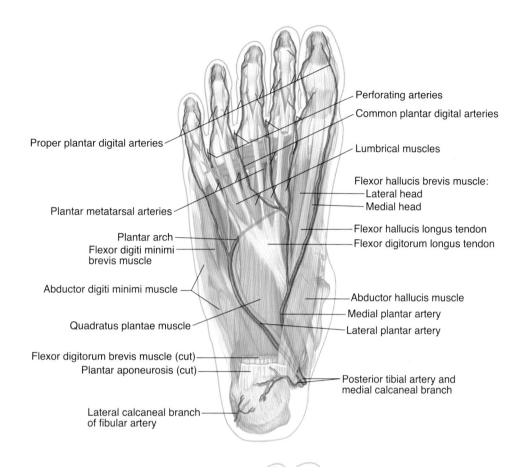

Perforating arteries

Common plantar digital arteries

Proper plantar digital arteries

Lumbrical muscles

Flexor hallucis brevis muscle:
Lateral head
Medial head

Plantar metatarsal arteries

Flexor hallucis longus tendon
Flexor digitorum longus tendon

Plantar arch
Flexor digiti minimi brevis muscle

Abductor digiti minimi muscle

Quadratus plantae muscle

Abductor hallucis muscle
Medial plantar artery
Lateral plantar artery

Flexor digitorum brevis muscle (cut)
Plantar aponeurosis (cut)

Posterior tibial artery and medial calcaneal branch

Lateral calcaneal branch of fibular artery

B. Nerves

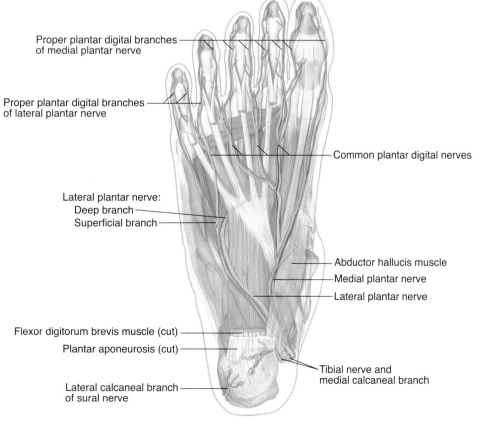

Proper plantar digital branches of medial plantar nerve

Proper plantar digital branches of lateral plantar nerve

Common plantar digital nerves

Lateral plantar nerve:
Deep branch
Superficial branch

Abductor hallucis muscle
Medial plantar nerve
Lateral plantar nerve

Flexor digitorum brevis muscle (cut)
Plantar aponeurosis (cut)

Tibial nerve and medial calcaneal branch

Lateral calcaneal branch of sural nerve

PLATE 3-54   Hip Joint, External Features

A. Anterior view

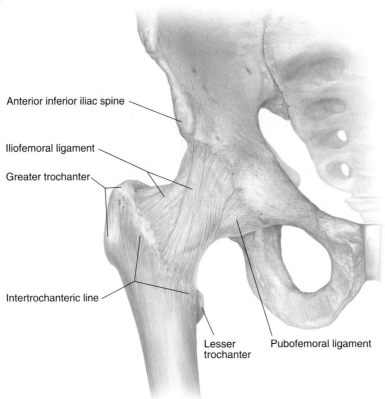

Anterior inferior iliac spine

Iliofemoral ligament

Greater trochanter

Intertrochanteric line

Lesser trochanter

Pubofemoral ligament

B. Posterior view

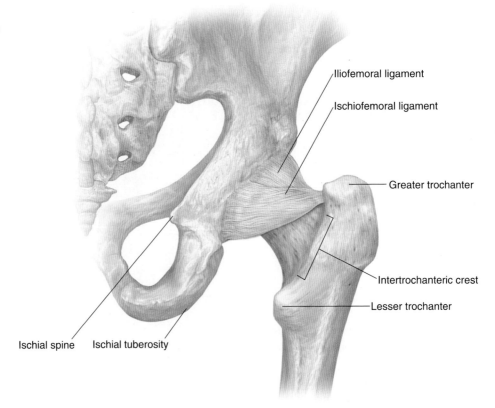

Iliofemoral ligament

Ischiofemoral ligament

Greater trochanter

Intertrochanteric crest

Lesser trochanter

Ischial spine   Ischial tuberosity

A. Lateral view, joint opened

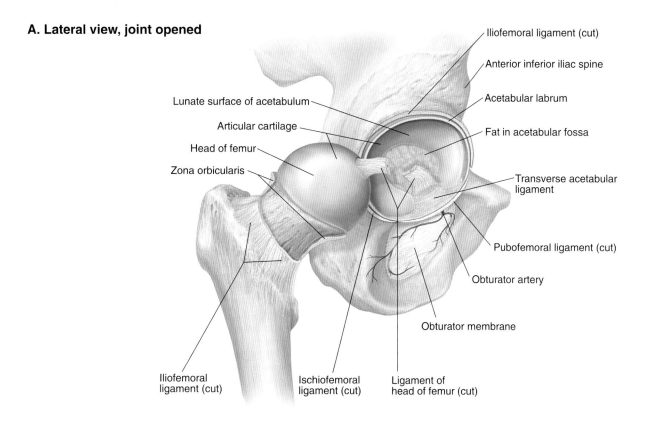

Iliofemoral ligament (cut)

Anterior inferior iliac spine

Acetabular labrum

Fat in acetabular fossa

Lunate surface of acetabulum

Articular cartilage

Head of femur

Zona orbicularis

Transverse acetabular ligament

Pubofemoral ligament (cut)

Obturator artery

Obturator membrane

Iliofemoral ligament (cut)

Ischiofemoral ligament (cut)

Ligament of head of femur (cut)

B. Blood supply

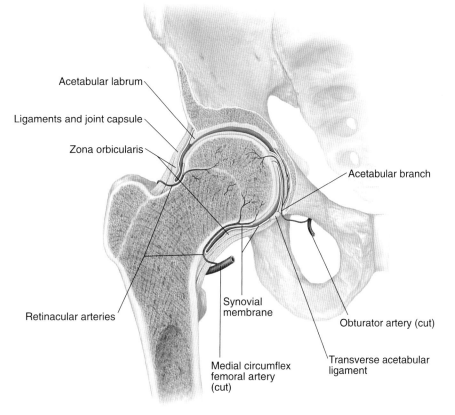

Acetabular labrum

Ligaments and joint capsule

Zona orbicularis

Acetabular branch

Retinacular arteries

Synovial membrane

Obturator artery (cut)

Transverse acetabular ligament

Medial circumflex femoral artery (cut)

PLATE 3-56   Knee Joint, Anterior and Posterior Views

A. Right knee, anterior view

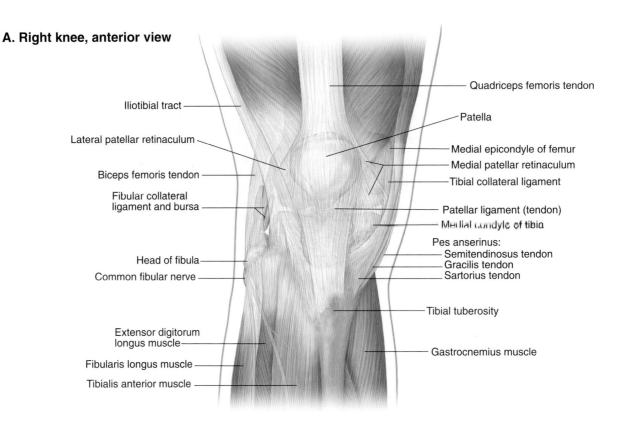

Iliotibial tract

Lateral patellar retinaculum

Biceps femoris tendon

Fibular collateral
ligament and bursa

Head of fibula

Common fibular nerve

Extensor digitorum
longus muscle

Fibularis longus muscle

Tibialis anterior muscle

Quadriceps femoris tendon

Patella

Medial epicondyle of femur

Medial patellar retinaculum

Tibial collateral ligament

Patellar ligament (tendon)

Medial condyle of tibia

Pes anserinus:
Semitendinosus tendon
Gracilis tendon
Sartorius tendon

Tibial tuberosity

Gastrocnemius muscle

B. Right knee, posterior view

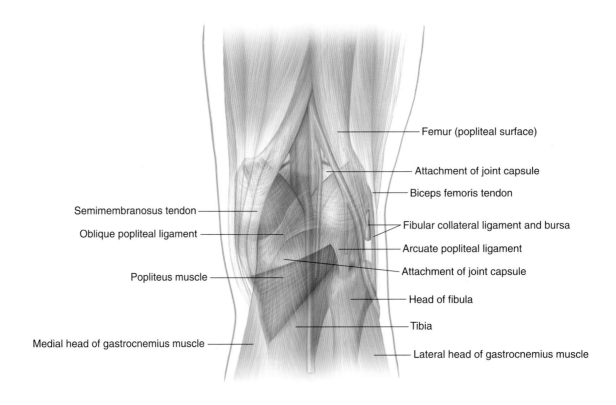

Semimembranosus tendon

Oblique popliteal ligament

Popliteus muscle

Medial head of gastrocnemius muscle

Femur (popliteal surface)

Attachment of joint capsule

Biceps femoris tendon

Fibular collateral ligament and bursa

Arcuate popliteal ligament

Attachment of joint capsule

Head of fibula

Tibia

Lateral head of gastrocnemius muscle

A. Right knee, medial view

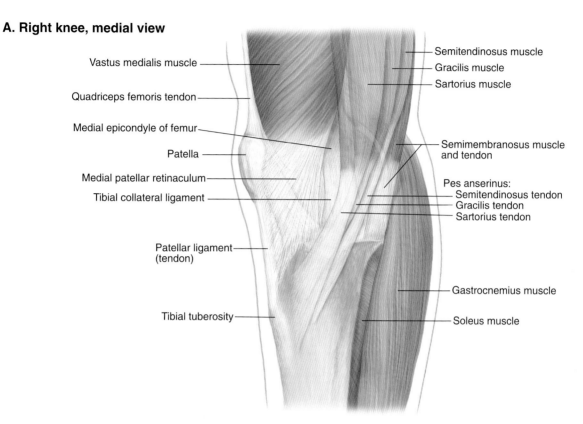

Vastus medialis muscle

Quadriceps femoris tendon

Medial epicondyle of femur

Patella

Medial patellar retinaculum

Tibial collateral ligament

Patellar ligament (tendon)

Tibial tuberosity

Semitendinosus muscle

Gracilis muscle

Sartorius muscle

Semimembranosus muscle and tendon

Pes anserinus:
Semitendinosus tendon
Gracilis tendon
Sartorius tendon

Gastrocnemius muscle

Soleus muscle

B. Right knee, lateral view

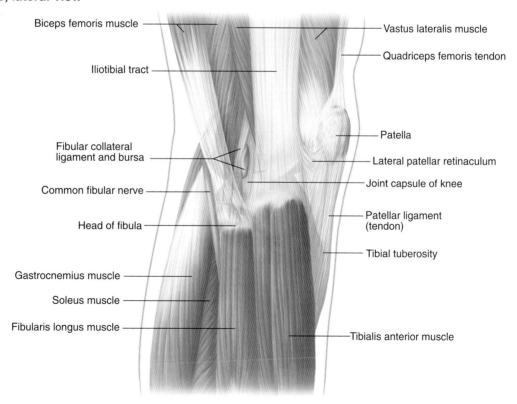

Biceps femoris muscle

Iliotibial tract

Fibular collateral ligament and bursa

Common fibular nerve

Head of fibula

Gastrocnemius muscle

Soleus muscle

Fibularis longus muscle

Vastus lateralis muscle

Quadriceps femoris tendon

Patella

Lateral patellar retinaculum

Joint capsule of knee

Patellar ligament (tendon)

Tibial tuberosity

Tibialis anterior muscle

PLATE 3-58   Knee Joint, Internal View

A. Anterior view, joint opened

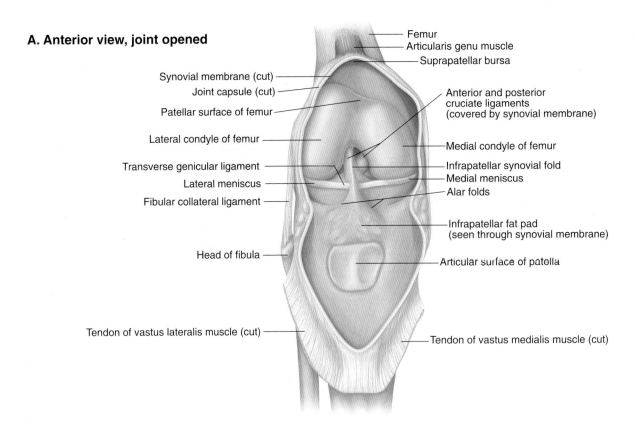

Femur
Articularis genu muscle
Suprapatellar bursa
Synovial membrane (cut)
Joint capsule (cut)
Patellar surface of femur
Anterior and posterior cruciate ligaments (covered by synovial membrane)
Lateral condyle of femur
Medial condyle of femur
Transverse genicular ligament
Infrapatellar synovial fold
Lateral meniscus
Medial meniscus
Fibular collateral ligament
Alar folds
Head of fibula
Infrapatellar fat pad (seen through synovial membrane)
Articular surface of patella
Tendon of vastus lateralis muscle (cut)
Tendon of vastus medialis muscle (cut)

B. Distal femur, inferior view

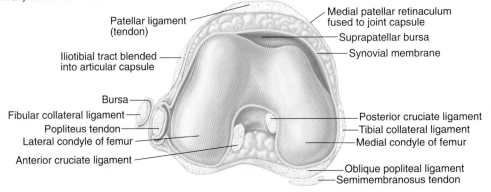

Patellar ligament (tendon)
Medial patellar retinaculum fused to joint capsule
Suprapatellar bursa
Synovial membrane
Iliotibial tract blended into articular capsule
Bursa
Fibular collateral ligament
Posterior cruciate ligament
Popliteus tendon
Tibial collateral ligament
Lateral condyle of femur
Medial condyle of femur
Anterior cruciate ligament
Oblique popliteal ligament
Semimembranosus tendon

C. Proximal tibia, superior view

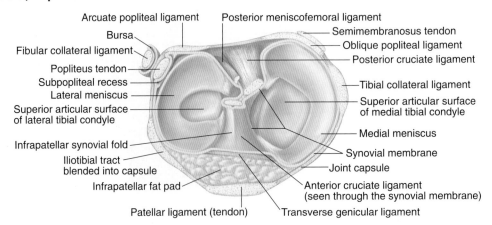

Arcuate popliteal ligament
Posterior meniscofemoral ligament
Bursa
Semimembranosus tendon
Fibular collateral ligament
Oblique popliteal ligament
Popliteus tendon
Posterior cruciate ligament
Subpopliteal recess
Lateral meniscus
Tibial collateral ligament
Superior articular surface of lateral tibial condyle
Superior articular surface of medial tibial condyle
Infrapatellar synovial fold
Medial meniscus
Iliotibial tract blended into capsule
Synovial membrane
Infrapatellar fat pad
Joint capsule
Anterior cruciate ligament (seen through the synovial membrane)
Patellar ligament (tendon)
Transverse genicular ligament

A. Ligaments, anterior view

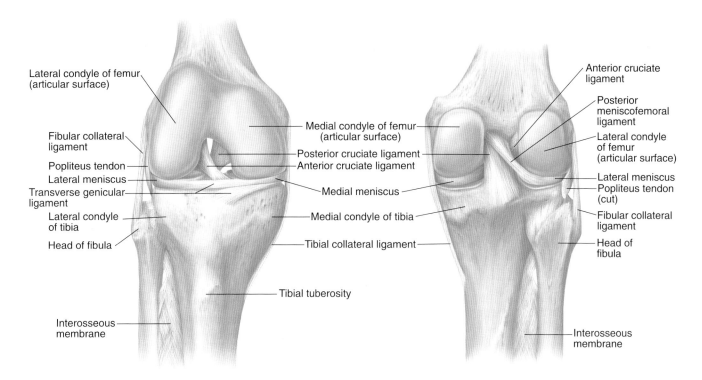

Lateral condyle of femur (articular surface)

Fibular collateral ligament

Popliteus tendon

Lateral meniscus

Transverse genicular ligament

Lateral condyle of tibia

Head of fibula

Interosseous membrane

Medial condyle of femur (articular surface)

Posterior cruciate ligament

Anterior cruciate ligament

Medial meniscus

Medial condyle of tibia

Tibial collateral ligament

Tibial tuberosity

B. Ligaments, posterior view

Anterior cruciate ligament

Posterior meniscofemoral ligament

Lateral condyle of femur (articular surface)

Lateral meniscus

Popliteus tendon (cut)

Fibular collateral ligament

Head of fibula

Interosseous membrane

C. Cruciate ligaments, lateral view, knee extended

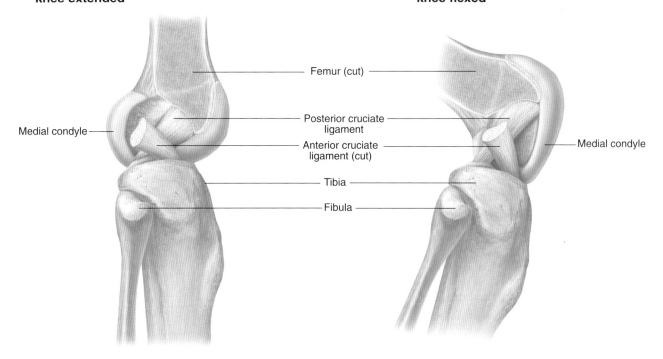

Medial condyle

Femur (cut)

Posterior cruciate ligament

Anterior cruciate ligament (cut)

Tibia

Fibula

D. Cruciate ligaments, lateral view, knee flexed

Medial condyle

PLATE 3-60   **Ankle Joint and Joints of the Foot**

A. Medial view

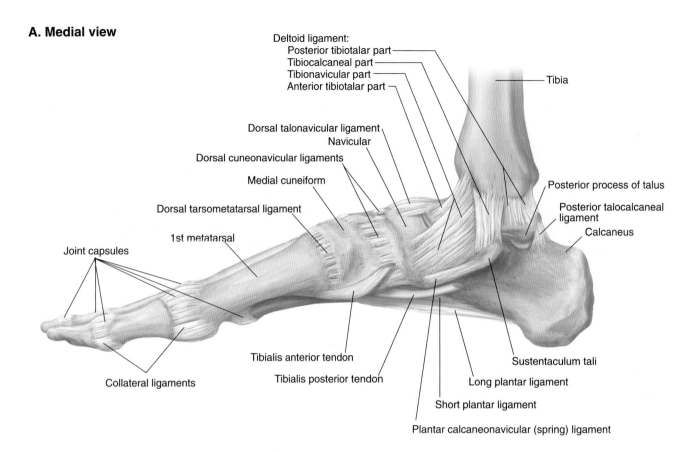

Deltoid ligament:
Posterior tibiotalar part
Tibiocalcaneal part
Tibionavicular part
Anterior tibiotalar part

Tibia

Dorsal talonavicular ligament
Navicular

Dorsal cuneonavicular ligaments

Medial cuneiform

Posterior process of talus

Dorsal tarsometatarsal ligament

Posterior talocalcaneal ligament

Calcaneus

1st metatarsal

Joint capsules

Tibialis anterior tendon

Tibialis posterior tendon

Sustentaculum tali

Long plantar ligament

Collateral ligaments

Short plantar ligament

Plantar calcaneonavicular (spring) ligament

B. Lateral view

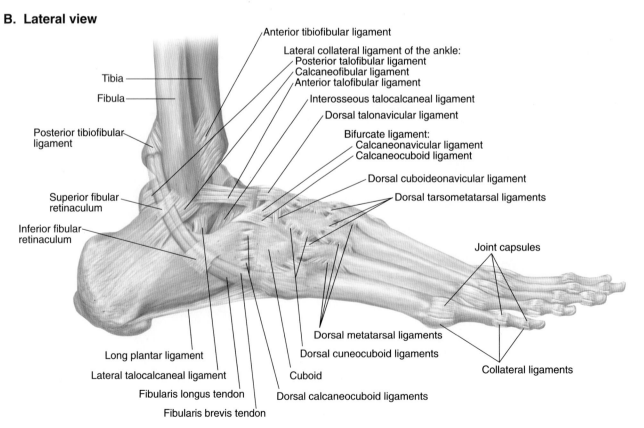

Anterior tibiofibular ligament

Lateral collateral ligament of the ankle:
Posterior talofibular ligament
Calcaneofibular ligament
Anterior talofibular ligament

Tibia

Fibula

Interosseous talocalcaneal ligament

Dorsal talonavicular ligament

Posterior tibiofibular ligament

Bifurcate ligament:
Calcaneonavicular ligament
Calcaneocuboid ligament

Dorsal cuboideonavicular ligament

Superior fibular retinaculum

Dorsal tarsometatarsal ligaments

Inferior fibular retinaculum

Joint capsules

Long plantar ligament

Lateral talocalcaneal ligament

Dorsal metatarsal ligaments

Collateral ligaments

Fibularis longus tendon

Dorsal cuneocuboid ligaments

Cuboid

Fibularis brevis tendon

Dorsal calcaneocuboid ligaments

A. Plantar view

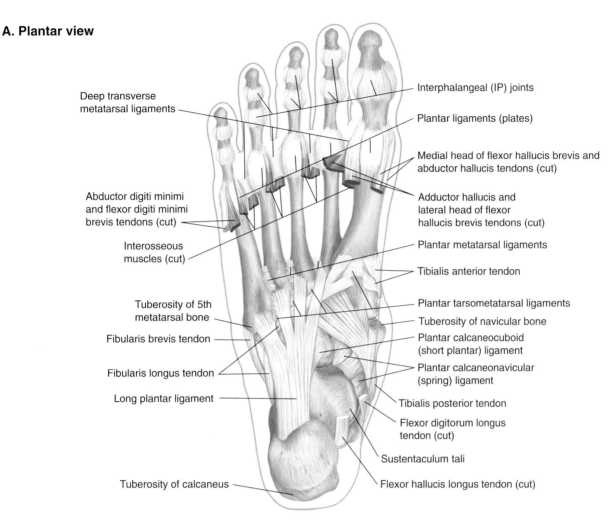

Deep transverse metatarsal ligaments

Abductor digiti minimi and flexor digiti minimi brevis tendons (cut)

Interosseous muscles (cut)

Tuberosity of 5th metatarsal bone

Fibularis brevis tendon

Fibularis longus tendon

Long plantar ligament

Tuberosity of calcaneus

Interphalangeal (IP) joints

Plantar ligaments (plates)

Medial head of flexor hallucis brevis and abductor hallucis tendons (cut)

Adductor hallucis and lateral head of flexor hallucis brevis tendons (cut)

Plantar metatarsal ligaments

Tibialis anterior tendon

Plantar tarsometatarsal ligaments

Tuberosity of navicular bone

Plantar calcaneocuboid (short plantar) ligament

Plantar calcaneonavicular (spring) ligament

Tibialis posterior tendon

Flexor digitorum longus tendon (cut)

Sustentaculum tali

Flexor hallucis longus tendon (cut)

B. Joints of inversion and eversion

C. Ligament attachments

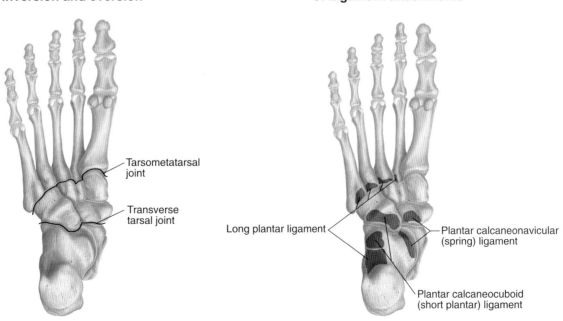

Tarsometatarsal joint

Transverse tarsal joint

Long plantar ligament

Plantar calcaneonavicular (spring) ligament

Plantar calcaneocuboid (short plantar) ligament

PLATE 3-62   **Arteries of the Lower Limb**

A. Anterior view

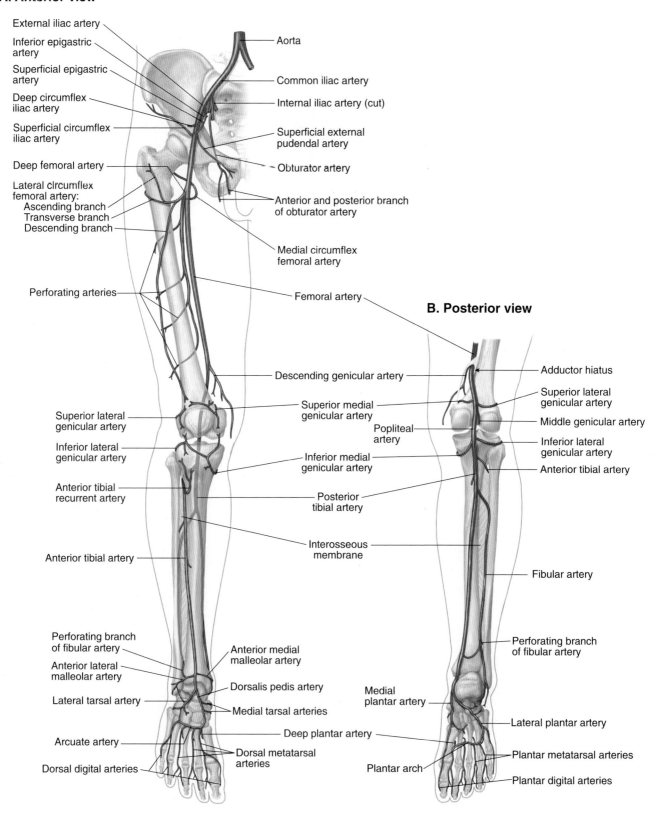

External iliac artery

Inferior epigastric artery

Superficial epigastric artery

Deep circumflex iliac artery

Superficial circumflex iliac artery

Deep femoral artery

Lateral circumflex femoral artery:
  Ascending branch
  Transverse branch
  Descending branch

Perforating arteries

Aorta

Common iliac artery

Internal iliac artery (cut)

Superficial external pudendal artery

Obturator artery

Anterior and posterior branch of obturator artery

Medial circumflex femoral artery

Femoral artery

B. Posterior view

Descending genicular artery

Superior medial genicular artery

Superior lateral genicular artery

Inferior lateral genicular artery

Anterior tibial recurrent artery

Anterior tibial artery

Inferior medial genicular artery

Posterior tibial artery

Interosseous membrane

Adductor hiatus

Superior lateral genicular artery

Middle genicular artery

Inferior lateral genicular artery

Anterior tibial artery

Popliteal artery

Fibular artery

Perforating branch of fibular artery

Anterior lateral malleolar artery

Lateral tarsal artery

Arcuate artery

Dorsal digital arteries

Anterior medial malleolar artery

Dorsalis pedis artery

Medial tarsal arteries

Deep plantar artery

Dorsal metatarsal arteries

Medial plantar artery

Lateral plantar artery

Plantar metatarsal arteries

Plantar arch

Plantar digital arteries

A. Anterior view

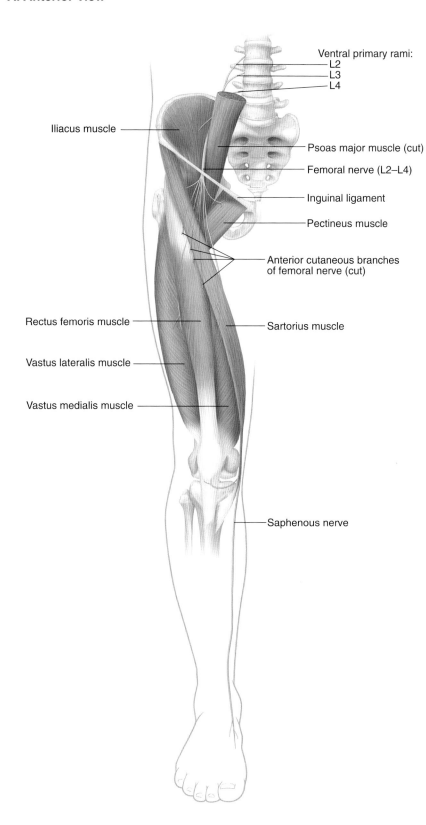

Ventral primary rami:
- L2
- L3
- L4

Iliacus muscle

Psoas major muscle (cut)

Femoral nerve (L2–L4)

Inguinal ligament

Pectineus muscle

Anterior cutaneous branches of femoral nerve (cut)

Rectus femoris muscle

Sartorius muscle

Vastus lateralis muscle

Vastus medialis muscle

Saphenous nerve

B. Cutaneous distribution, anterior view

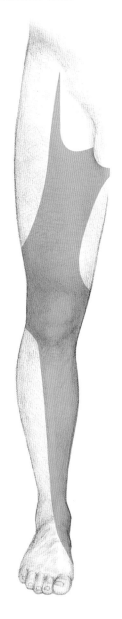

PLATE 3-64 | Obturator Nerve

A. Anterior view

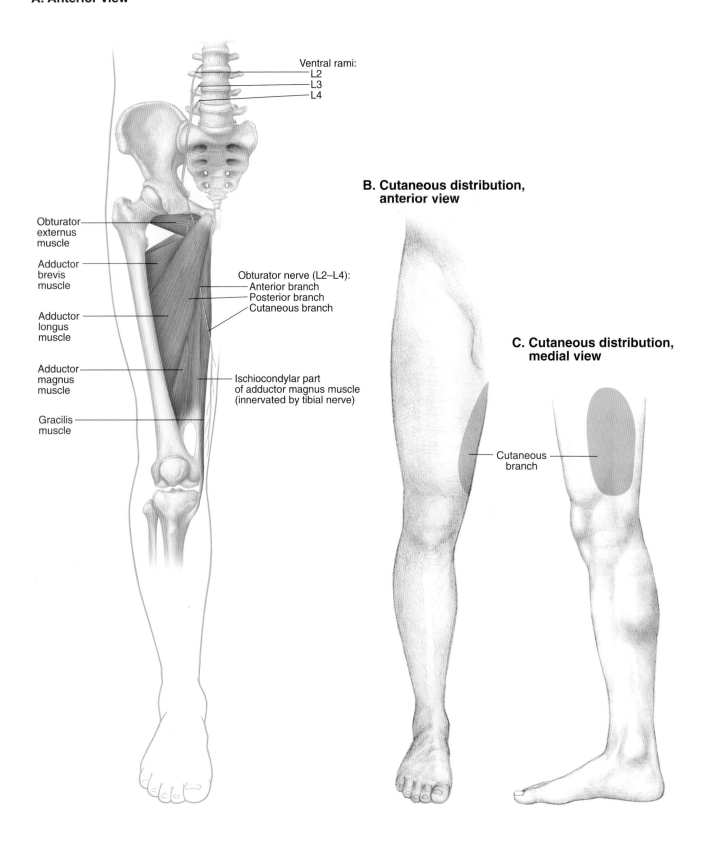

Ventral rami:
L2
L3
L4

Obturator externus muscle

Adductor brevis muscle

Adductor longus muscle

Adductor magnus muscle

Gracilis muscle

Obturator nerve (L2–L4):
Anterior branch
Posterior branch
Cutaneous branch

Ischiocondylar part of adductor magnus muscle (innervated by tibial nerve)

B. Cutaneous distribution, anterior view

C. Cutaneous distribution, medial view

Cutaneous branch

A. Posterior view

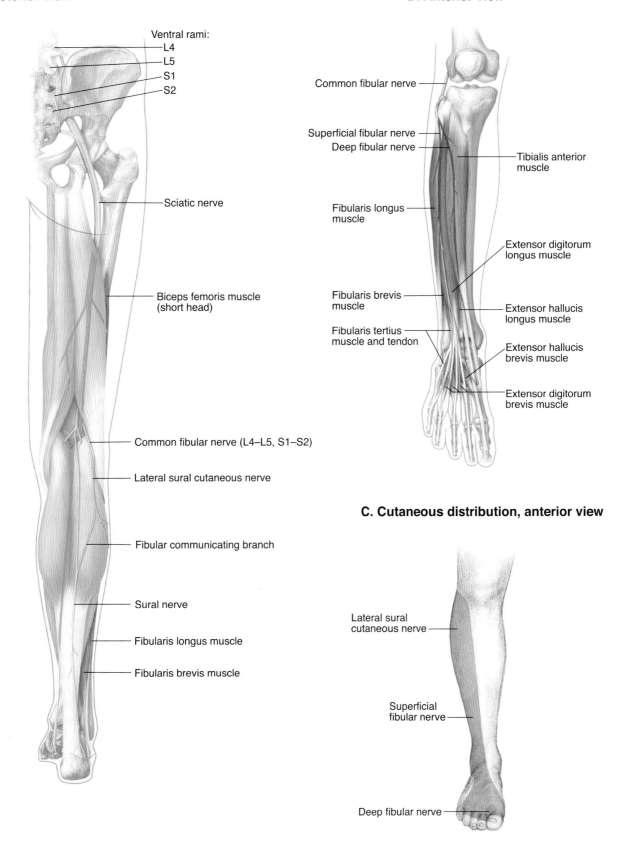

Ventral rami:
— L4
— L5
— S1
— S2

Sciatic nerve

Biceps femoris muscle (short head)

Common fibular nerve (L4–L5, S1–S2)

Lateral sural cutaneous nerve

Fibular communicating branch

Sural nerve

Fibularis longus muscle

Fibularis brevis muscle

B. Anterior view

Common fibular nerve

Superficial fibular nerve
Deep fibular nerve

Tibialis anterior muscle

Fibularis longus muscle

Extensor digitorum longus muscle

Fibularis brevis muscle

Extensor hallucis longus muscle

Fibularis tertius muscle and tendon

Extensor hallucis brevis muscle

Extensor digitorum brevis muscle

C. Cutaneous distribution, anterior view

Lateral sural cutaneous nerve

Superficial fibular nerve

Deep fibular nerve

Tibial Division of Sciatic Nerve, Superficial and Deep Views

A. Superficial view

B. Deep view

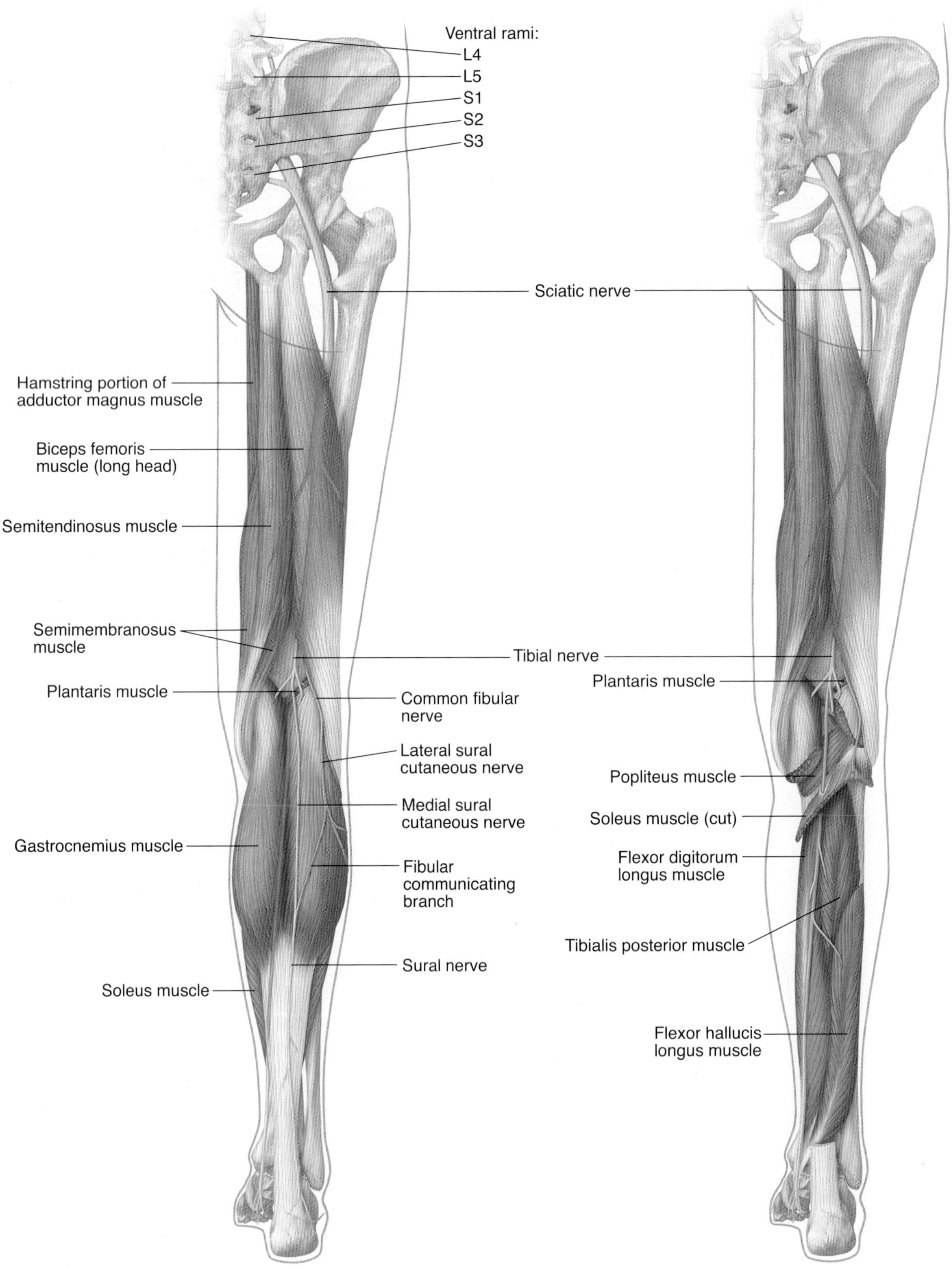
Ventral rami:
L4
L5
S1
S2
S3
Sciatic nerve
Hamstring portion of adductor magnus muscle
Biceps femoris muscle (long head)
Semitendinosus muscle
Semimembranosus muscle
Tibial nerve
Plantaris muscle
Common fibular nerve
Lateral sural cutaneous nerve
Medial sural cutaneous nerve
Gastrocnemius muscle
Fibular communicating branch
Sural nerve
Soleus muscle
Plantaris muscle
Popliteus muscle
Soleus muscle (cut)
Flexor digitorum longus muscle
Tibialis posterior muscle
Flexor hallucis longus muscle

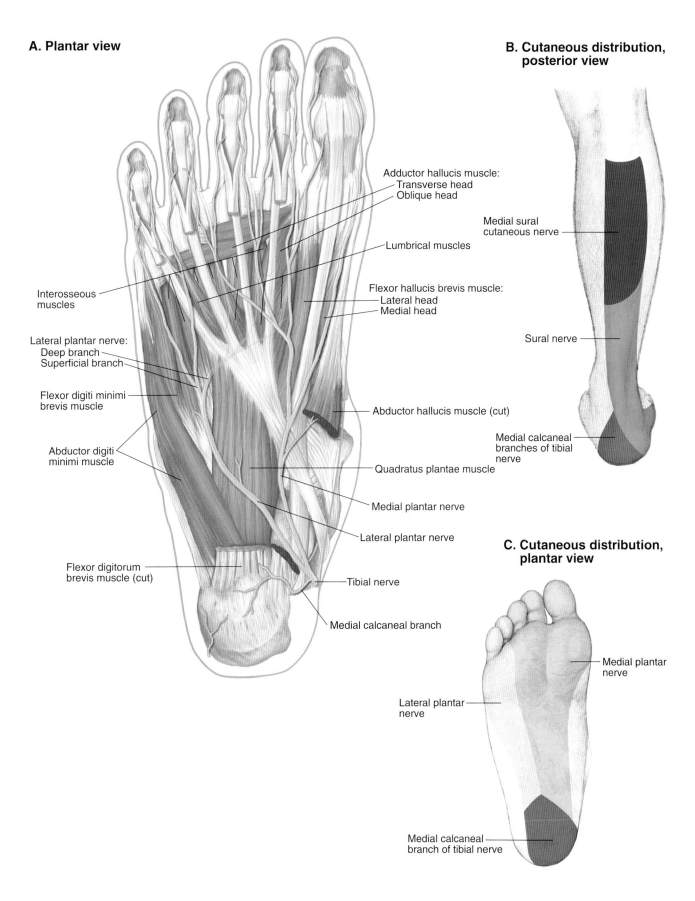

A. Plantar view

Interosseous muscles

Lateral plantar nerve:
Deep branch
Superficial branch

Flexor digiti minimi brevis muscle

Abductor digiti minimi muscle

Flexor digitorum brevis muscle (cut)

Adductor hallucis muscle:
Transverse head
Oblique head

Lumbrical muscles

Flexor hallucis brevis muscle:
Lateral head
Medial head

Abductor hallucis muscle (cut)

Quadratus plantae muscle

Medial plantar nerve

Lateral plantar nerve

Tibial nerve

Medial calcaneal branch

B. Cutaneous distribution, posterior view

Medial sural cutaneous nerve

Sural nerve

Medial calcaneal branches of tibial nerve

C. Cutaneous distribution, plantar view

Medial plantar nerve

Lateral plantar nerve

Medial calcaneal branch of tibial nerve

PLATE 3-68 | **Cutaneous Innervation of the Lower Limb**

A. Anterior view

B. Posterior view

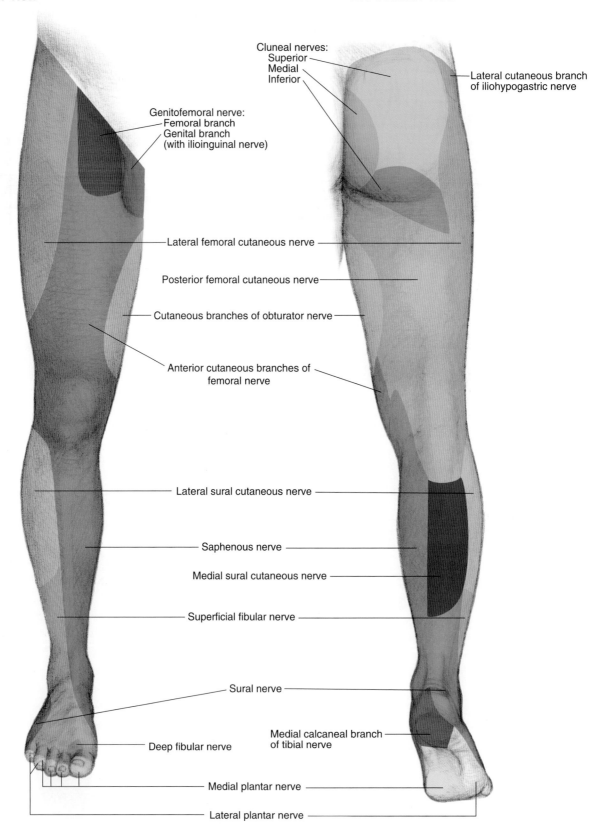

Cluneal nerves:
Superior
Medial
Inferior

Lateral cutaneous branch
of iliohypogastric nerve

Genitofemoral nerve:
Femoral branch
Genital branch
(with ilioinguinal nerve)

Lateral femoral cutaneous nerve

Posterior femoral cutaneous nerve

Cutaneous branches of obturator nerve

Anterior cutaneous branches of
femoral nerve

Lateral sural cutaneous nerve

Saphenous nerve

Medial sural cutaneous nerve

Superficial fibular nerve

Sural nerve

Medial calcaneal branch
of tibial nerve

Deep fibular nerve

Medial plantar nerve

Lateral plantar nerve

A. Anterior view

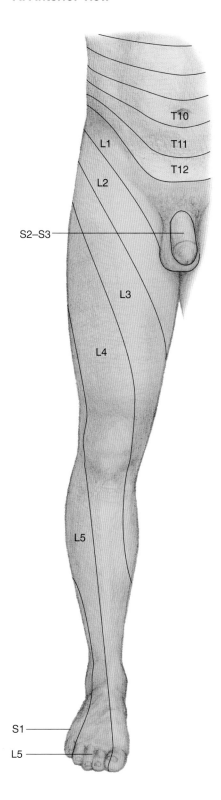

B. Posterior view

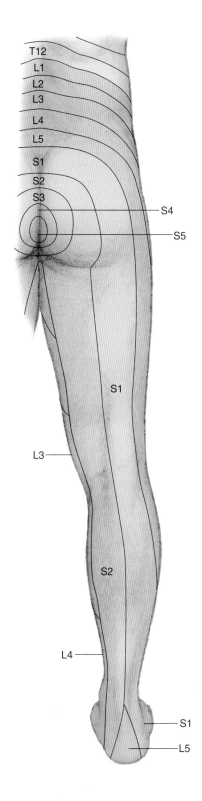

PLATE 3-70 | Lymphatics of the Lower Limb

A. Anterior view

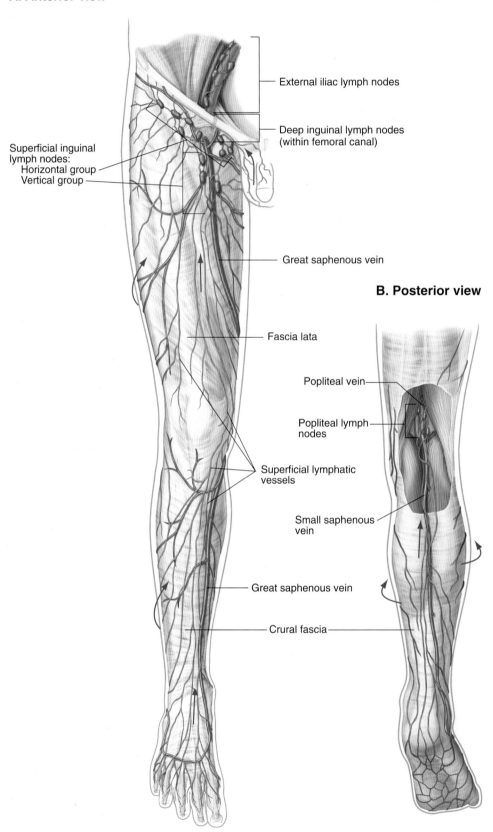

External iliac lymph nodes

Deep inguinal lymph nodes (within femoral canal)

Superficial inguinal lymph nodes:
Horizontal group
Vertical group

Great saphenous vein

Fascia lata

B. Posterior view

Popliteal vein

Popliteal lymph nodes

Superficial lymphatic vessels

Small saphenous vein

Great saphenous vein

Crural fascia

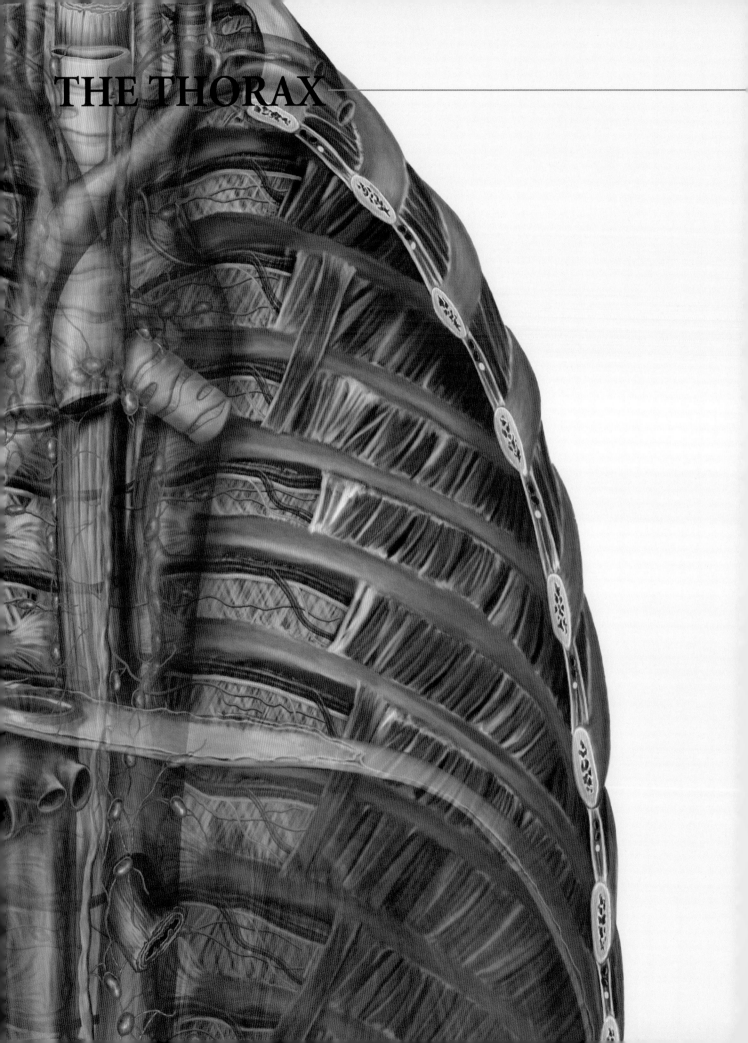

PLATE 4-01   **Palpable Features and Landmarks of the Thorax**

A. Anterior view

Palpable bony structures

Clavicle

Sternum:
Jugular notch
Manubrium
Sternal angle
Body
Xiphisternal joint
Xiphoid process

Anterior axillary fold

Costal cartilages

Costal margin

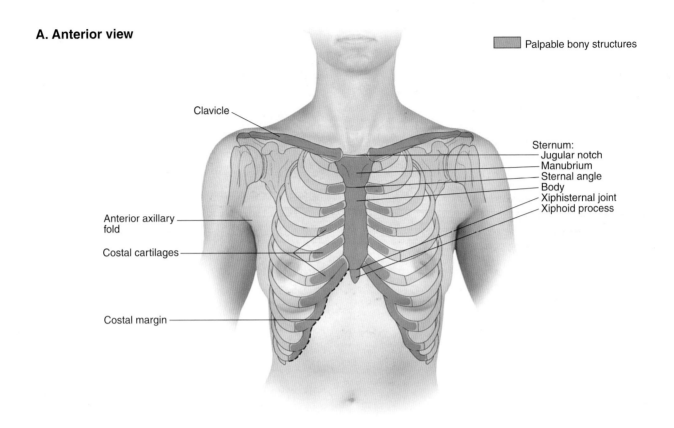

B. Landmarks, anterior view

Midclavicular line

Nipple in 4th intercostal space

C. Landmarks, lateral view

Clavicle

Outline of shoulder and axilla

Sternal angle

Anterior axillary line

Midaxillary line

Posterior axillary line

D. Landmarks, posterior view

Spine of scapula

Thoracic vertebrae:
Transverse processes
Spinous processes

Inferior angle of scapula

Paravertebral line

Scapular line

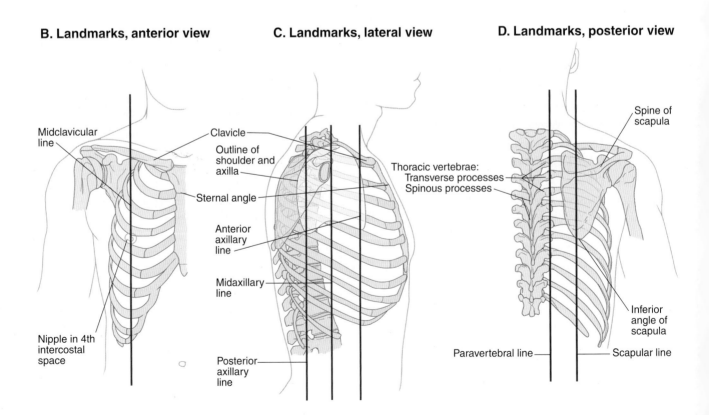

A. Anterior view, female

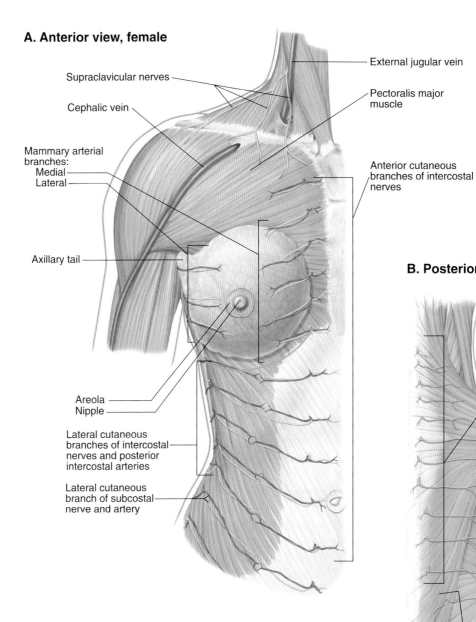

Supraclavicular nerves

Cephalic vein

Mammary arterial branches:
Medial
Lateral

Axillary tail

Areola
Nipple

Lateral cutaneous branches of intercostal nerves and posterior intercostal arteries

Lateral cutaneous branch of subcostal nerve and artery

External jugular vein

Pectoralis major muscle

Anterior cutaneous branches of intercostal nerves

B. Posterior view

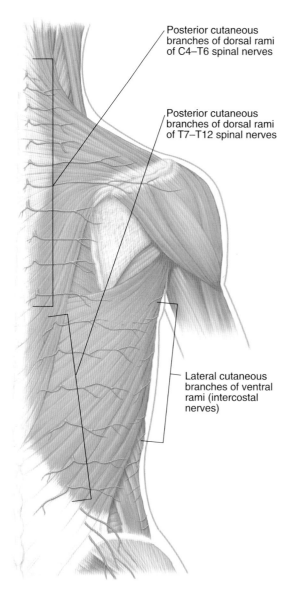

Posterior cutaneous branches of dorsal rami of C4–T6 spinal nerves

Posterior cutaneous branches of dorsal rami of T7–T12 spinal nerves

Lateral cutaneous branches of ventral rami (intercostal nerves)

PLATE 4-03   **Dermatomes of the Thorax**

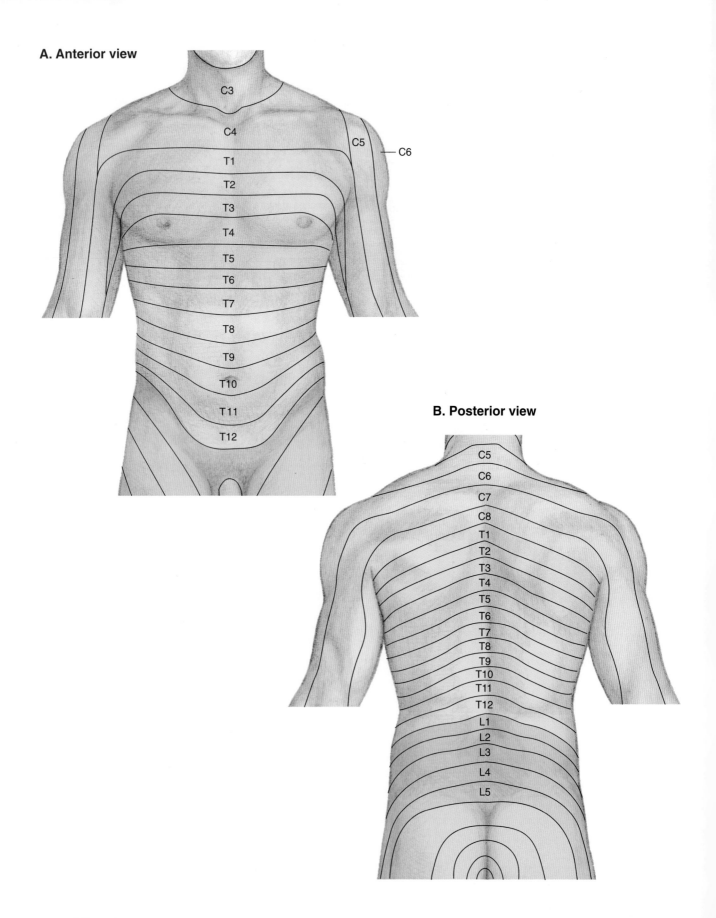

A. Anterior view

C3
C4
C5 — C6
T1
T2
T3
T4
T5
T6
T7
T8
T9
T10
T11
T12

B. Posterior view

C5
C6
C7
C8
T1
T2
T3
T4
T5
T6
T7
T8
T9
T10
T11
T12
L1
L2
L3
L4
L5

A. Anterior view

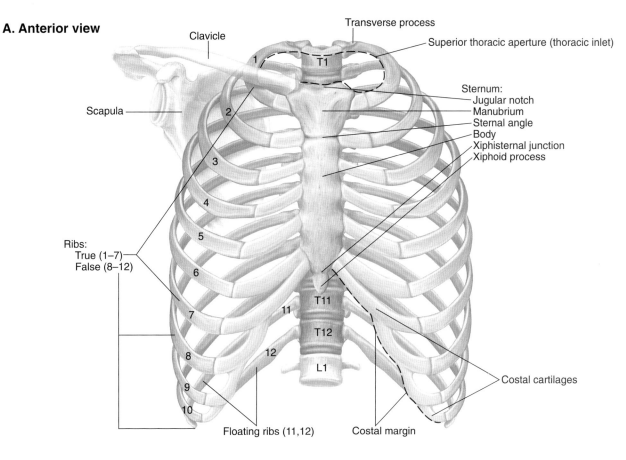

Clavicle

Transverse process

Superior thoracic aperture (thoracic inlet)

Scapula

T1

Sternum:
Jugular notch
Manubrium
Sternal angle
Body
Xiphisternal junction
Xiphoid process

Ribs:
True (1–7)
False (8–12)

1
2
3
4
5
6
7
8
9
10
11
12

T11
T12
L1

Costal cartilages

Floating ribs (11,12)

Costal margin

B. Posterior view

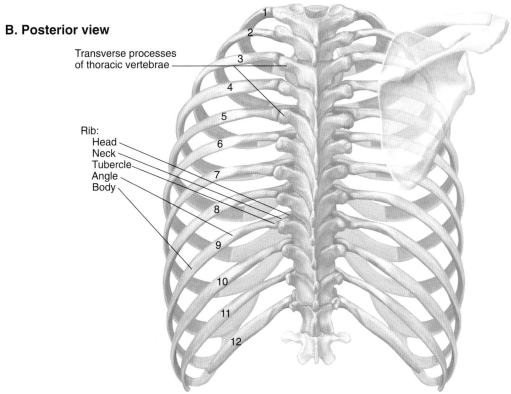

Transverse processes
of thoracic vertebrae

Rib:
Head
Neck
Tubercle
Angle
Body

1
2
3
4
5
6
7
8
9
10
11
12

PLATE 4-05   Ribs

A. First rib, posterior view

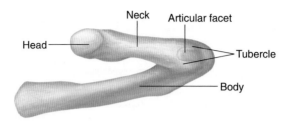

Neck   Articular facet

Head

Tubercle

Body

B. Sixth rib, posterior view

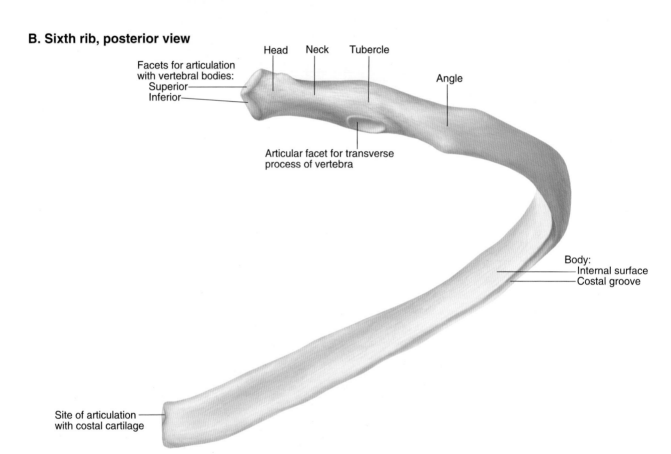

Head   Neck   Tubercle

Facets for articulation
with vertebral bodies:
Superior
Inferior

Angle

Articular facet for transverse
process of vertebra

Body:
Internal surface
Costal groove

Site of articulation
with costal cartilage

C. Twelfth rib, posterior view

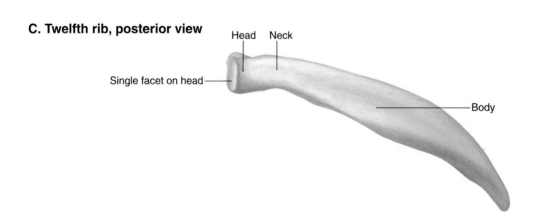

Head   Neck

Single facet on head

Body

A. Posterior view

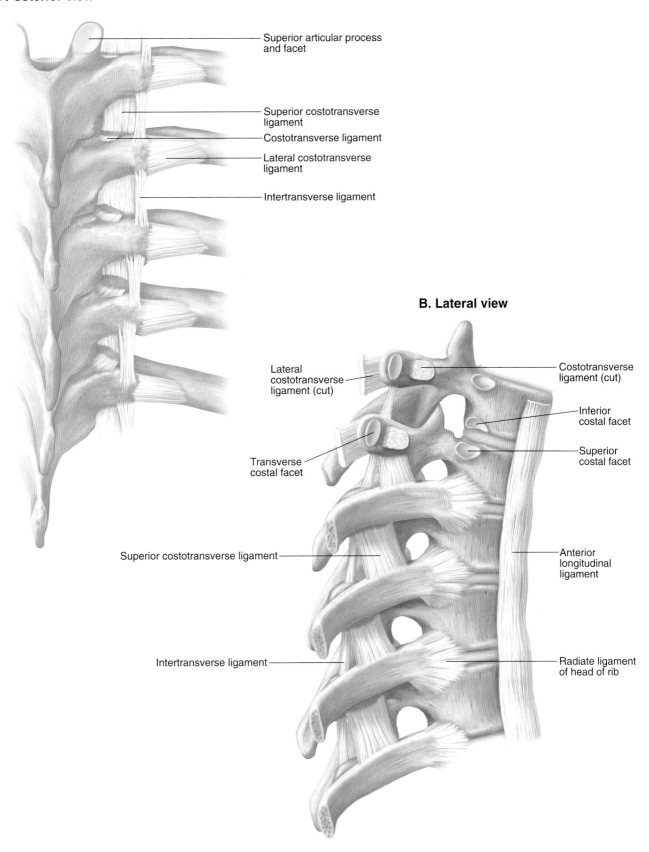

Superior articular process and facet

Superior costotransverse ligament

Costotransverse ligament

Lateral costotransverse ligament

Intertransverse ligament

B. Lateral view

Lateral costotransverse ligament (cut)

Costotransverse ligament (cut)

Inferior costal facet

Superior costal facet

Transverse costal facet

Superior costotransverse ligament

Anterior longitudinal ligament

Intertransverse ligament

Radiate ligament of head of rib

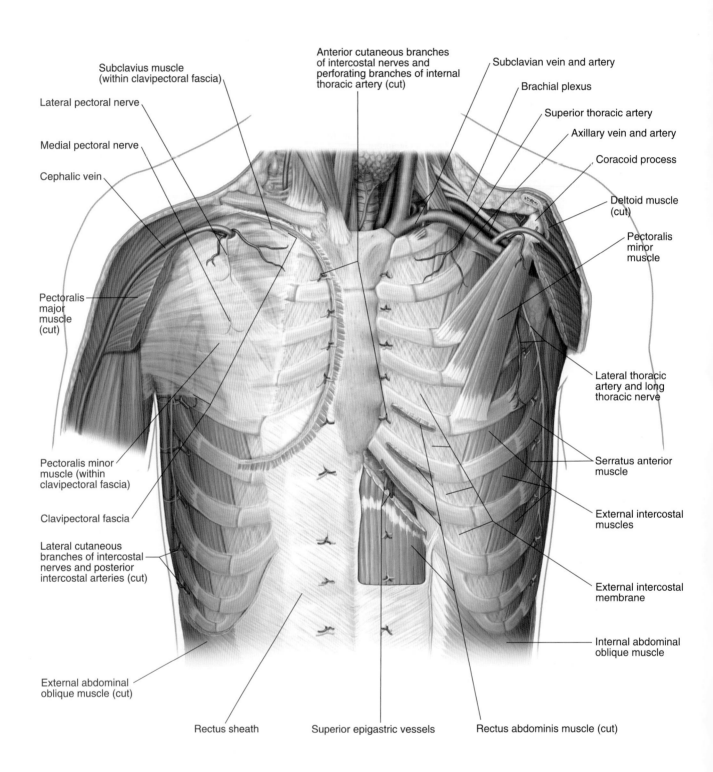

Subclavius muscle
(within clavipectoral fascia)

Lateral pectoral nerve

Medial pectoral nerve

Cephalic vein

Pectoralis
major
muscle
(cut)

Pectoralis minor
muscle (within
clavipectoral fascia)

Clavipectoral fascia

Lateral cutaneous
branches of intercostal
nerves and posterior
intercostal arteries (cut)

External abdominal
oblique muscle (cut)

Anterior cutaneous branches
of intercostal nerves and
perforating branches of internal
thoracic artery (cut)

Subclavian vein and artery

Brachial plexus

Superior thoracic artery

Axillary vein and artery

Coracoid process

Deltoid muscle
(cut)

Pectoralis
minor
muscle

Lateral thoracic
artery and long
thoracic nerve

Serratus anterior
muscle

External intercostal
muscles

External intercostal
membrane

Internal abdominal
oblique muscle

Rectus sheath

Superior epigastric vessels

Rectus abdominis muscle (cut)

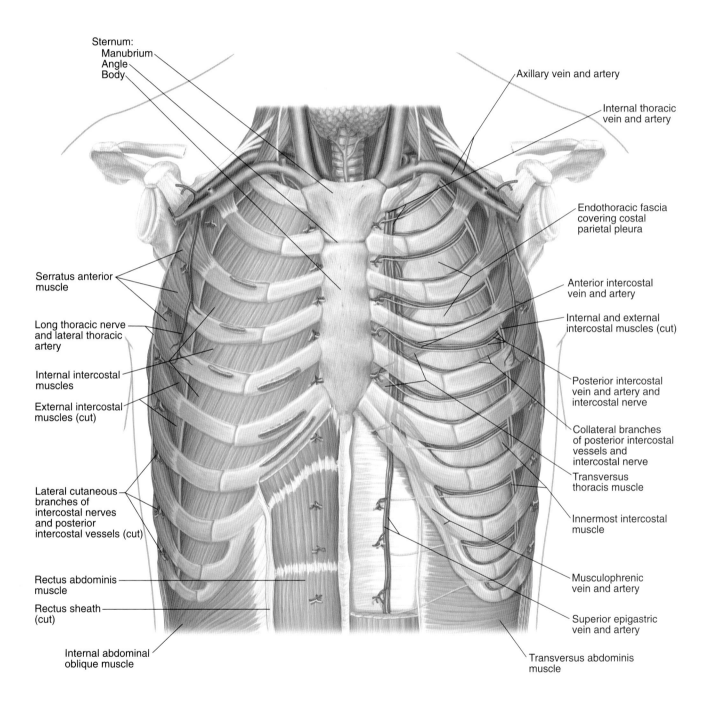

Sternum:
Manubrium
Angle
Body

Axillary vein and artery

Internal thoracic
vein and artery

Endothoracic fascia
covering costal
parietal pleura

Serratus anterior
muscle

Anterior intercostal
vein and artery

Long thoracic nerve
and lateral thoracic
artery

Internal and external
intercostal muscles (cut)

Internal intercostal
muscles

Posterior intercostal
vein and artery and
intercostal nerve

External intercostal
muscles (cut)

Collateral branches
of posterior intercostal
vessels and
intercostal nerve

Transversus
thoracis muscle

Lateral cutaneous
branches of
intercostal nerves
and posterior
intercostal vessels (cut)

Innermost intercostal
muscle

Rectus abdominis
muscle

Musculophrenic
vein and artery

Rectus sheath
(cut)

Superior epigastric
vein and artery

Internal abdominal
oblique muscle

Transversus abdominis
muscle

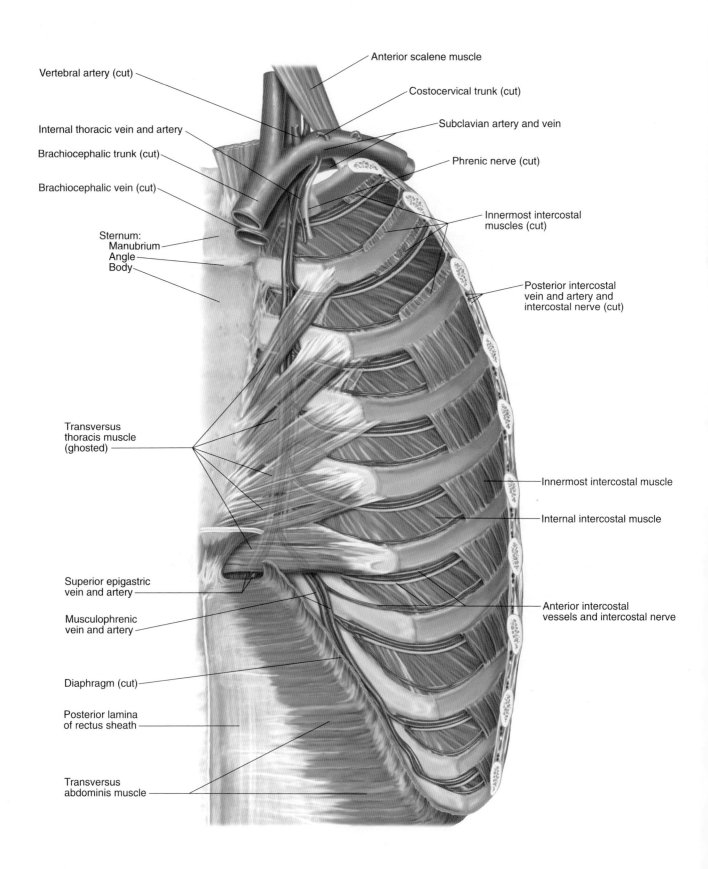

Vertebral artery (cut)

Internal thoracic vein and artery

Brachiocephalic trunk (cut)

Brachiocephalic vein (cut)

Sternum:
Manubrium
Angle
Body

Transversus
thoracis muscle
(ghosted)

Superior epigastric
vein and artery

Musculophrenic
vein and artery

Diaphragm (cut)

Posterior lamina
of rectus sheath

Transversus
abdominis muscle

Anterior scalene muscle

Costocervical trunk (cut)

Subclavian artery and vein

Phrenic nerve (cut)

Innermost intercostal
muscles (cut)

Posterior intercostal
vein and artery and
intercostal nerve (cut)

Innermost intercostal muscle

Internal intercostal muscle

Anterior intercostal
vessels and intercostal nerve

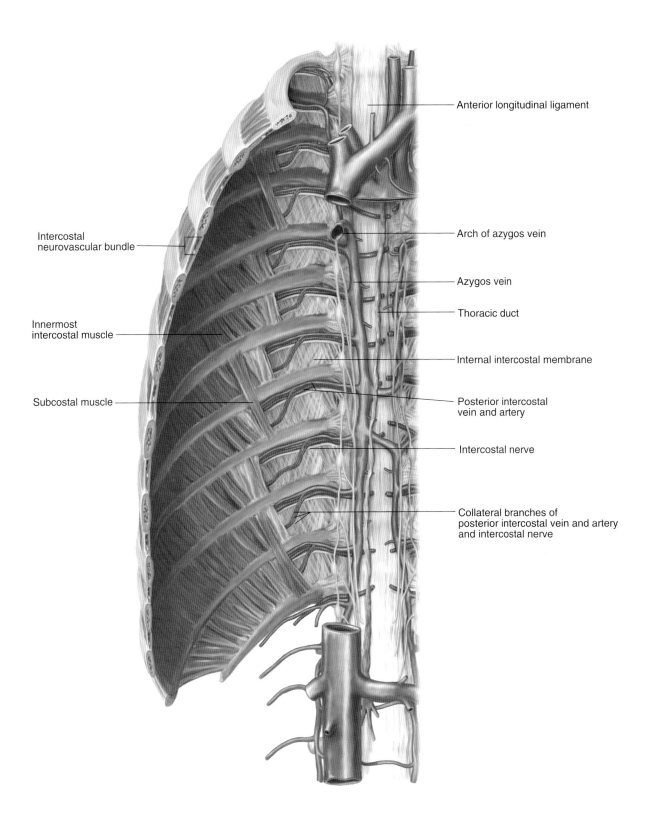

Intercostal
neurovascular bundle

Innermost
intercostal muscle

Subcostal muscle

Anterior longitudinal ligament

Arch of azygos vein

Azygos vein

Thoracic duct

Internal intercostal membrane

Posterior intercostal
vein and artery

Intercostal nerve

Collateral branches of
posterior intercostal vein and artery
and intercostal nerve

PLATE 4-11   Pattern of the 4th Intercostal Nerve

A. Orientation

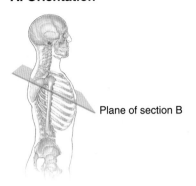

Plane of section B

B. Oblique section through 4th intercostal space

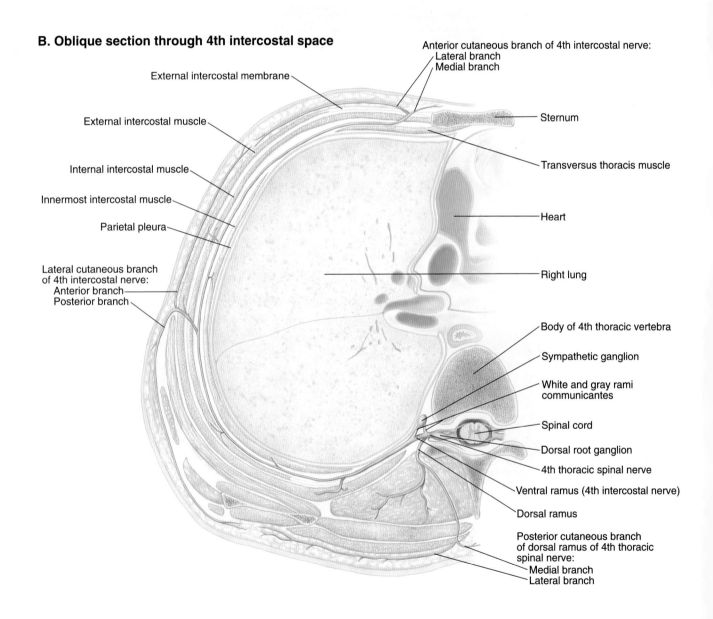

External intercostal membrane

External intercostal muscle

Internal intercostal muscle

Innermost intercostal muscle

Parietal pleura

Lateral cutaneous branch
of 4th intercostal nerve:
  Anterior branch
  Posterior branch

Anterior cutaneous branch of 4th intercostal nerve:
  Lateral branch
  Medial branch

Sternum

Transversus thoracis muscle

Heart

Right lung

Body of 4th thoracic vertebra

Sympathetic ganglion

White and gray rami
communicantes

Spinal cord

Dorsal root ganglion

4th thoracic spinal nerve

Ventral ramus (4th intercostal nerve)

Dorsal ramus

Posterior cutaneous branch
of dorsal ramus of 4th thoracic
spinal nerve:
  Medial branch
  Lateral branch

A. Orientation

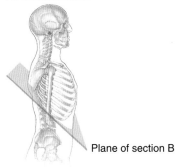

Plane of section B

B. Oblique section through 10th intercostal space

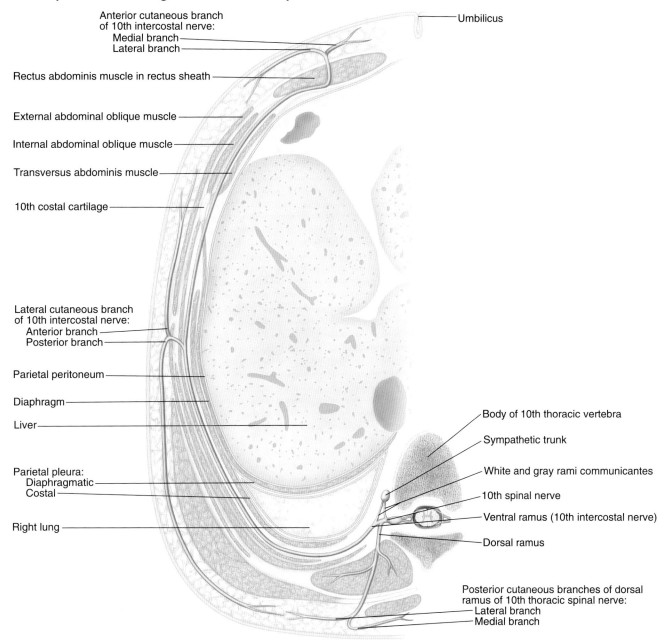

Anterior cutaneous branch
of 10th intercostal nerve:
Medial branch
Lateral branch

Umbilicus

Rectus abdominis muscle in rectus sheath

External abdominal oblique muscle

Internal abdominal oblique muscle

Transversus abdominis muscle

10th costal cartilage

Lateral cutaneous branch
of 10th intercostal nerve:
Anterior branch
Posterior branch

Parietal peritoneum

Diaphragm

Liver

Parietal pleura:
Diaphragmatic
Costal

Right lung

Body of 10th thoracic vertebra

Sympathetic trunk

White and gray rami communicantes

10th spinal nerve

Ventral ramus (10th intercostal nerve)

Dorsal ramus

Posterior cutaneous branches of dorsal
ramus of 10th thoracic spinal nerve:
Lateral branch
Medial branch

PLATE 4-13   **Surface Projection of the Lungs and Pleurae**

A. Anterior view

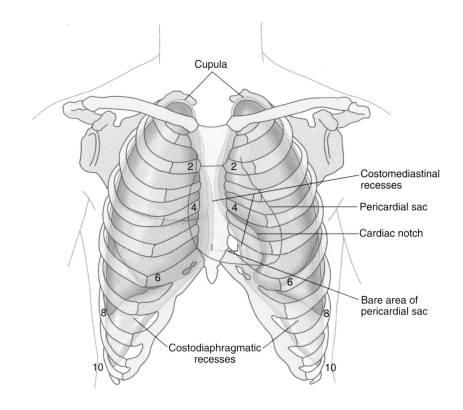

Cupula

Costomediastinal recesses

Pericardial sac

Cardiac notch

Bare area of pericardial sac

Costodiaphragmatic recesses

B. Posterior view

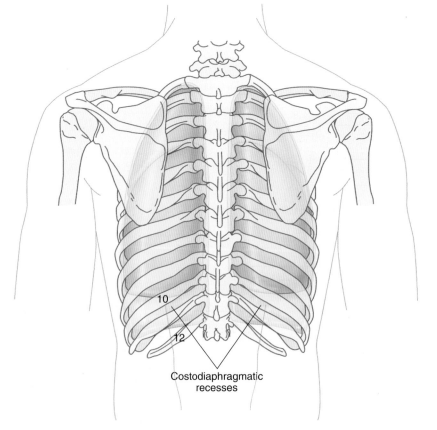

Costodiaphragmatic recesses

A. Heart and heart valves

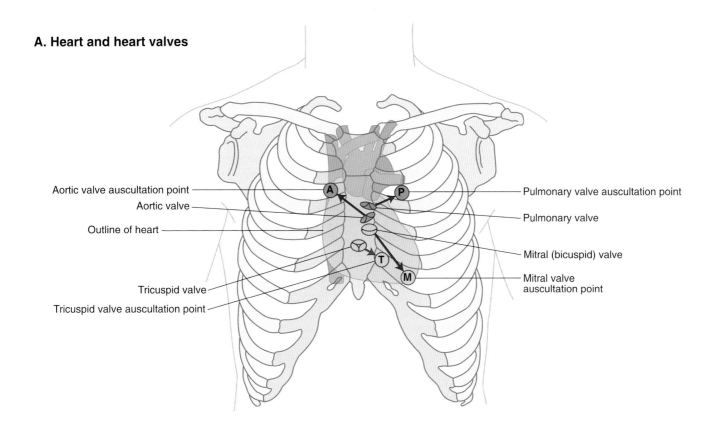

Aortic valve auscultation point

Aortic valve

Outline of heart

Tricuspid valve

Tricuspid valve auscultation point

Pulmonary valve auscultation point

Pulmonary valve

Mitral (bicuspid) valve

Mitral valve auscultation point

B. Mediastinum, anterior view

C. Mediastinum, right lateral view

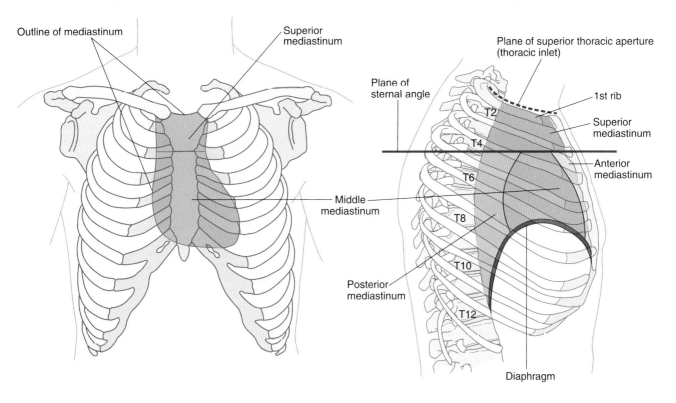

Outline of mediastinum

Superior mediastinum

Middle mediastinum

Posterior mediastinum

Plane of superior thoracic aperture (thoracic inlet)

Plane of sternal angle

1st rib

Superior mediastinum

Anterior mediastinum

T2

T4

T6

T8

T10

T12

Diaphragm

PLATE 4-15   **Projection of the Thoracic Viscera, Anterior View**

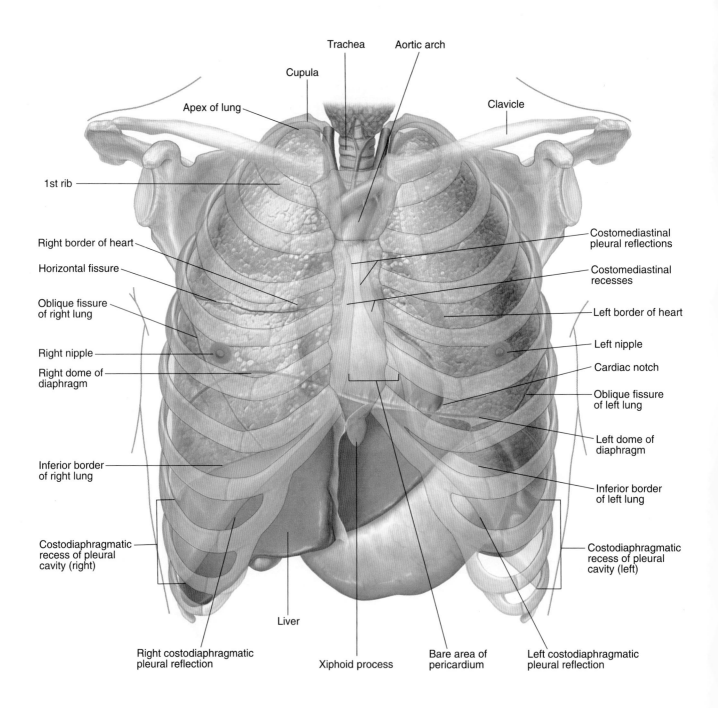

Trachea

Aortic arch

Cupula

Apex of lung

Clavicle

1st rib

Right border of heart

Horizontal fissure

Oblique fissure
of right lung

Right nipple

Right dome of
diaphragm

Inferior border
of right lung

Costodiaphragmatic
recess of pleural
cavity (right)

Costomediastinal
pleural reflections

Costomediastinal
recesses

Left border of heart

Left nipple

Cardiac notch

Oblique fissure
of left lung

Left dome of
diaphragm

Inferior border
of left lung

Costodiaphragmatic
recess of pleural
cavity (left)

Right costodiaphragmatic
pleural reflection

Liver

Xiphoid process

Bare area of
pericardium

Left costodiaphragmatic
pleural reflection

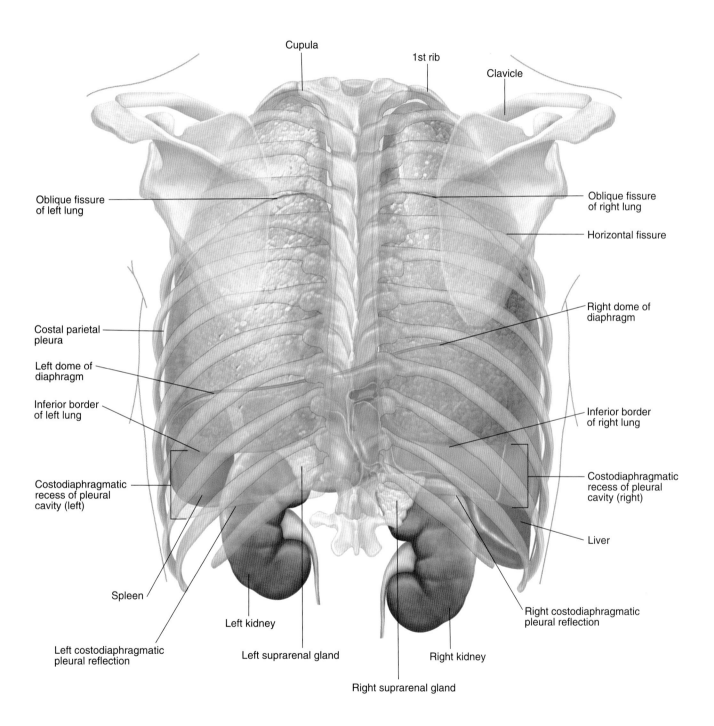

Cupula

1st rib

Clavicle

Oblique fissure
of left lung

Oblique fissure
of right lung

Horizontal fissure

Right dome of
diaphragm

Costal parietal
pleura

Left dome of
diaphragm

Inferior border
of left lung

Inferior border
of right lung

Costodiaphragmatic
recess of pleural
cavity (left)

Costodiaphragmatic
recess of pleural
cavity (right)

Liver

Spleen

Right costodiaphragmatic
pleural reflection

Left kidney

Left costodiaphragmatic
pleural reflection

Left suprarenal gland

Right kidney

Right suprarenal gland

PLATE 4-17   **Thoracic Viscera, Pleural Cavities**

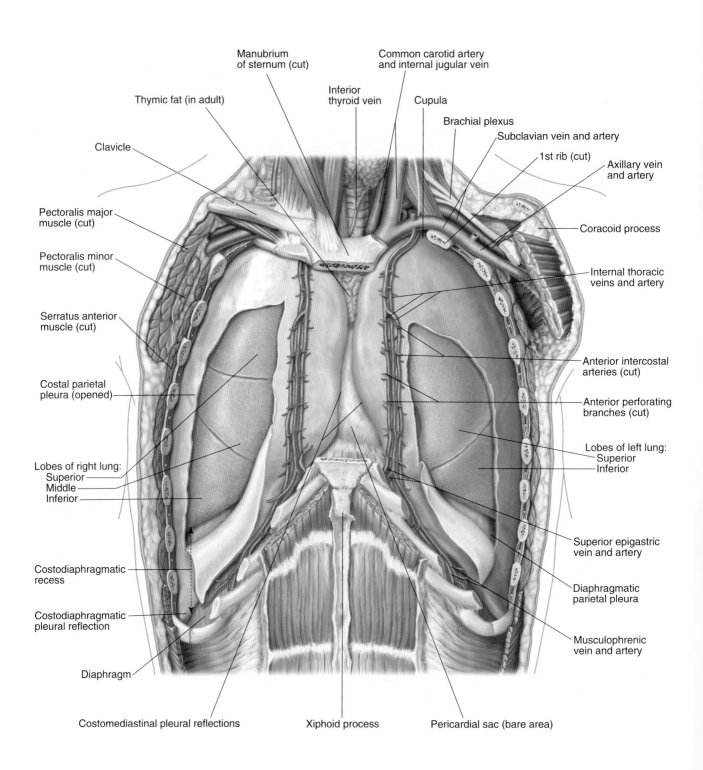

Manubrium
of sternum (cut)

Common carotid artery
and internal jugular vein

Thymic fat (in adult)

Inferior
thyroid vein

Cupula

Brachial plexus

Clavicle

Subclavian vein and artery

1st rib (cut)

Axillary vein
and artery

Pectoralis major
muscle (cut)

Coracoid process

Pectoralis minor
muscle (cut)

Internal thoracic
veins and artery

Serratus anterior
muscle (cut)

Costal parietal
pleura (opened)

Anterior intercostal
arteries (cut)

Anterior perforating
branches (cut)

Lobes of left lung:
Superior
Inferior

Lobes of right lung:
Superior
Middle
Inferior

Superior epigastric
vein and artery

Costodiaphragmatic
recess

Diaphragmatic
parietal pleura

Costodiaphragmatic
pleural reflection

Musculophrenic
vein and artery

Diaphragm

Costomediastinal pleural reflections

Xiphoid process

Pericardial sac (bare area)

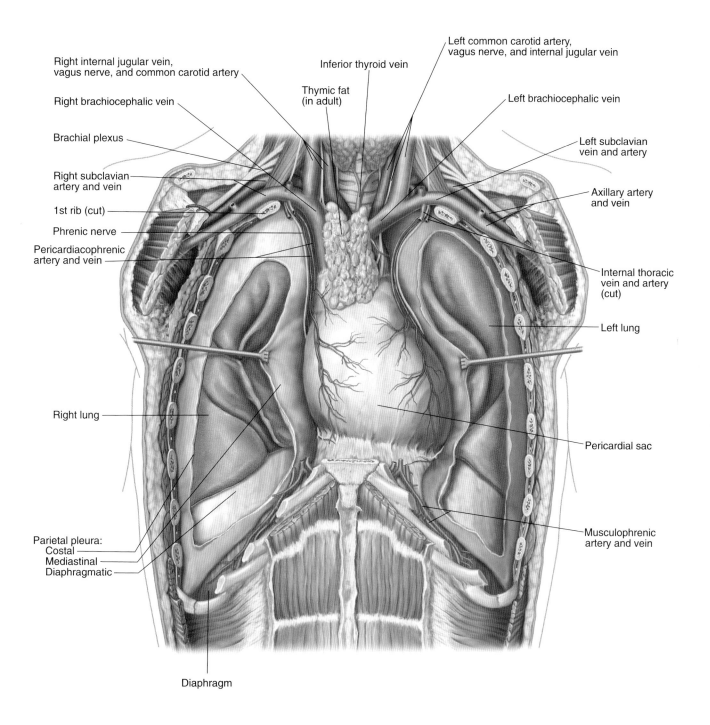

Right internal jugular vein, vagus nerve, and common carotid artery

Inferior thyroid vein

Left common carotid artery, vagus nerve, and internal jugular vein

Right brachiocephalic vein

Thymic fat (in adult)

Left brachiocephalic vein

Brachial plexus

Left subclavian vein and artery

Right subclavian artery and vein

Axillary artery and vein

1st rib (cut)

Phrenic nerve

Pericardiacophrenic artery and vein

Internal thoracic vein and artery (cut)

Left lung

Right lung

Pericardial sac

Parietal pleura:
Costal
Mediastinal
Diaphragmatic

Musculophrenic artery and vein

Diaphragm

PLATE 4-19 **Thoracic Viscera, Heart in Pericardial Sac**

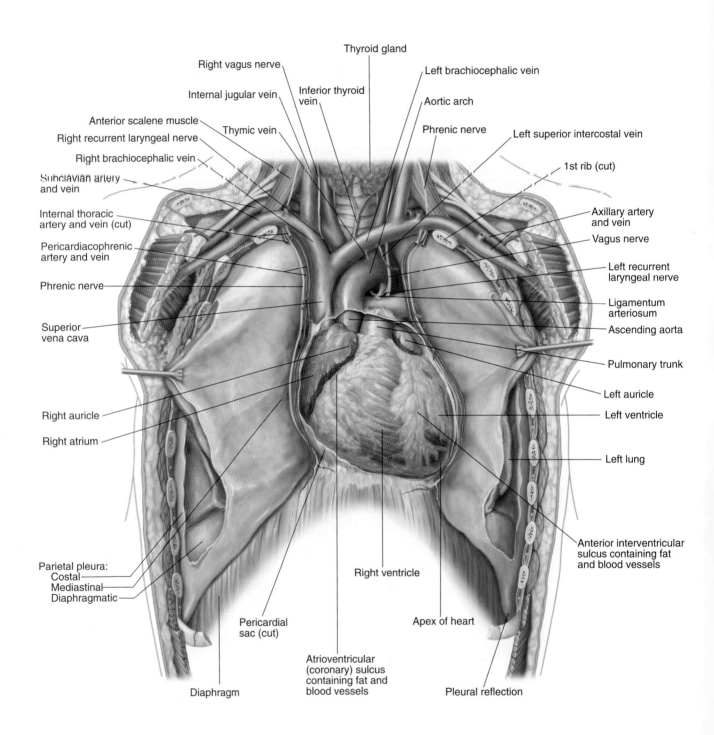

Thyroid gland

Right vagus nerve

Internal jugular vein

Inferior thyroid vein

Left brachiocephalic vein

Aortic arch

Phrenic nerve

Left superior intercostal vein

Anterior scalene muscle

Thymic vein

Right recurrent laryngeal nerve

Right brachiocephalic vein

Subclavian artery and vein

1st rib (cut)

Internal thoracic artery and vein (cut)

Axillary artery and vein

Vagus nerve

Pericardiacophrenic artery and vein

Left recurrent laryngeal nerve

Phrenic nerve

Ligamentum arteriosum

Superior vena cava

Ascending aorta

Pulmonary trunk

Left auricle

Right auricle

Left ventricle

Right atrium

Left lung

Parietal pleura:
Costal
Mediastinal
Diaphragmatic

Anterior interventricular sulcus containing fat and blood vessels

Right ventricle

Pericardial sac (cut)

Apex of heart

Diaphragm

Atrioventricular (coronary) sulcus containing fat and blood vessels

Pleural reflection

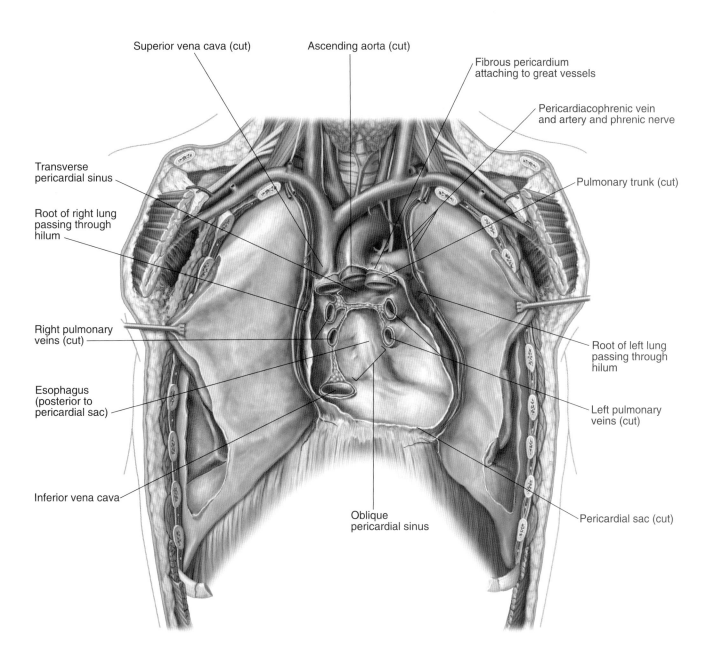

Superior vena cava (cut)

Ascending aorta (cut)

Fibrous pericardium attaching to great vessels

Pericardiacophrenic vein and artery and phrenic nerve

Transverse pericardial sinus

Pulmonary trunk (cut)

Root of right lung passing through hilum

Right pulmonary veins (cut)

Root of left lung passing through hilum

Esophagus (posterior to pericardial sac)

Left pulmonary veins (cut)

Inferior vena cava

Oblique pericardial sinus

Pericardial sac (cut)

PLATE 4-21   **Heart, External Features**

A. Anterior view

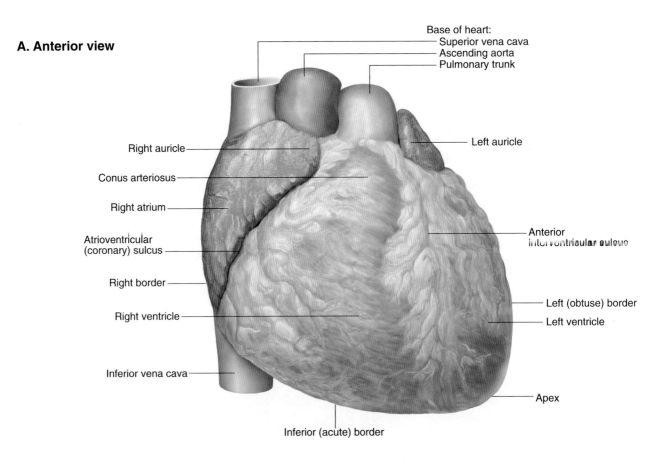

Base of heart:
Superior vena cava
Ascending aorta
Pulmonary trunk

Right auricle

Conus arteriosus

Right atrium

Atrioventricular
(coronary) sulcus

Right border

Right ventricle

Inferior vena cava

Left auricle

Anterior
interventricular sulcus

Left (obtuse) border
Left ventricle

Apex

Inferior (acute) border

B. Posteroinferior view (diaphragmatic surface)

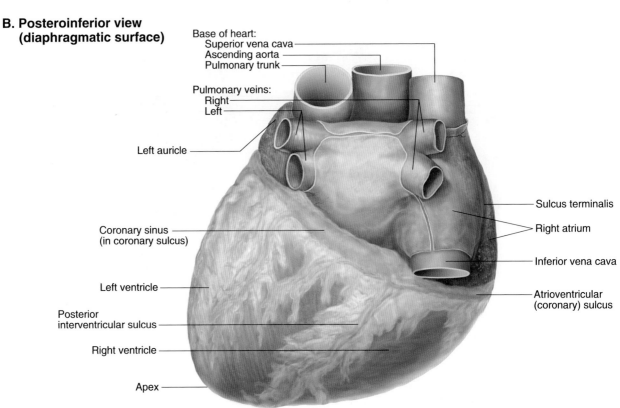

Base of heart:
Superior vena cava
Ascending aorta
Pulmonary trunk

Pulmonary veins:
Right
Left

Left auricle

Coronary sinus
(in coronary sulcus)

Left ventricle

Posterior
interventricular sulcus

Right ventricle

Apex

Sulcus terminalis

Right atrium

Inferior vena cava

Atrioventricular
(coronary) sulcus

A. Anterior view

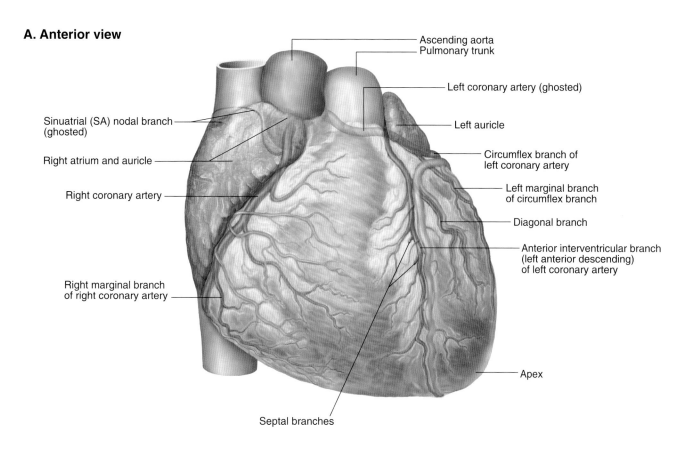

Ascending aorta
Pulmonary trunk
Left coronary artery (ghosted)
Sinuatrial (SA) nodal branch (ghosted)
Left auricle
Right atrium and auricle
Circumflex branch of left coronary artery
Right coronary artery
Left marginal branch of circumflex branch
Diagonal branch
Anterior interventricular branch (left anterior descending) of left coronary artery
Right marginal branch of right coronary artery
Apex
Septal branches

B. Posteroinferior view

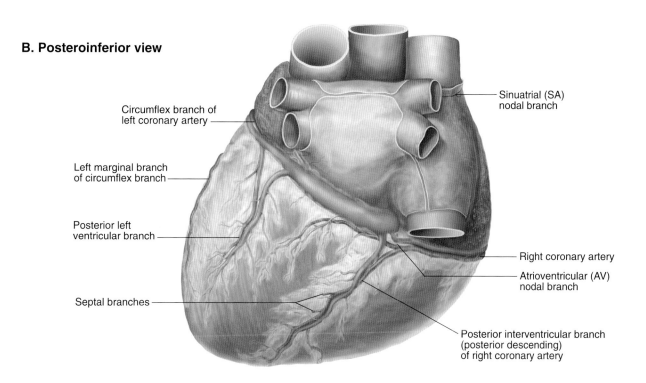

Circumflex branch of left coronary artery
Sinuatrial (SA) nodal branch
Left marginal branch of circumflex branch
Posterior left ventricular branch
Right coronary artery
Atrioventricular (AV) nodal branch
Septal branches
Posterior interventricular branch (posterior descending) of right coronary artery

PLATE 4-23   Coronary Arteries, Normal Patterns and Variations

A. Normal arterial pattern, anterior view

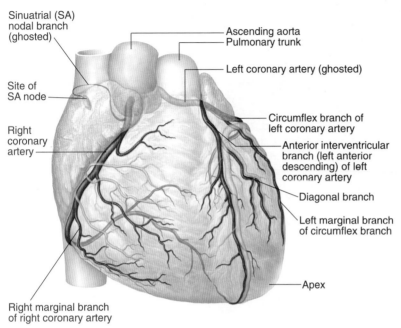

Sinuatrial (SA) nodal branch (ghosted)

Site of SA node

Right coronary artery

Right marginal branch of right coronary artery

Ascending aorta
Pulmonary trunk
Left coronary artery (ghosted)
Circumflex branch of left coronary artery
Anterior interventricular branch (left anterior descending) of left coronary artery
Diagonal branch
Left marginal branch of circumflex branch
Apex

B. Variation, anterior view

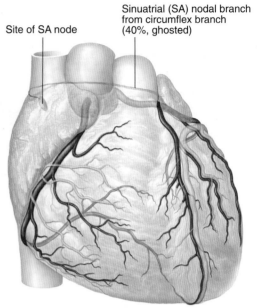

Site of SA node

Sinuatrial (SA) nodal branch from circumflex branch (40%, ghosted)

C. Normal arterial pattern, posteroinferior view

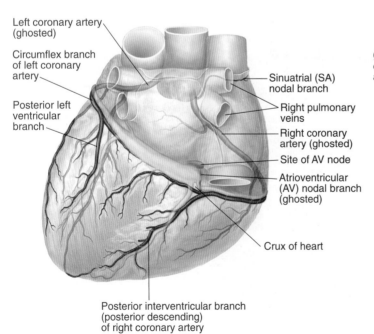

Left coronary artery (ghosted)

Circumflex branch of left coronary artery

Posterior left ventricular branch

Sinuatrial (SA) nodal branch
Right pulmonary veins
Right coronary artery (ghosted)
Site of AV node
Atrioventricular (AV) nodal branch (ghosted)
Crux of heart

Posterior interventricular branch (posterior descending) of right coronary artery

D. Variation, posteroinferior view

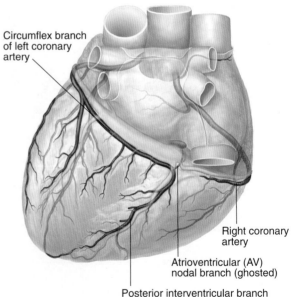

Circumflex branch of left coronary artery

Right coronary artery
Atrioventricular (AV) nodal branch (ghosted)

Posterior interventricular branch from circumflex branch (left dominance, 15%)

A. Anterior view

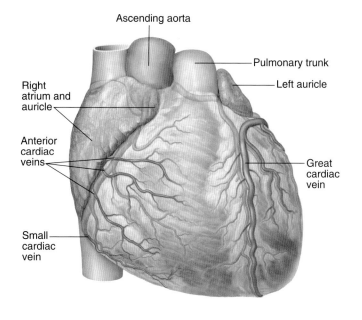

Ascending aorta

Pulmonary trunk

Left auricle

Right atrium and auricle

Anterior cardiac veins

Great cardiac vein

Small cardiac vein

B. Normal venous pattern, anterior view

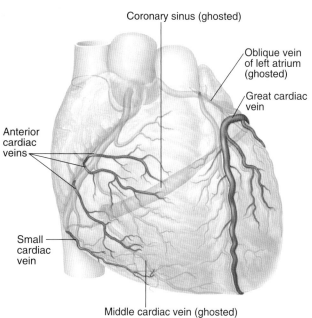

Coronary sinus (ghosted)

Oblique vein of left atrium (ghosted)

Great cardiac vein

Anterior cardiac veins

Small cardiac vein

Middle cardiac vein (ghosted)

C. Posteroinferior view

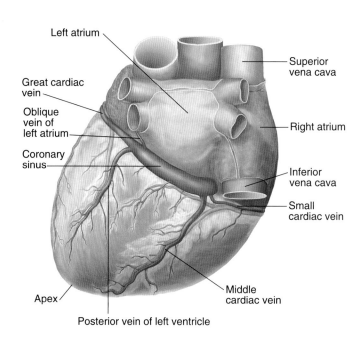

Left atrium

Superior vena cava

Great cardiac vein

Oblique vein of left atrium

Right atrium

Coronary sinus

Inferior vena cava

Small cardiac vein

Apex

Middle cardiac vein

Posterior vein of left ventricle

D. Normal venous pattern, posteroinferior view

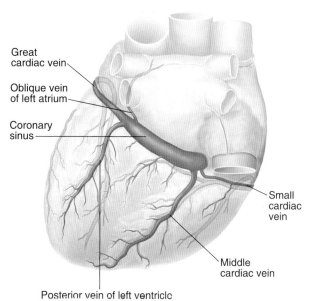

Great cardiac vein

Oblique vein of left atrium

Coronary sinus

Small cardiac vein

Middle cardiac vein

Posterior vein of left ventricle

PLATE 4-25   Heart, Internal Features, Right Chambers

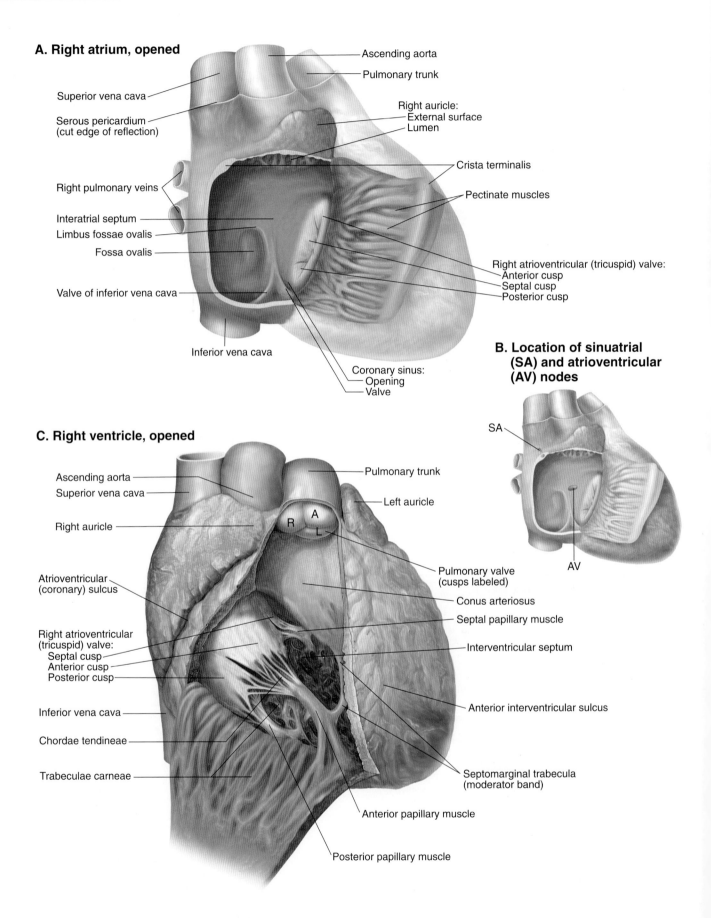

A. Right atrium, opened

Ascending aorta

Pulmonary trunk

Superior vena cava

Serous pericardium
(cut edge of reflection)

Right auricle:
External surface
Lumen

Crista terminalis

Right pulmonary veins

Pectinate muscles

Interatrial septum

Limbus fossae ovalis

Fossa ovalis

Right atrioventricular (tricuspid) valve:
Anterior cusp
Septal cusp
Posterior cusp

Valve of inferior vena cava

Inferior vena cava

Coronary sinus:
Opening
Valve

B. Location of sinuatrial (SA) and atrioventricular (AV) nodes

SA

AV

C. Right ventricle, opened

Ascending aorta

Superior vena cava

Right auricle

Pulmonary trunk

Left auricle

R A
L

Pulmonary valve
(cusps labeled)

Conus arteriosus

Septal papillary muscle

Atrioventricular
(coronary) sulcus

Interventricular septum

Right atrioventricular
(tricuspid) valve:
Septal cusp
Anterior cusp
Posterior cusp

Anterior interventricular sulcus

Inferior vena cava

Chordae tendineae

Trabeculae carneae

Septomarginal trabecula
(moderator band)

Anterior papillary muscle

Posterior papillary muscle

A. Left atrium, opened

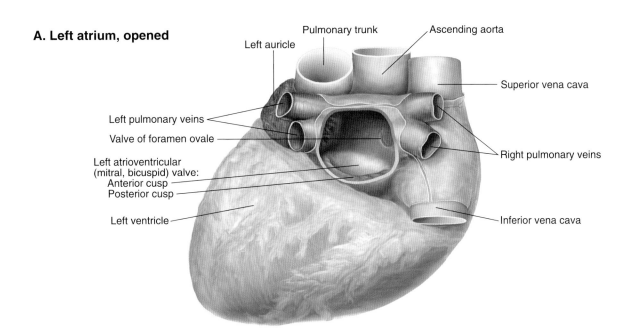

Left auricle
Pulmonary trunk
Ascending aorta
Superior vena cava
Left pulmonary veins
Valve of foramen ovale
Right pulmonary veins
Left atrioventricular
(mitral, bicuspid) valve:
Anterior cusp
Posterior cusp
Left ventricle
Inferior vena cava

B. Left ventricle, opened

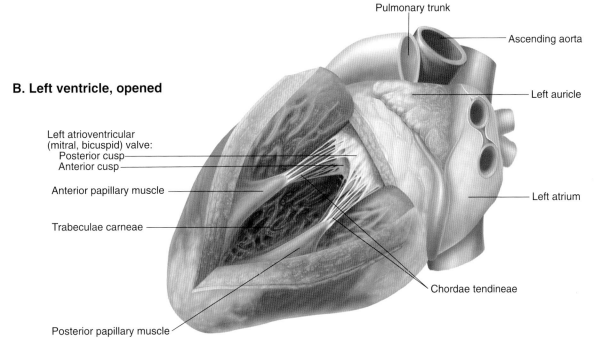

Pulmonary trunk
Ascending aorta
Left auricle
Left atrioventricular
(mitral, bicuspid) valve:
Posterior cusp
Anterior cusp
Anterior papillary muscle
Left atrium
Trabeculae carneae
Posterior papillary muscle
Chordae tendineae

C. Aortic valve seen through the mitral valve

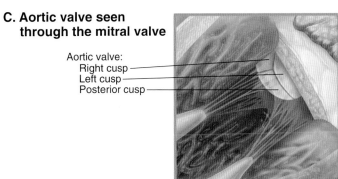

Aortic valve:
Right cusp
Left cusp
Posterior cusp

PLATE 4-27   **Sectional View of the Heart**

A. Plane of section

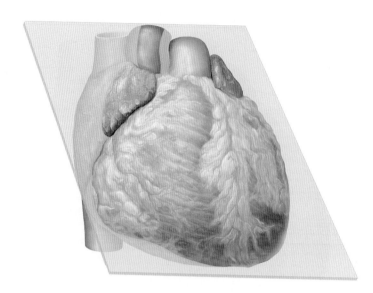

B. Section through the heart showing the posteroinferior portion

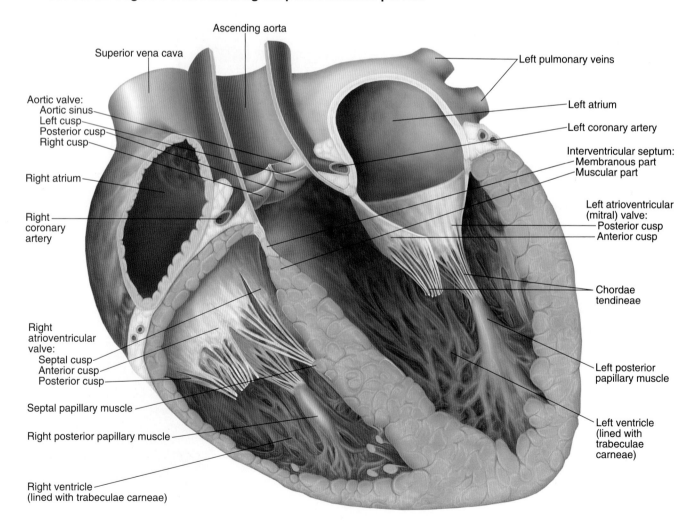

Ascending aorta

Superior vena cava

Left pulmonary veins

Aortic valve:
Aortic sinus
Left cusp
Posterior cusp
Right cusp

Left atrium

Left coronary artery

Right atrium

Interventricular septum:
Membranous part
Muscular part

Right
coronary
artery

Left atrioventricular
(mitral) valve:
Posterior cusp
Anterior cusp

Chordae
tendineae

Right
atrioventricular
valve:
Septal cusp
Anterior cusp
Posterior cusp

Left posterior
papillary muscle

Septal papillary muscle

Right posterior papillary muscle

Left ventricle
(lined with
trabeculae
carneae)

Right ventricle
(lined with trabeculae carneae)

A. Anterior view

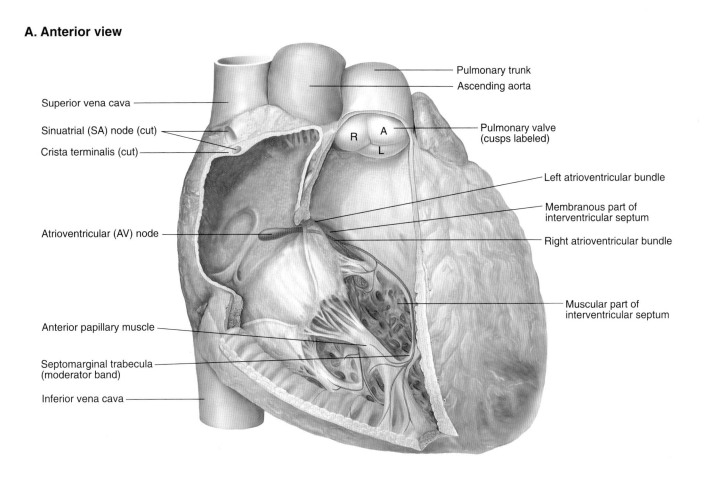

Pulmonary trunk
Ascending aorta
Superior vena cava
Sinuatrial (SA) node (cut)
Crista terminalis (cut)
Pulmonary valve
(cusps labeled)
R   A
L
Left atrioventricular bundle
Membranous part of
interventricular septum
Atrioventricular (AV) node
Right atrioventricular bundle
Muscular part of
interventricular septum
Anterior papillary muscle
Septomarginal trabecula
(moderator band)
Inferior vena cava

B. Left lateral view

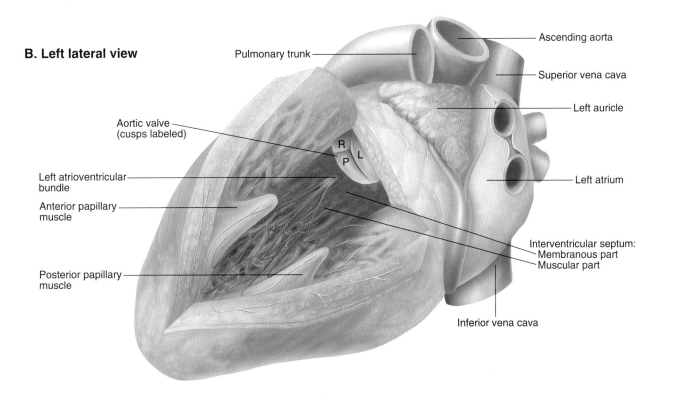

Pulmonary trunk
Ascending aorta
Superior vena cava
Left auricle
Aortic valve
(cusps labeled)
R   L
P
Left atrioventricular
bundle
Anterior papillary
muscle
Left atrium
Interventricular septum:
Membranous part
Muscular part
Posterior papillary
muscle
Inferior vena cava

PLATE 4-29   Thoracic Viscera, Lungs

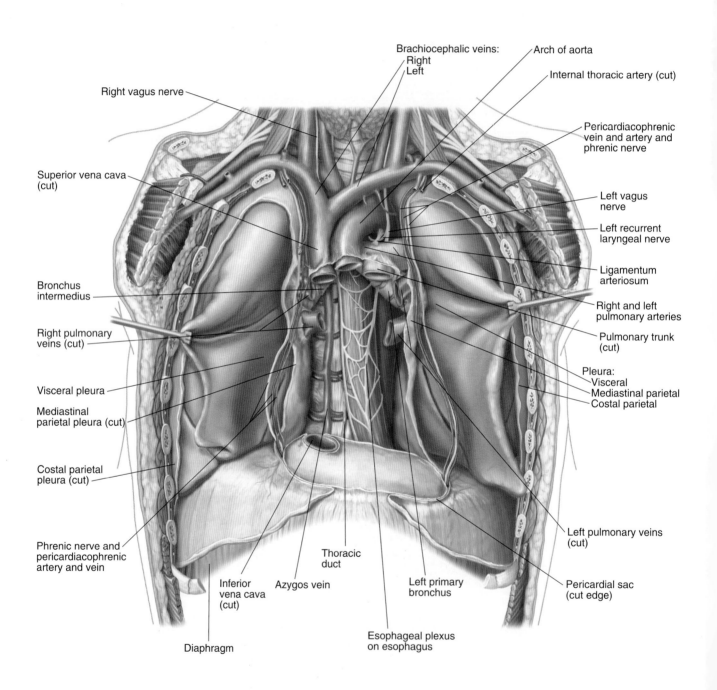

Brachiocephalic veins:
Right
Left

Arch of aorta

Internal thoracic artery (cut)

Right vagus nerve

Pericardiacophrenic
vein and artery and
phrenic nerve

Superior vena cava
(cut)

Left vagus
nerve

Left recurrent
laryngeal nerve

Ligamentum
arteriosum

Bronchus
intermedius

Right and left
pulmonary arteries

Right pulmonary
veins (cut)

Pulmonary trunk
(cut)

Pleura:
Visceral
Mediastinal parietal
Costal parietal

Visceral pleura

Mediastinal
parietal pleura (cut)

Costal parietal
pleura (cut)

Left pulmonary veins
(cut)

Phrenic nerve and
pericardiacophrenic
artery and vein

Pericardial sac
(cut edge)

Inferior
vena cava
(cut)

Azygos vein

Thoracic
duct

Left primary
bronchus

Diaphragm

Esophageal plexus
on esophagus

A. Right lung

Apex

Superior
lobe

Anterior border

Posterior
border

Horizontal
fissure

Middle
lobe

Inferior
lobe

Oblique fissure

Inferior border

B. Left lung

Apex

Superior
lobe

Posterior
border

Oblique
fissure

Inferior
lobe

Cardiac
notch

Lingula

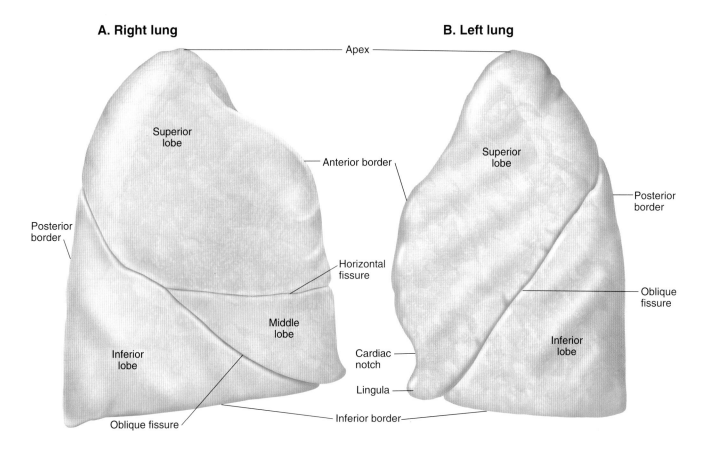

C. Radiograph, anterior view

Apex of
right lung

Trachea

Apex of
left lung

Horizontal
(minor)
fissure

Aortic
arch

Right border
of heart

Left border
of heart

Right
hemidiaphragm

Left
hemidiaphragm

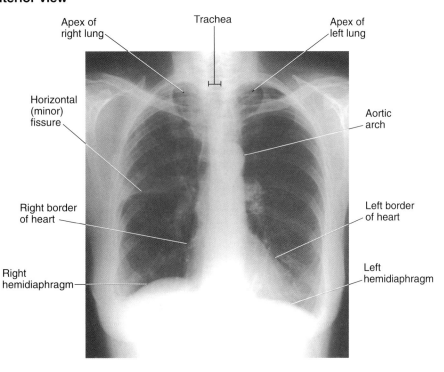

PLATE 4-31   Lungs, Medial View

A. Right lung

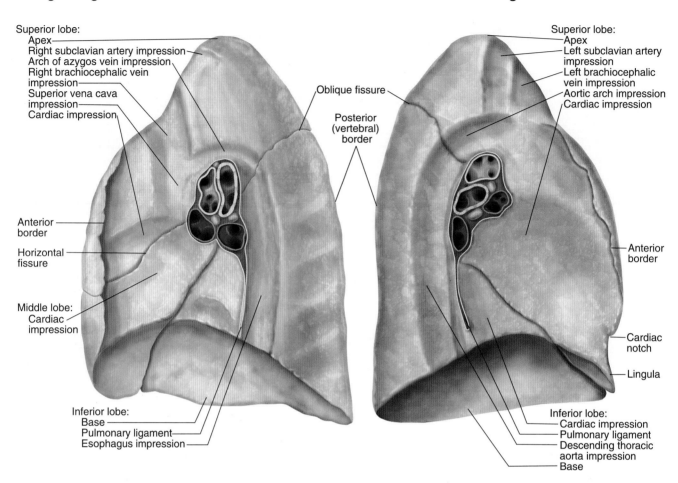

Superior lobe:
Apex
Right subclavian artery impression
Arch of azygos vein impression
Right brachiocephalic vein impression
Superior vena cava impression
Cardiac impression

Anterior border

Horizontal fissure

Middle lobe:
Cardiac impression

Inferior lobe:
Base
Pulmonary ligament
Esophagus impression

B. Left lung

Oblique fissure

Posterior (vertebral) border

Superior lobe:
Apex
Left subclavian artery impression
Left brachiocephalic vein impression
Aortic arch impression
Cardiac impression

Anterior border

Cardiac notch

Lingula

Inferior lobe:
Cardiac impression
Pulmonary ligament
Descending thoracic aorta impression
Base

C. Structures in right hilum

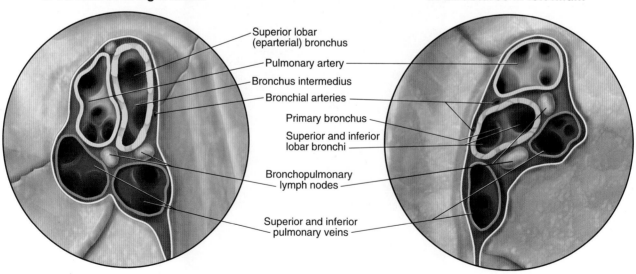

D. Structures in left hilum

Superior lobar (eparterial) bronchus

Pulmonary artery

Bronchus intermedius

Bronchial arteries

Primary bronchus

Superior and inferior lobar bronchi

Bronchopulmonary lymph nodes

Superior and inferior pulmonary veins

A. Right lung, medial view

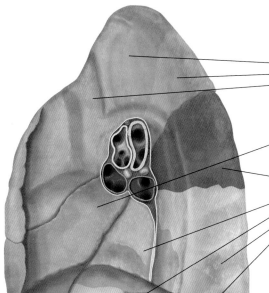

B. Left lung, medial view

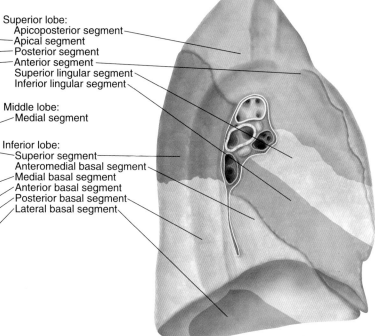

Superior lobe:
Apicoposterior segment
Apical segment
Posterior segment
Anterior segment
Superior lingular segment
Inferior lingular segment

Middle lobe:
Medial segment

Inferior lobe:
Superior segment
Anteromedial basal segment
Medial basal segment
Anterior basal segment
Posterior basal segment
Lateral basal segment

C. Right lung, lateral view

D. Left lung, lateral view

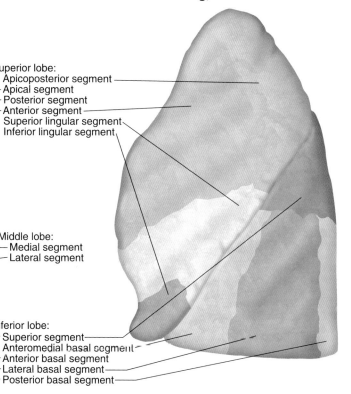

Superior lobe:
Apicoposterior segment
Apical segment
Posterior segment
Anterior segment
Superior lingular segment
Inferior lingular segment

Middle lobe:
Medial segment
Lateral segment

Inferior lobe:
Superior segment
Anteromedial basal segment
Anterior basal segment
Lateral basal segment
Posterior basal segment

PLATE 4-33   **Trachea and Bronchial Tree**

A. Anterior view

B. Cross section

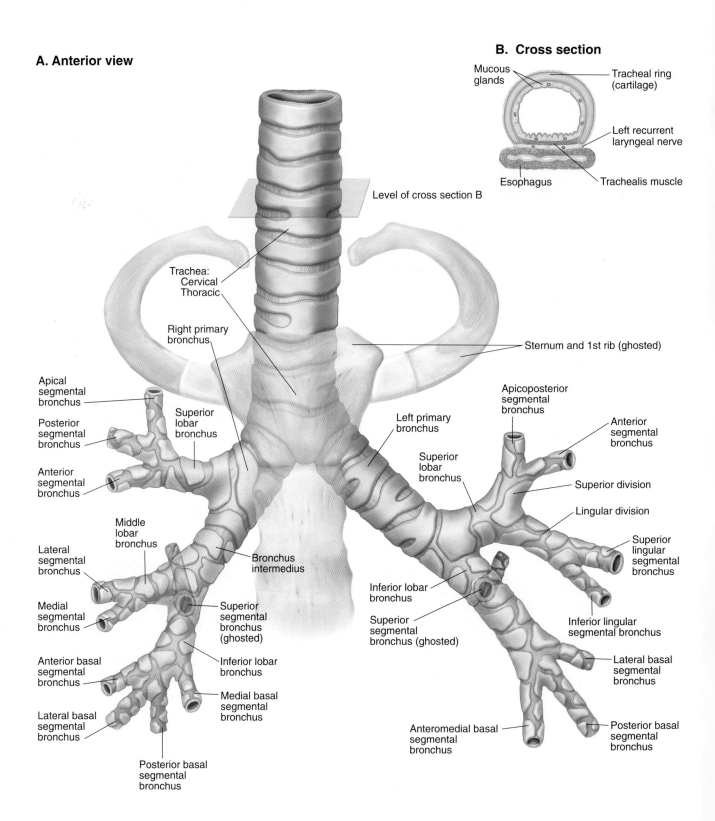

Mucous glands

Tracheal ring (cartilage)

Left recurrent laryngeal nerve

Esophagus

Trachealis muscle

Level of cross section B

Trachea:
Cervical
Thoracic

Right primary bronchus

Sternum and 1st rib (ghosted)

Apical segmental bronchus

Apicoposterior segmental bronchus

Anterior segmental bronchus

Posterior segmental bronchus

Superior lobar bronchus

Left primary bronchus

Superior division

Anterior segmental bronchus

Superior lobar bronchus

Lingular division

Middle lobar bronchus

Superior lingular segmental bronchus

Lateral segmental bronchus

Bronchus intermedius

Inferior lobar bronchus

Medial segmental bronchus

Superior segmental bronchus (ghosted)

Superior segmental bronchus (ghosted)

Inferior lingular segmental bronchus

Anterior basal segmental bronchus

Inferior lobar bronchus

Lateral basal segmental bronchus

Lateral basal segmental bronchus

Medial basal segmental bronchus

Anteromedial basal segmental bronchus

Posterior basal segmental bronchus

Posterior basal segmental bronchus

A. Pulmonary vessels

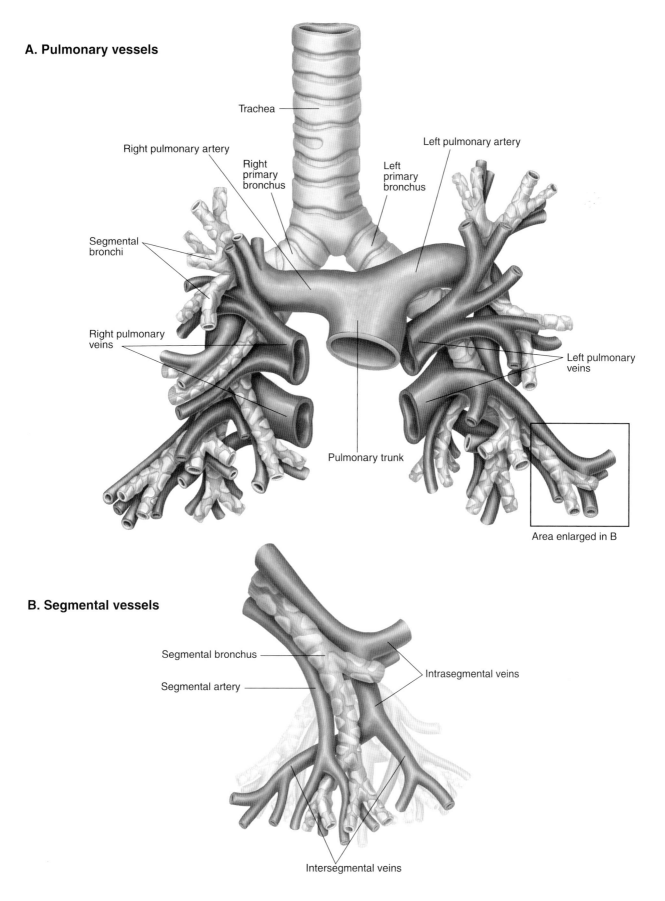

Trachea

Right pulmonary artery

Right primary bronchus

Left pulmonary artery

Left primary bronchus

Segmental bronchi

Right pulmonary veins

Left pulmonary veins

Pulmonary trunk

Area enlarged in B

B. Segmental vessels

Segmental bronchus

Segmental artery

Intrasegmental veins

Intersegmental veins

PLATE 4-35   Mediastinum, Right Lateral View

A. Parts of the mediastinum

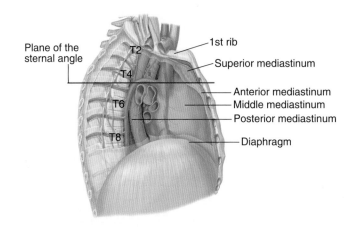

Plane of the sternal angle

T2
T4
T6
T8

1st rib
Superior mediastinum
Anterior mediastinum
Middle mediastinum
Posterior mediastinum
Diaphragm

B. Dissection

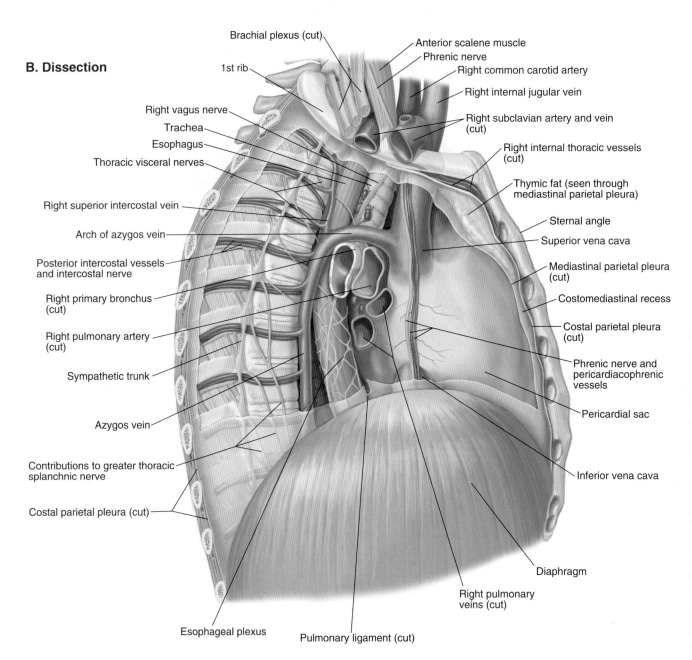

Brachial plexus (cut)
1st rib
Right vagus nerve
Trachea
Esophagus
Thoracic visceral nerves
Right superior intercostal vein
Arch of azygos vein
Posterior intercostal vessels and intercostal nerve
Right primary bronchus (cut)
Right pulmonary artery (cut)
Sympathetic trunk
Azygos vein
Contributions to greater thoracic splanchnic nerve
Costal parietal pleura (cut)
Esophageal plexus
Pulmonary ligament (cut)

Anterior scalene muscle
Phrenic nerve
Right common carotid artery
Right internal jugular vein
Right subclavian artery and vein (cut)
Right internal thoracic vessels (cut)
Thymic fat (seen through mediastinal parietal pleura)
Sternal angle
Superior vena cava
Mediastinal parietal pleura (cut)
Costomediastinal recess
Costal parietal pleura (cut)
Phrenic nerve and pericardiacophrenic vessels
Pericardial sac
Inferior vena cava
Diaphragm
Right pulmonary veins (cut)

A. Parts of the mediastinum

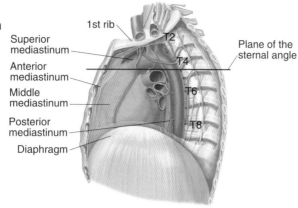

1st rib
Superior mediastinum
Anterior mediastinum
Middle mediastinum
Posterior mediastinum
Diaphragm
T2
T4
T6
T8
Plane of the sternal angle

B. Dissection

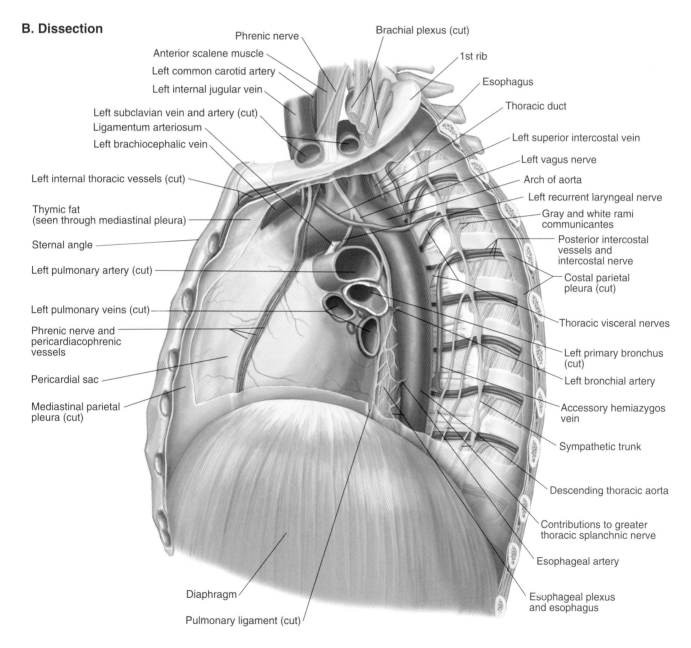

Phrenic nerve
Anterior scalene muscle
Left common carotid artery
Left internal jugular vein
Left subclavian vein and artery (cut)
Ligamentum arteriosum
Left brachiocephalic vein
Left internal thoracic vessels (cut)
Thymic fat (seen through mediastinal pleura)
Sternal angle
Left pulmonary artery (cut)
Left pulmonary veins (cut)
Phrenic nerve and pericardiacophrenic vessels
Pericardial sac
Mediastinal parietal pleura (cut)
Diaphragm
Pulmonary ligament (cut)

Brachial plexus (cut)
1st rib
Esophagus
Thoracic duct
Left superior intercostal vein
Left vagus nerve
Arch of aorta
Left recurrent laryngeal nerve
Gray and white rami communicantes
Posterior intercostal vessels and intercostal nerve
Costal parietal pleura (cut)
Thoracic visceral nerves
Left primary bronchus (cut)
Left bronchial artery
Accessory hemiazygos vein
Sympathetic trunk
Descending thoracic aorta
Contributions to greater thoracic splanchnic nerve
Esophageal artery
Esophageal plexus and esophagus

PLATE 4-37   Mediastinum, Anterior View

A. Parts of the mediastinum

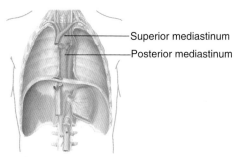

Superior mediastinum
Posterior mediastinum

B. Dissection

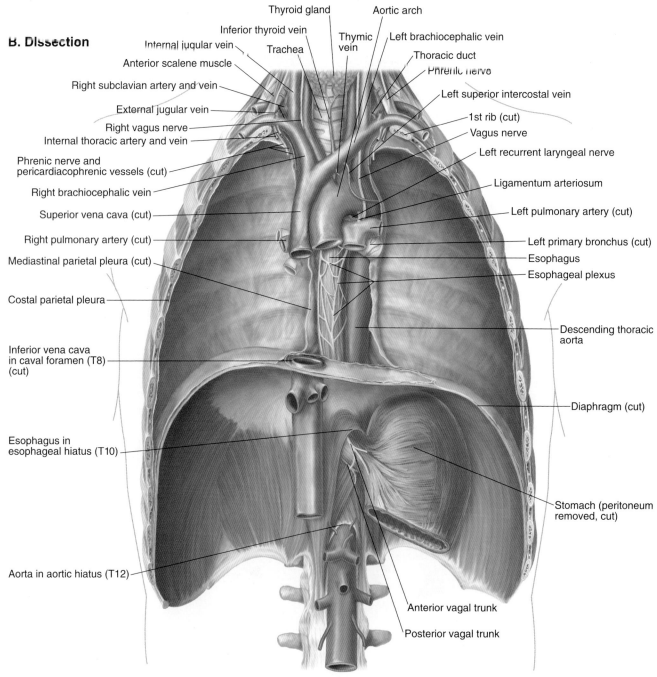

Thyroid gland
Aortic arch
Inferior thyroid vein
Thymic vein
Left brachiocephalic vein
Internal jugular vein
Trachea
Thoracic duct
Anterior scalene muscle
Phrenic nerve
Right subclavian artery and vein
Left superior intercostal vein
External jugular vein
1st rib (cut)
Right vagus nerve
Vagus nerve
Internal thoracic artery and vein
Left recurrent laryngeal nerve
Phrenic nerve and pericardiacophrenic vessels (cut)
Ligamentum arteriosum
Right brachiocephalic vein
Left pulmonary artery (cut)
Superior vena cava (cut)
Left primary bronchus (cut)
Right pulmonary artery (cut)
Esophagus
Mediastinal parietal pleura (cut)
Esophageal plexus
Costal parietal pleura
Descending thoracic aorta
Inferior vena cava in caval foramen (T8) (cut)
Diaphragm (cut)
Esophagus in esophageal hiatus (T10)
Stomach (peritoneum removed, cut)
Aorta in aortic hiatus (T12)
Anterior vagal trunk
Posterior vagal trunk

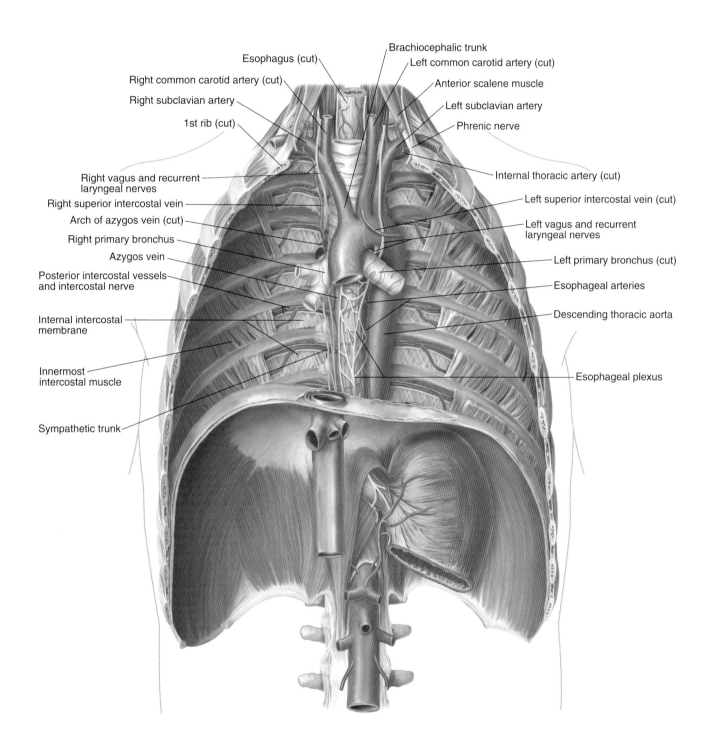

Esophagus (cut)

Brachiocephalic trunk

Left common carotid artery (cut)

Right common carotid artery (cut)

Anterior scalene muscle

Right subclavian artery

Left subclavian artery

1st rib (cut)

Phrenic nerve

Right vagus and recurrent laryngeal nerves

Internal thoracic artery (cut)

Right superior intercostal vein

Left superior intercostal vein (cut)

Arch of azygos vein (cut)

Left vagus and recurrent laryngeal nerves

Right primary bronchus

Azygos vein

Left primary bronchus (cut)

Posterior intercostal vessels and intercostal nerve

Esophageal arteries

Internal intercostal membrane

Descending thoracic aorta

Innermost intercostal muscle

Esophageal plexus

Sympathetic trunk

PLATE 4-39 | **Arteries of the Posterior Thoracic Wall**

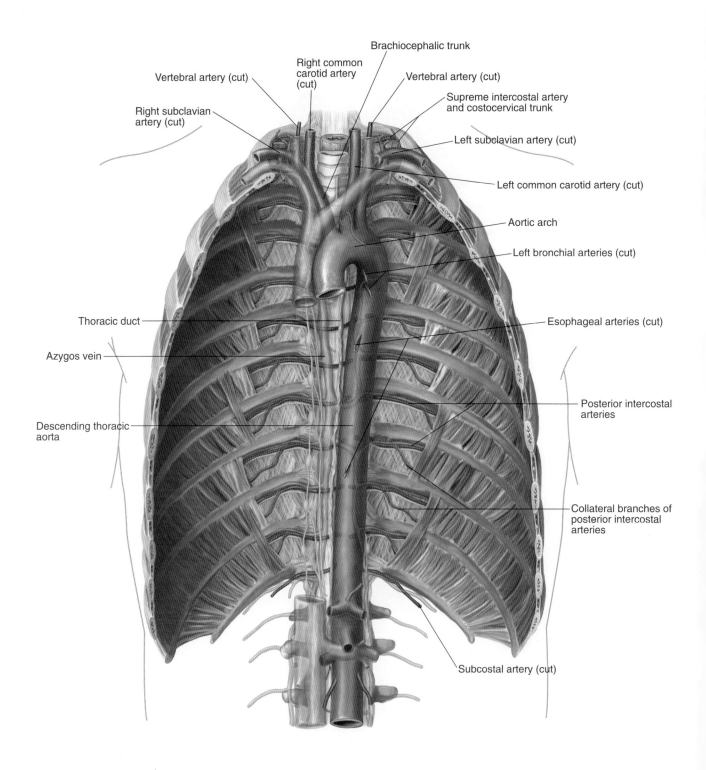

Brachiocephalic trunk

Right common carotid artery (cut)

Vertebral artery (cut)

Vertebral artery (cut)

Right subclavian artery (cut)

Supreme intercostal artery and costocervical trunk

Left subclavian artery (cut)

Left common carotid artery (cut)

Aortic arch

Left bronchial arteries (cut)

Thoracic duct

Esophageal arteries (cut)

Azygos vein

Posterior intercostal arteries

Descending thoracic aorta

Collateral branches of posterior intercostal arteries

Subcostal artery (cut)

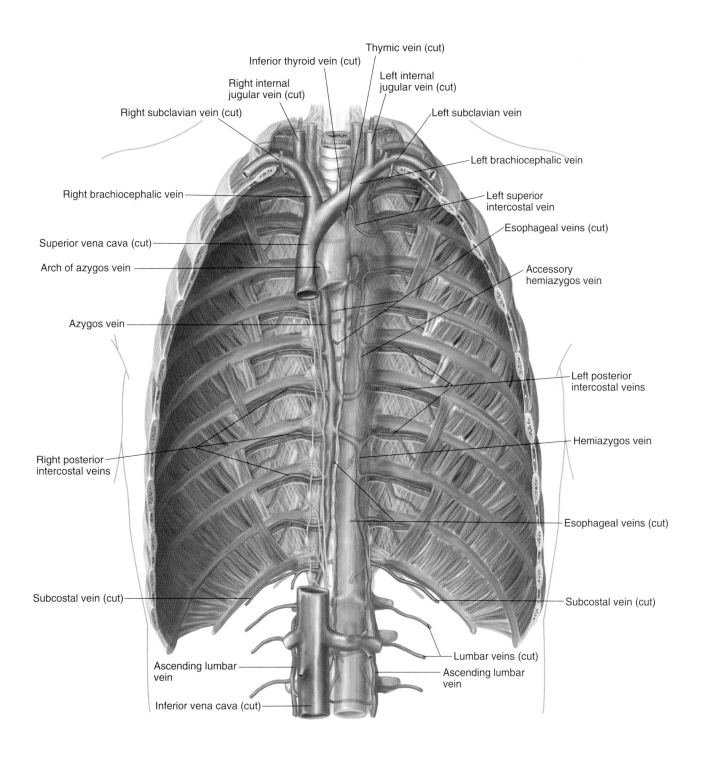

Thymic vein (cut)

Inferior thyroid vein (cut)

Right internal
jugular vein (cut)

Left internal
jugular vein (cut)

Right subclavian vein (cut)

Left subclavian vein

Left brachiocephalic vein

Right brachiocephalic vein

Left superior
intercostal vein

Superior vena cava (cut)

Esophageal veins (cut)

Arch of azygos vein

Accessory
hemiazygos vein

Azygos vein

Left posterior
intercostal veins

Hemiazygos vein

Right posterior
intercostal veins

Esophageal veins (cut)

Subcostal vein (cut)

Subcostal vein (cut)

Lumbar veins (cut)

Ascending lumbar
vein

Ascending lumbar
vein

Inferior vena cava (cut)

PLATE 4-41   **Muscles and Ligaments of the Posterior Thoracic Wall**

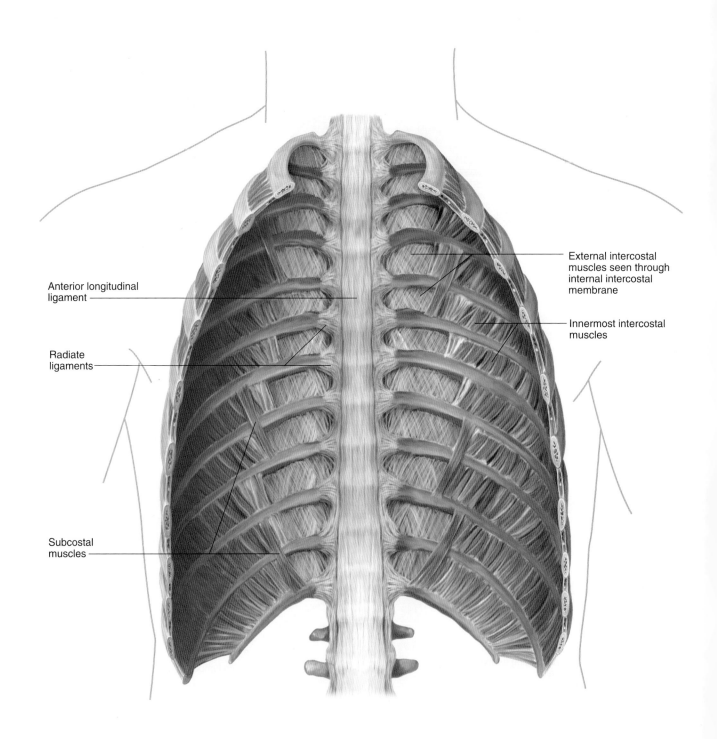

Anterior longitudinal
ligament

Radiate
ligaments

Subcostal
muscles

External intercostal
muscles seen through
internal intercostal
membrane

Innermost intercostal
muscles

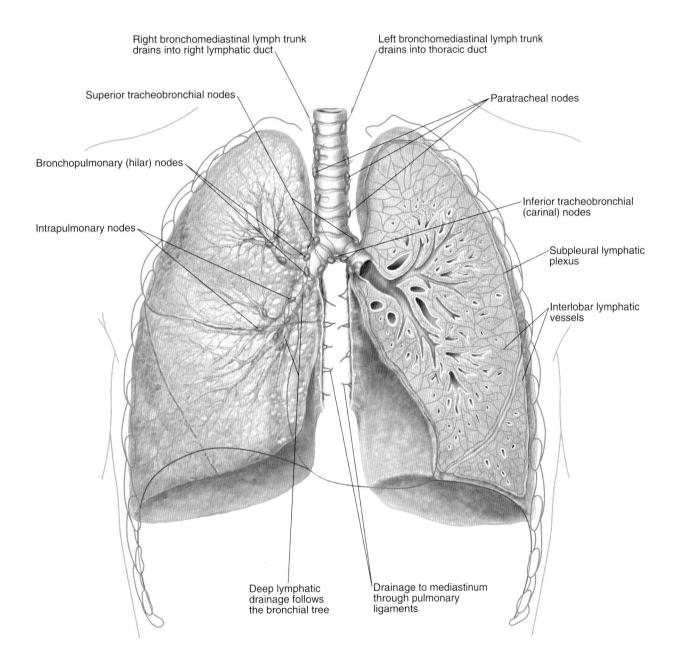

Right bronchomediastinal lymph trunk drains into right lymphatic duct

Left bronchomediastinal lymph trunk drains into thoracic duct

Superior tracheobronchial nodes

Paratracheal nodes

Bronchopulmonary (hilar) nodes

Inferior tracheobronchial (carinal) nodes

Intrapulmonary nodes

Subpleural lymphatic plexus

Interlobar lymphatic vessels

Deep lymphatic drainage follows the bronchial tree

Drainage to mediastinum through pulmonary ligaments

PLATE 4-43   **Lymphatics of the Anterior Thoracic Wall**

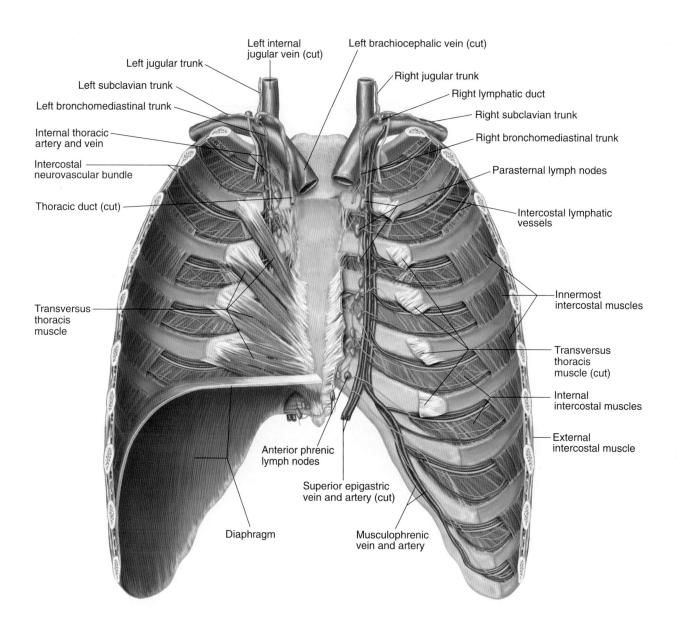

Left internal
jugular vein (cut)

Left brachiocephalic vein (cut)

Left jugular trunk

Right jugular trunk

Left subclavian trunk

Right lymphatic duct

Left bronchomediastinal trunk

Right subclavian trunk

Internal thoracic
artery and vein

Right bronchomediastinal trunk

Intercostal
neurovascular bundle

Parasternal lymph nodes

Thoracic duct (cut)

Intercostal lymphatic
vessels

Innermost
intercostal muscles

Transversus
thoracis
muscle

Transversus
thoracis
muscle (cut)

Internal
intercostal muscles

External
intercostal muscle

Anterior phrenic
lymph nodes

Superior epigastric
vein and artery (cut)

Diaphragm

Musculophrenic
vein and artery

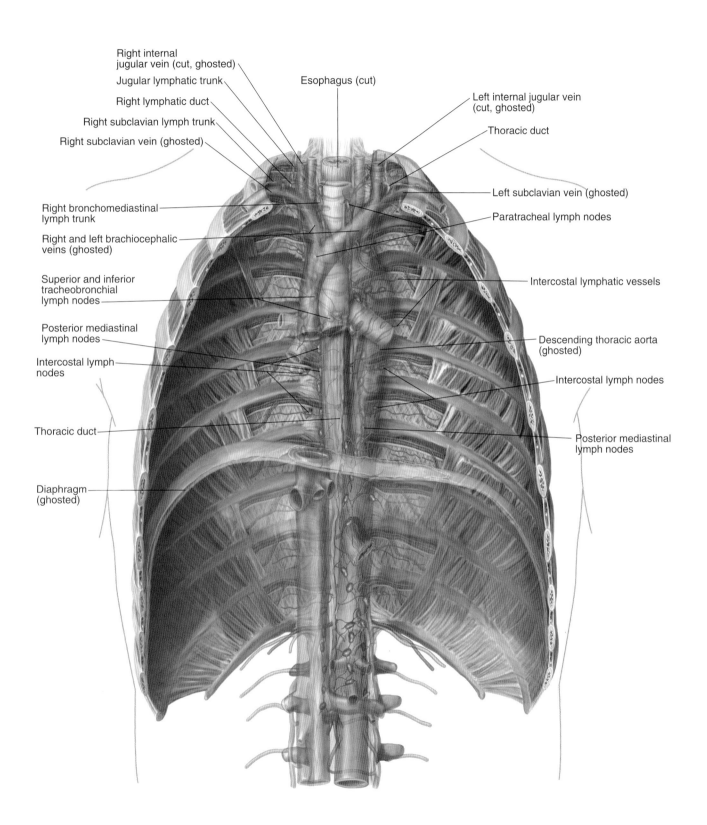

Right internal
jugular vein (cut, ghosted)

Jugular lymphatic trunk

Right lymphatic duct

Right subclavian lymph trunk

Right subclavian vein (ghosted)

Esophagus (cut)

Left internal jugular vein
(cut, ghosted)

Thoracic duct

Right bronchomediastinal
lymph trunk

Right and left brachiocephalic
veins (ghosted)

Superior and inferior
tracheobronchial
lymph nodes

Posterior mediastinal
lymph nodes

Intercostal lymph
nodes

Thoracic duct

Diaphragm
(ghosted)

Left subclavian vein (ghosted)

Paratracheal lymph nodes

Intercostal lymphatic vessels

Descending thoracic aorta
(ghosted)

Intercostal lymph nodes

Posterior mediastinal
lymph nodes

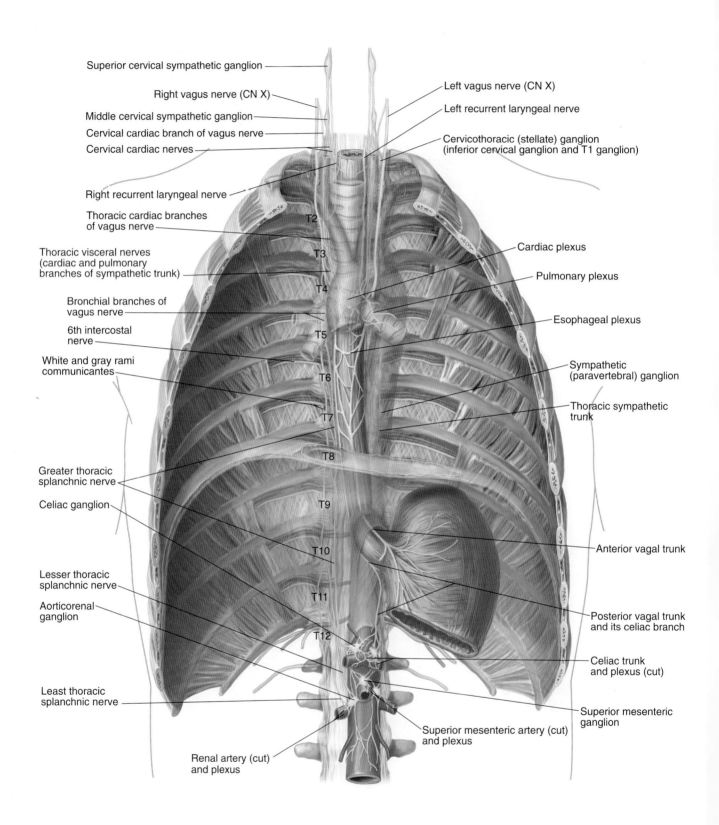

Superior cervical sympathetic ganglion

Right vagus nerve (CN X)

Middle cervical sympathetic ganglion

Cervical cardiac branch of vagus nerve

Cervical cardiac nerves

Right recurrent laryngeal nerve

Thoracic cardiac branches of vagus nerve

Thoracic visceral nerves (cardiac and pulmonary branches of sympathetic trunk)

Bronchial branches of vagus nerve

6th intercostal nerve

White and gray rami communicantes

Greater thoracic splanchnic nerve

Celiac ganglion

Lesser thoracic splanchnic nerve

Aorticorenal ganglion

Least thoracic splanchnic nerve

Renal artery (cut) and plexus

Left vagus nerve (CN X)

Left recurrent laryngeal nerve

Cervicothoracic (stellate) ganglion (inferior cervical ganglion and T1 ganglion)

Cardiac plexus

Pulmonary plexus

Esophageal plexus

Sympathetic (paravertebral) ganglion

Thoracic sympathetic trunk

Anterior vagal trunk

Posterior vagal trunk and its celiac branch

Celiac trunk and plexus (cut)

Superior mesenteric ganglion

Superior mesenteric artery (cut) and plexus

T2

T3

T4

T5

T6

T7

T8

T9

T10

T11

T12

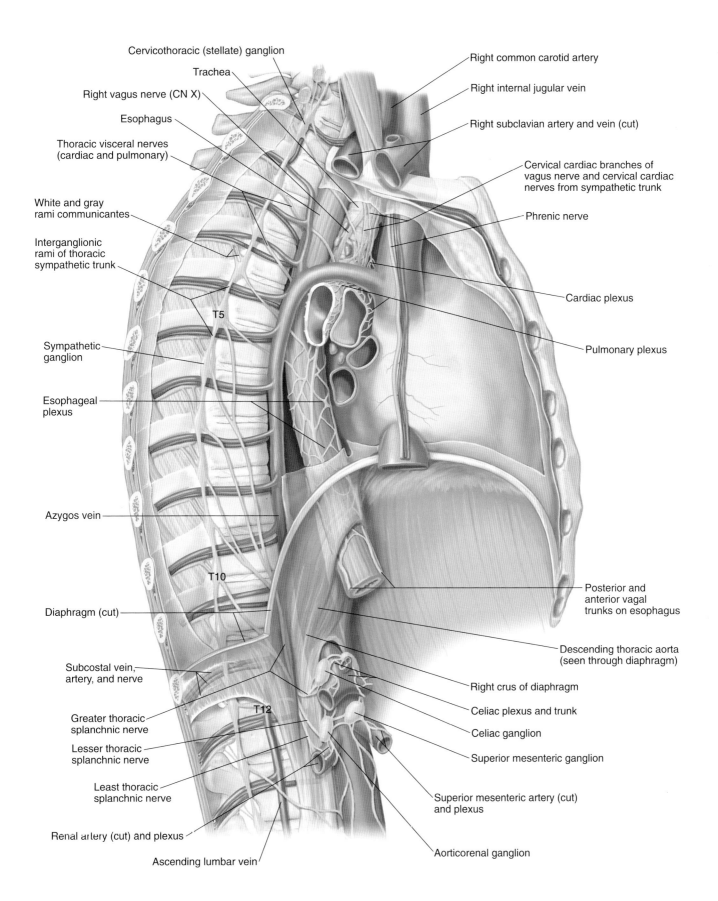

Cervicothoracic (stellate) ganglion

Trachea

Right vagus nerve (CN X)

Esophagus

Thoracic visceral nerves (cardiac and pulmonary)

White and gray rami communicantes

Interganglionic rami of thoracic sympathetic trunk

T5

Sympathetic ganglion

Esophageal plexus

Azygos vein

T10

Diaphragm (cut)

Subcostal vein, artery, and nerve

Greater thoracic splanchnic nerve

T12

Lesser thoracic splanchnic nerve

Least thoracic splanchnic nerve

Renal artery (cut) and plexus

Ascending lumbar vein

Right common carotid artery

Right internal jugular vein

Right subclavian artery and vein (cut)

Cervical cardiac branches of vagus nerve and cervical cardiac nerves from sympathetic trunk

Phrenic nerve

Cardiac plexus

Pulmonary plexus

Posterior and anterior vagal trunks on esophagus

Descending thoracic aorta (seen through diaphragm)

Right crus of diaphragm

Celiac plexus and trunk

Celiac ganglion

Superior mesenteric ganglion

Superior mesenteric artery (cut) and plexus

Aorticorenal ganglion

PLATE 4-47   **Cross Section of the Thorax at the T2 Vertebral Level**

A. Orientation

B. Cross section

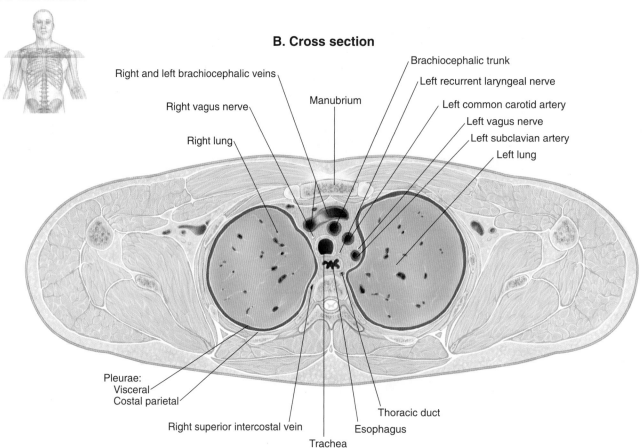

Right and left brachiocephalic veins

Brachiocephalic trunk

Left recurrent laryngeal nerve

Right vagus nerve

Manubrium

Left common carotid artery

Left vagus nerve

Right lung

Left subclavian artery

Left lung

Pleurae:
Visceral
Costal parietal

Right superior intercostal vein

Thoracic duct

Esophagus

Trachea

C. CT view

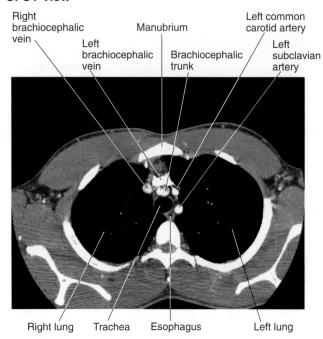

Right brachiocephalic vein

Left brachiocephalic vein

Manubrium

Brachiocephalic trunk

Left common carotid artery

Left subclavian artery

Right lung   Trachea   Esophagus   Left lung

D. CT view with lung window

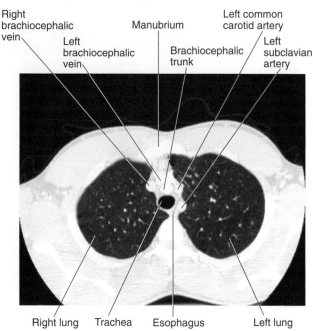

Right brachiocephalic vein

Left brachiocephalic vein

Manubrium

Brachiocephalic trunk

Left common carotid artery

Left subclavian artery

Right lung   Trachea   Esophagus   Left lung

A. Orientation

B. Cross section

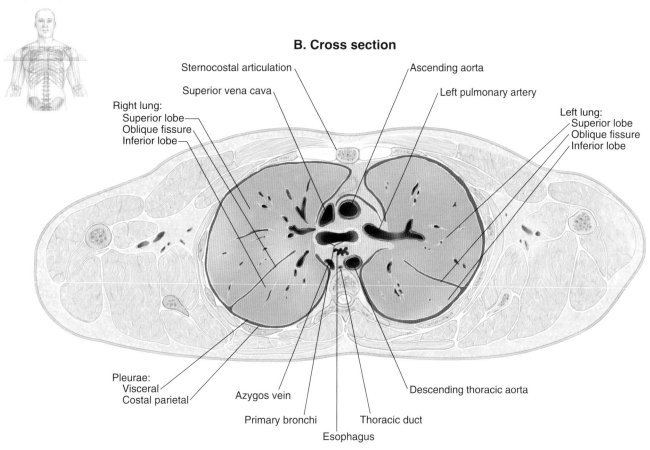

Sternocostal articulation

Ascending aorta

Superior vena cava

Left pulmonary artery

Right lung:
Superior lobe
Oblique fissure
Inferior lobe

Left lung:
Superior lobe
Oblique fissure
Inferior lobe

Pleurae:
Visceral
Costal parietal

Azygos vein

Descending thoracic aorta

Primary bronchi

Thoracic duct

Esophagus

C. CT view

D. CT view with lung window

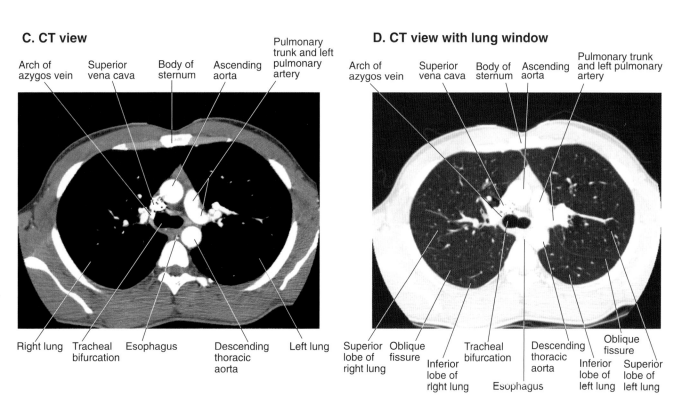

Arch of
azygos vein

Superior
vena cava

Body of
sternum

Ascending
aorta

Pulmonary
trunk and left
pulmonary
artery

Right lung   Tracheal
bifurcation

Esophagus

Descending
thoracic
aorta

Left lung

Arch of
azygos vein

Superior
vena cava

Body of
sternum

Ascending
aorta

Pulmonary trunk
and left pulmonary
artery

Superior
lobe of
right lung

Oblique
fissure

Inferior
lobe of
right lung

Tracheal
bifurcation

Descending
thoracic
aorta

Oblique
fissure

Inferior
lobe of
left lung

Superior
lobe of
left lung

Esophagus

PLATE 4-49   **Cross Section of the Thorax at the T7 Vertebral Level**

A. Orientation

B. Cross section

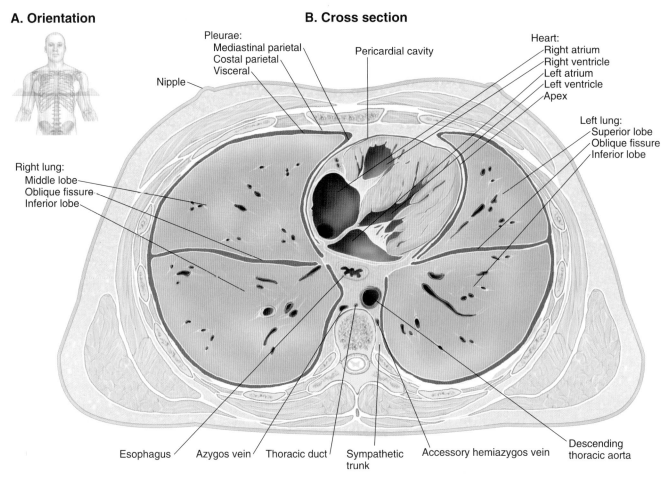

Pleurae:
Mediastinal parietal
Costal parietal
Visceral

Nipple

Pericardial cavity

Heart:
Right atrium
Right ventricle
Left atrium
Left ventricle
Apex

Left lung:
Superior lobe
Oblique fissure
Inferior lobe

Right lung:
Middle lobe
Oblique fissure
Inferior lobe

Esophagus   Azygos vein   Thoracic duct   Sympathetic trunk   Accessory hemiazygos vein   Descending thoracic aorta

C. CT view

Right atrium
Right atrioventricular valve
Right ventricle
Xiphoid process
Interventricular septum
Left ventricle

Right lung   Left atrium   Esophagus   Descending thoracic aorta   Left atrioventricular valve   Left lung

D. CT view with lung window

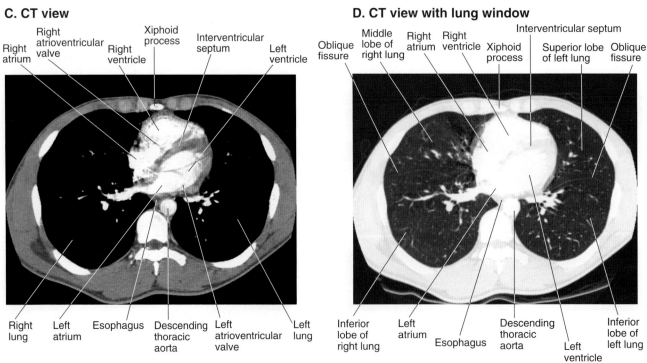

Oblique fissure
Middle lobe of right lung
Right atrium
Right ventricle
Xiphoid process
Interventricular septum
Superior lobe of left lung
Oblique fissure

Inferior lobe of right lung   Left atrium   Esophagus   Descending thoracic aorta   Left ventricle   Inferior lobe of left lung

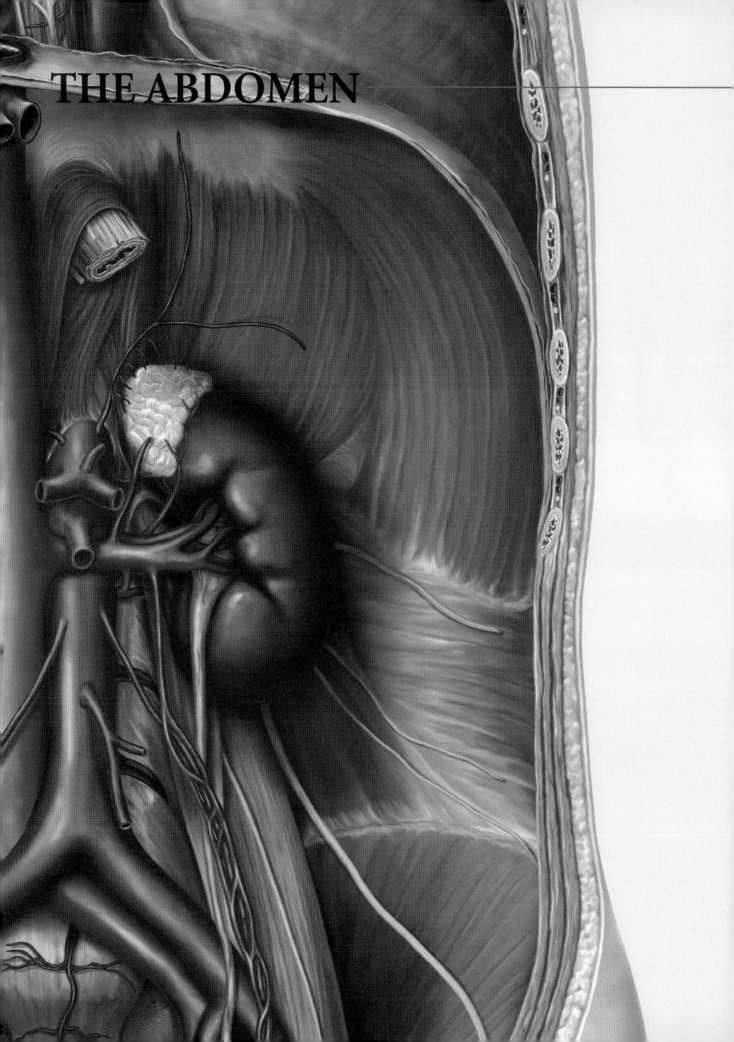

THE ABDOMEN

A. Palpable structures

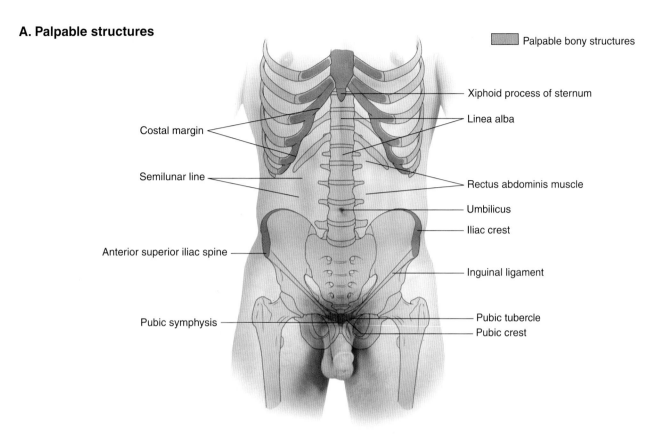

Palpable bony structures

Xiphoid process of sternum

Linea alba

Costal margin

Semilunar line

Rectus abdominis muscle

Umbilicus

Iliac crest

Anterior superior iliac spine

Inguinal ligament

Pubic symphysis

Pubic tubercle

Pubic crest

B. Abdominal quadrants

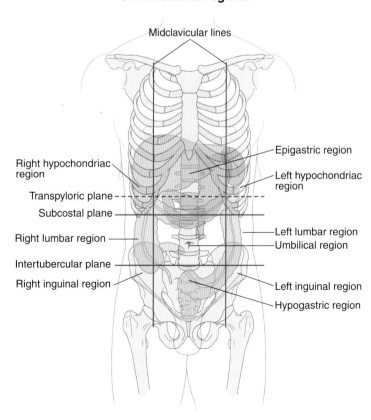

Median plane

Right upper quadrant

Umbilicus

Transumbilical plane

Right lower quadrant

Left upper quadrant

Left lower quadrant

C. Abdominal regions

Midclavicular lines

Right hypochondriac region

Epigastric region

Left hypochondriac region

Transpyloric plane

Subcostal plane

Right lumbar region

Left lumbar region

Umbilical region

Intertubercular plane

Right inguinal region

Left inguinal region

Hypogastric region

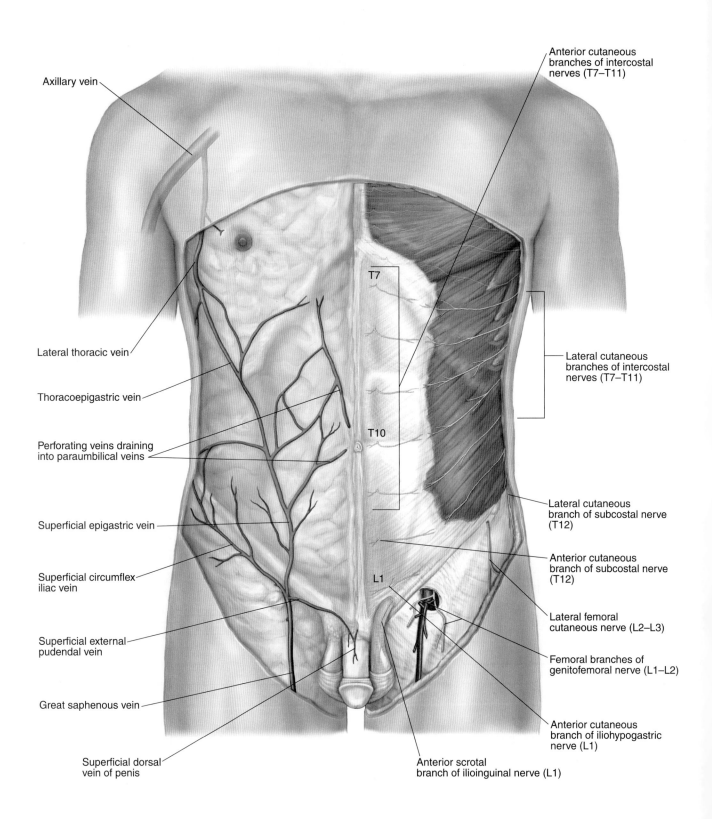

Axillary vein

Anterior cutaneous
branches of intercostal
nerves (T7–T11)

Lateral thoracic vein

T7

Lateral cutaneous
branches of intercostal
nerves (T7–T11)

Thoracoepigastric vein

T10

Perforating veins draining
into paraumbilical veins

Superficial epigastric vein

Lateral cutaneous
branch of subcostal nerve
(T12)

Anterior cutaneous
branch of subcostal nerve
(T12)

L1

Superficial circumflex
iliac vein

Lateral femoral
cutaneous nerve (L2–L3)

Superficial external
pudendal vein

Femoral branches of
genitofemoral nerve (L1–L2)

Great saphenous vein

Anterior cutaneous
branch of iliohypogastric
nerve (L1)

Superficial dorsal
vein of penis

Anterior scrotal
branch of ilioinguinal nerve (L1)

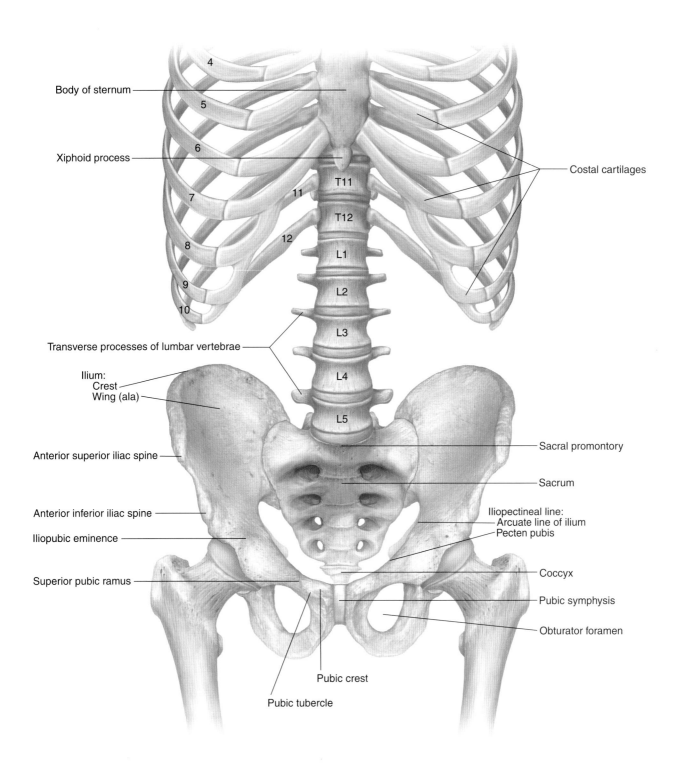

Body of sternum

Xiphoid process

4

5

6

Costal cartilages

T11

11

T12

7

12

8

L1

9

L2

10

L3

Transverse processes of lumbar vertebrae

L4

Ilium:
Crest
Wing (ala)

L5

Anterior superior iliac spine

Sacral promontory

Sacrum

Anterior inferior iliac spine

Iliopectineal line:
Arcuate line of ilium
Pecten pubis

Iliopubic eminence

Coccyx

Superior pubic ramus

Pubic symphysis

Obturator foramen

Pubic crest

Pubic tubercle

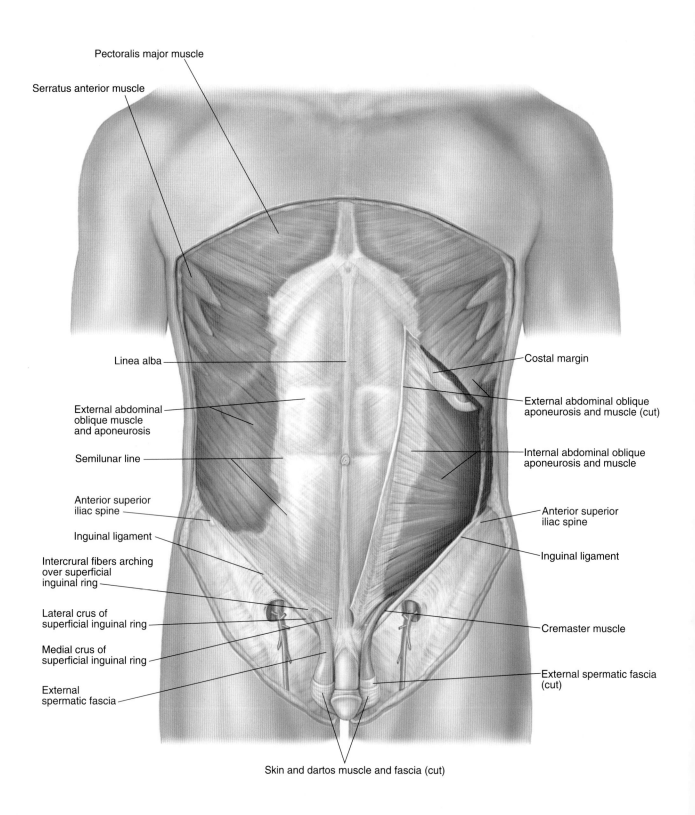

Pectoralis major muscle

Serratus anterior muscle

Linea alba

External abdominal oblique muscle and aponeurosis

Semilunar line

Anterior superior iliac spine

Inguinal ligament

Intercrural fibers arching over superficial inguinal ring

Lateral crus of superficial inguinal ring

Medial crus of superficial inguinal ring

External spermatic fascia

Costal margin

External abdominal oblique aponeurosis and muscle (cut)

Internal abdominal oblique aponeurosis and muscle

Anterior superior iliac spine

Inguinal ligament

Cremaster muscle

External spermatic fascia (cut)

Skin and dartos muscle and fascia (cut)

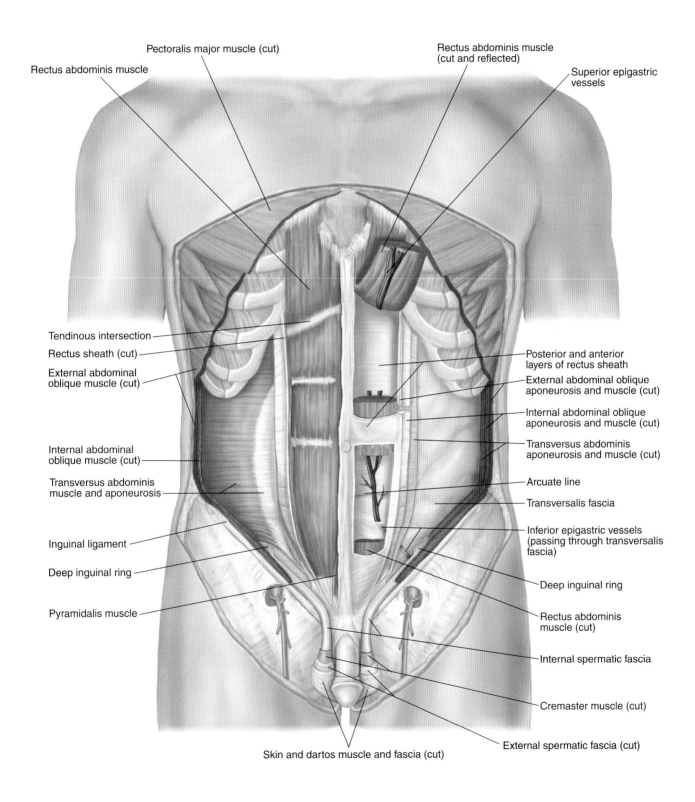

Pectoralis major muscle (cut)

Rectus abdominis muscle

Rectus abdominis muscle (cut and reflected)

Superior epigastric vessels

Tendinous intersection

Rectus sheath (cut)

External abdominal oblique muscle (cut)

Internal abdominal oblique muscle (cut)

Transversus abdominis muscle and aponeurosis

Inguinal ligament

Deep inguinal ring

Pyramidalis muscle

Posterior and anterior layers of rectus sheath

External abdominal oblique aponeurosis and muscle (cut)

Internal abdominal oblique aponeurosis and muscle (cut)

Transversus abdominis aponeurosis and muscle (cut)

Arcuate line

Transversalis fascia

Inferior epigastric vessels (passing through transversalis fascia)

Deep inguinal ring

Rectus abdominis muscle (cut)

Internal spermatic fascia

Cremaster muscle (cut)

External spermatic fascia (cut)

Skin and dartos muscle and fascia (cut)

PLATE 5-06   Rectus Sheath

A. Orientation

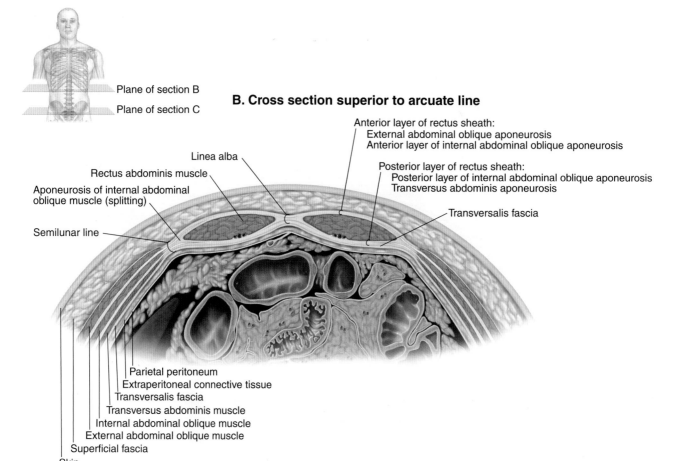

Plane of section B
Plane of section C

B. Cross section superior to arcuate line

Anterior layer of rectus sheath:
External abdominal oblique aponeurosis
Anterior layer of internal abdominal oblique aponeurosis

Posterior layer of rectus sheath:
Posterior layer of internal abdominal oblique aponeurosis
Transversus abdominis aponeurosis

Transversalis fascia

Linea alba

Rectus abdominis muscle

Aponeurosis of internal abdominal
oblique muscle (splitting)

Semilunar line

Parietal peritoneum
Extraperitoneal connective tissue
Transversalis fascia
Transversus abdominis muscle
Internal abdominal oblique muscle
External abdominal oblique muscle
Superficial fascia
Skin

C. Cross section inferior to arcuate line

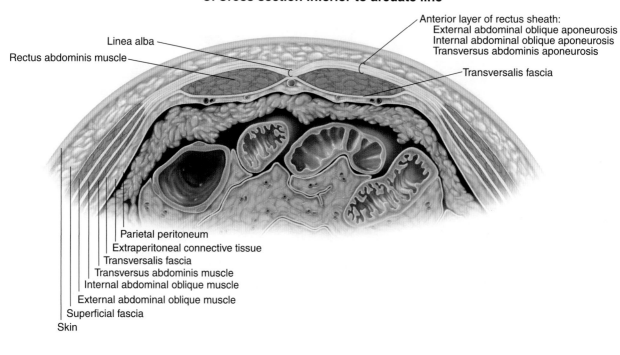

Anterior layer of rectus sheath:
External abdominal oblique aponeurosis
Internal abdominal oblique aponeurosis
Transversus abdominis aponeurosis

Transversalis fascia

Linea alba

Rectus abdominis muscle

Parietal peritoneum
Extraperitoneal connective tissue
Transversalis fascia
Transversus abdominis muscle
Internal abdominal oblique muscle
External abdominal oblique muscle
Superficial fascia
Skin

A. Male

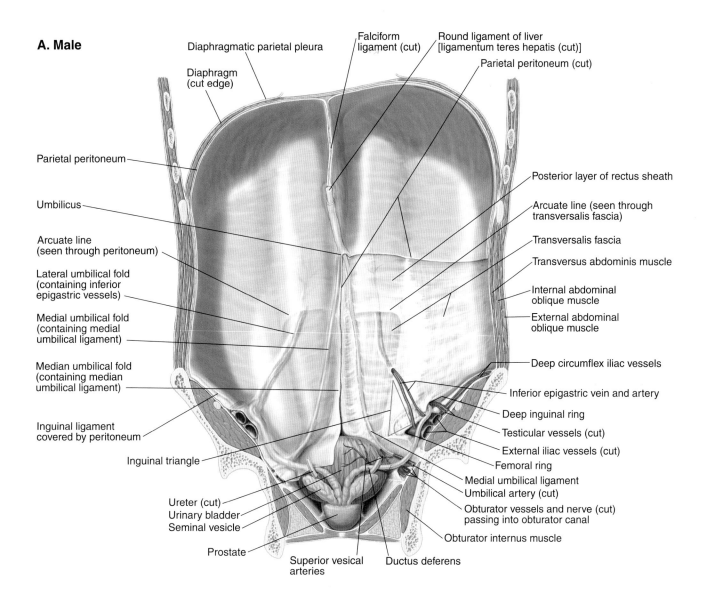

Falciform ligament (cut)

Round ligament of liver [ligamentum teres hepatis (cut)]

Diaphragmatic parietal pleura

Parietal peritoneum (cut)

Diaphragm (cut edge)

Parietal peritoneum

Umbilicus

Arcuate line (seen through peritoneum)

Lateral umbilical fold (containing inferior epigastric vessels)

Medial umbilical fold (containing medial umbilical ligament)

Median umbilical fold (containing median umbilical ligament)

Inguinal ligament covered by peritoneum

Inguinal triangle

Ureter (cut)

Urinary bladder

Seminal vesicle

Prostate

Superior vesical arteries

Ductus deferens

Posterior layer of rectus sheath

Arcuate line (seen through transversalis fascia)

Transversalis fascia

Transversus abdominis muscle

Internal abdominal oblique muscle

External abdominal oblique muscle

Deep circumflex iliac vessels

Inferior epigastric vein and artery

Deep inguinal ring

Testicular vessels (cut)

External iliac vessels (cut)

Femoral ring

Medial umbilical ligament

Umbilical artery (cut)

Obturator vessels and nerve (cut) passing into obturator canal

Obturator internus muscle

B. Female

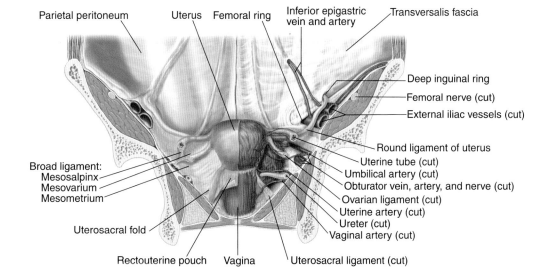

Parietal peritoneum

Uterus

Femoral ring

Inferior epigastric vein and artery

Transversalis fascia

Deep inguinal ring

Femoral nerve (cut)

External iliac vessels (cut)

Round ligament of uterus

Uterine tube (cut)

Umbilical artery (cut)

Obturator vein, artery, and nerve (cut)

Ovarian ligament (cut)

Uterine artery (cut)

Ureter (cut)

Vaginal artery (cut)

Broad ligament:
Mesosalpinx
Mesovarium
Mesometrium

Uterosacral fold

Rectouterine pouch

Vagina

Uterosacral ligament (cut)

PLATE 5-08   Inguinal Region, Male I

A. Superficial layer

External abdominal oblique muscle and aponeurosis

Anterior superior iliac spine

Intercrural fibers arching over superficial inguinal ring

Inguinal ligament and lateral crus

Anterior scrotal nerve

Anterior cutaneous branch of iliohypogastric nerve

Medial crus of superficial inguinal ring

Spermatic cord

External spermatic fascia

Skin and dartos muscle and fascia (cut)

B. Intermediate layer

Internal abdominal oblique muscle and aponeurosis

Anterior superior iliac spine

Inguinal ligament

Ilioinguinal nerve (cut)

Cremaster muscle and fascia

Iliohypogastric nerve

Falx inguinalis (conjoint tendon)

External spermatic fascia (cut)

Skin and dartos muscle and fascia (cut)

C. Deep layer

Transversus abdominis muscle and aponeurosis

Ilioinguinal nerve (cut)

Anterior superior iliac spine

Inguinal ligament

Deep inguinal ring

Spermatic cord

Iliohypogastric nerve (cut)

Inferior epigastric vessels (passing through transversalis fascia)

Transversalis fascia

Internal spermatic fascia

Cremasteric muscle and fascia (cut)

External spermatic fascia (cut)

Skin and dartos muscle and fascia (cut)

D. Internal view

Arcuate line

Deep inguinal ring

Rectus abdominis muscle (seen through transversalis fascia)

Inferior epigastric vessels

Falx inguinalis (conjoint tendon)

Lacunar ligament

Pectineal ligament

Transversus abdominis muscle (seen through transversalis fascia)

Inguinal ligament

Internal abdominal oblique muscle

Testicular vessels (cut)

Genitofemoral nerve:
Genital branch
Femoral branch

External iliac vessels (cut)

Femoral ring

Ductus deferens (cut)

Obturator artery and nerve entering obturator canal

A. Superficial layer

External abdominal oblique muscle and aponeurosis

Anterior superior iliac spine

Intercrural fibers arching over superficial inguinal ring

Inguinal ligament and lateral crus of superficial inguinal ring

Anterior labial nerve

Anterior cutaneous branch of iliohypogastric nerve

Medial crus of superficial inguinal ring

Round ligament of uterus

Skin and dartos muscle and fascia of labium majus

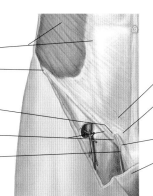

B. Intermediate layer

Internal abdominal oblique muscle and aponeurosis

Anterior superior iliac spine

Inguinal ligament

Ilioinguinal nerve (cut)*

Cremaster muscle and fascia

Iliohypogastric nerve

Transversalis fascia

Falx inguinalis (conjoint tendon)

Round ligament of uterus

*Ilioinguinal nerve unites with genitofemoral nerve in 35% of cases

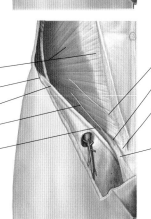

C. Deep layer

Transversus abdominis muscle and aponeurosis

Ilioinguinal nerve (cut)

Anterior superior iliac spine

Inguinal ligament

Deep inguinal ring

Round ligament of the uterus

Iliohypogastric nerve (cut)

Inferior epigastric vessels (passing through transversalis fascia)

Transversalis fascia

Falx inguinalis (conjoint tendon)

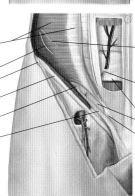

D. Internal view

Arcuate line

Deep inguinal ring

Rectus abdominis muscle (seen through transversalis fascia)

Inferior epigastric vessels

Falx inguinalis (conjoint tendon)

Lacunar ligament

Pectineal ligament

Transversus abdominis muscle (seen through transversalis fascia)

Inguinal ligament

Internal abdominal oblique muscle

Genitofemoral nerve:
Genital branch
Femoral branch

External iliac vessels (cut)

Femoral ring

Round ligament of uterus (cut)

Obturator artery and nerve entering obturator canal

PLATE 5-10   Inguinal Region, Male II

A. Dissection

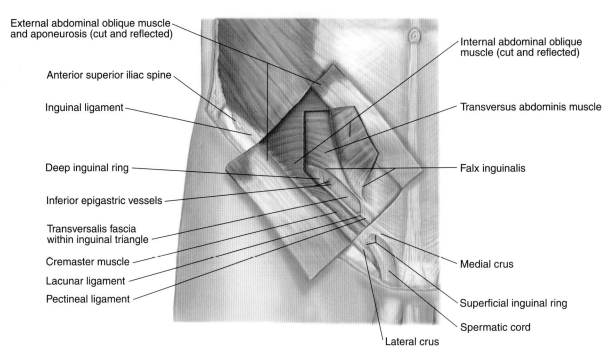

External abdominal oblique muscle and aponeurosis (cut and reflected)

Anterior superior iliac spine

Inguinal ligament

Deep inguinal ring

Inferior epigastric vessels

Transversalis fascia within inguinal triangle

Cremaster muscle

Lacunar ligament

Pectineal ligament

Internal abdominal oblique muscle (cut and reflected)

Transversus abdominis muscle

Falx inguinalis

Medial crus

Superficial inguinal ring

Spermatic cord

Lateral crus

B. Layers separated for visibility

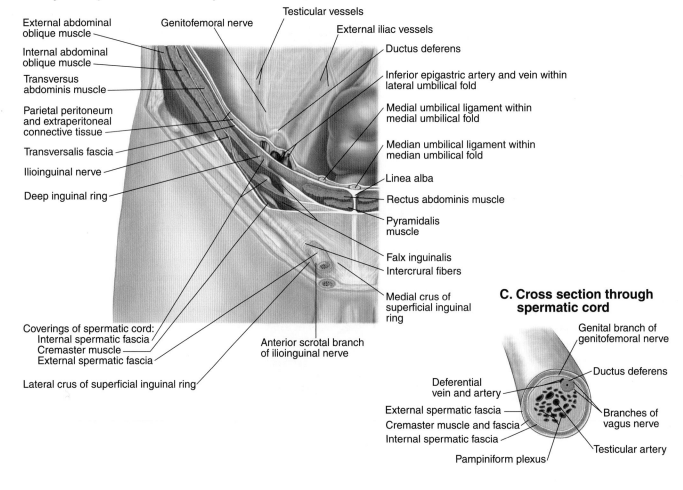

External abdominal oblique muscle

Internal abdominal oblique muscle

Transversus abdominis muscle

Parietal peritoneum and extraperitoneal connective tissue

Transversalis fascia

Ilioinguinal nerve

Deep inguinal ring

Genitofemoral nerve

Testicular vessels

External iliac vessels

Ductus deferens

Inferior epigastric artery and vein within lateral umbilical fold

Medial umbilical ligament within medial umbilical fold

Median umbilical ligament within median umbilical fold

Linea alba

Rectus abdominis muscle

Pyramidalis muscle

Falx inguinalis

Intercrural fibers

Medial crus of superficial inguinal ring

Coverings of spermatic cord:
Internal spermatic fascia
Cremaster muscle
External spermatic fascia

Lateral crus of superficial inguinal ring

Anterior scrotal branch of ilioinguinal nerve

C. Cross section through spermatic cord

Genital branch of genitofemoral nerve

Ductus deferens

Branches of vagus nerve

Testicular artery

Pampiniform plexus

Internal spermatic fascia

Cremaster muscle and fascia

External spermatic fascia

Deferential vein and artery

A. Surface projection of inguinal hernias

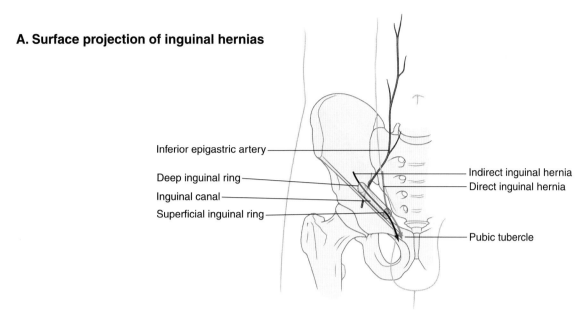

Inferior epigastric artery

Deep inguinal ring

Inguinal canal

Superficial inguinal ring

Indirect inguinal hernia

Direct inguinal hernia

Pubic tubercle

B. Indirect inguinal hernia

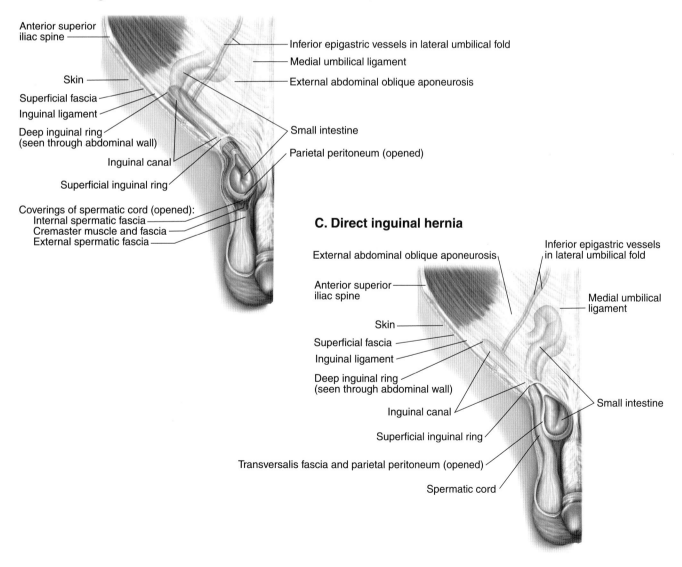

Anterior superior iliac spine

Skin

Superficial fascia

Inguinal ligament

Deep inguinal ring (seen through abdominal wall)

Inguinal canal

Superficial inguinal ring

Coverings of spermatic cord (opened):
Internal spermatic fascia
Cremaster muscle and fascia
External spermatic fascia

Inferior epigastric vessels in lateral umbilical fold

Medial umbilical ligament

External abdominal oblique aponeurosis

Small intestine

Parietal peritoneum (opened)

C. Direct inguinal hernia

External abdominal oblique aponeurosis

Anterior superior iliac spine

Skin

Superficial fascia

Inguinal ligament

Deep inguinal ring (seen through abdominal wall)

Inguinal canal

Superficial inguinal ring

Transversalis fascia and parietal peritoneum (opened)

Spermatic cord

Inferior epigastric vessels in lateral umbilical fold

Medial umbilical ligament

Small intestine

PLATE 5-12 | **Peritoneum and Peritoneal Cavity**

A. Greater omentum

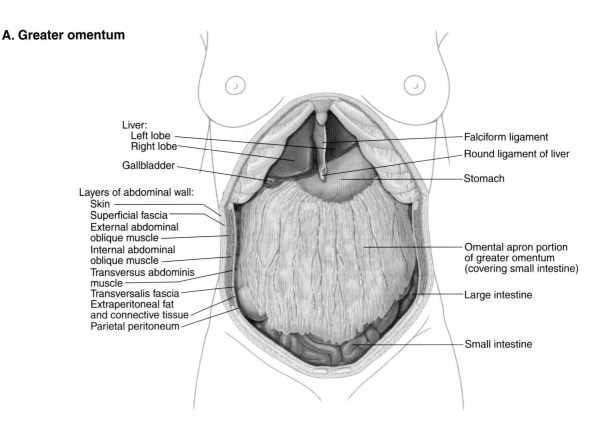

Liver:
Left lobe
Right lobe
Gallbladder

Falciform ligament
Round ligament of liver
Stomach

Layers of abdominal wall:
Skin
Superficial fascia
External abdominal oblique muscle
Internal abdominal oblique muscle
Transversus abdominis muscle
Transversalis fascia
Extraperitoneal fat and connective tissue
Parietal peritoneum

Omental apron portion of greater omentum (covering small intestine)
Large intestine
Small intestine

B. Large and small intestines

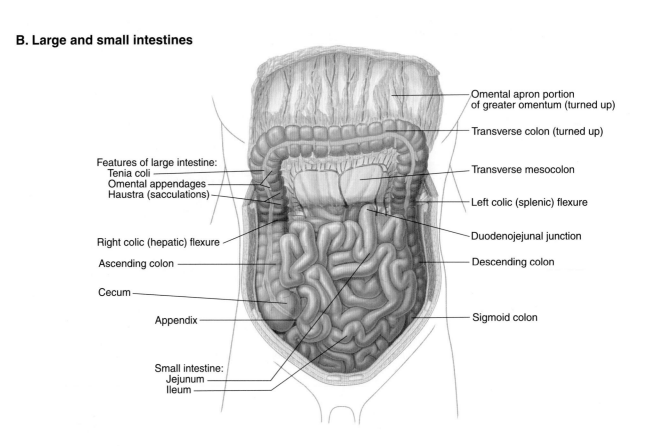

Features of large intestine:
Tenia coli
Omental appendages
Haustra (sacculations)

Right colic (hepatic) flexure
Ascending colon
Cecum
Appendix

Small intestine:
Jejunum
Ileum

Omental apron portion of greater omentum (turned up)
Transverse colon (turned up)
Transverse mesocolon
Left colic (splenic) flexure
Duodenojejunal junction
Descending colon
Sigmoid colon

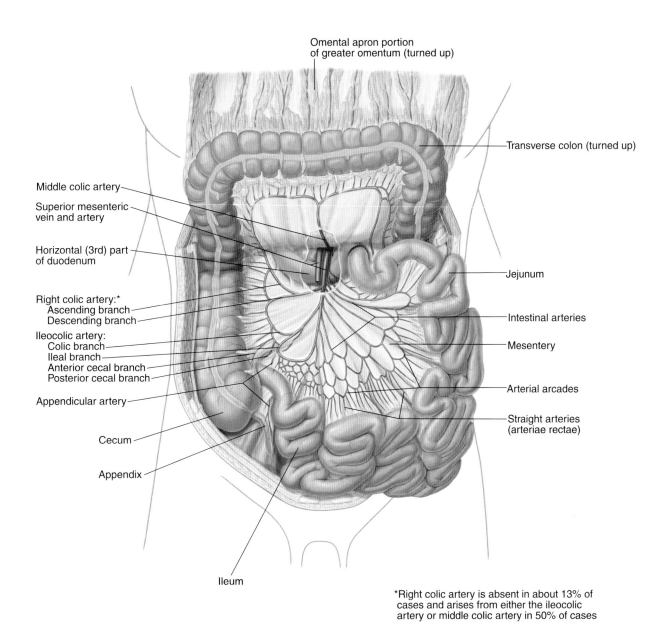

Omental apron portion
of greater omentum (turned up)

Transverse colon (turned up)

Middle colic artery

Superior mesenteric
vein and artery

Horizontal (3rd) part
of duodenum

Jejunum

Right colic artery:*
    Ascending branch
    Descending branch

Intestinal arteries

Mesentery

Ileocolic artery:
    Colic branch
    Ileal branch
    Anterior cecal branch
    Posterior cecal branch

Arterial arcades

Appendicular artery

Straight arteries
(arteriae rectae)

Cecum

Appendix

Ileum

*Right colic artery is absent in about 13% of
cases and arises from either the ileocolic
artery or middle colic artery in 50% of cases

PLATE 5-14   Inferior Mesenteric Artery

A. Dissection

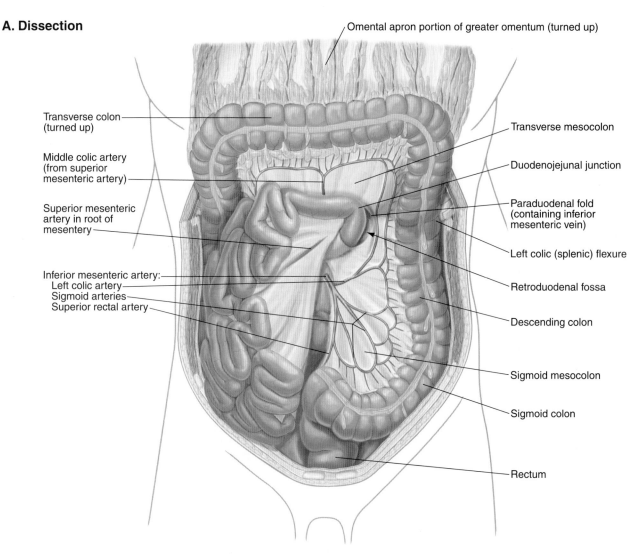

Omental apron portion of greater omentum (turned up)

Transverse colon (turned up)

Middle colic artery (from superior mesenteric artery)

Superior mesenteric artery in root of mesentery

Inferior mesenteric artery:
Left colic artery
Sigmoid arteries
Superior rectal artery

Transverse mesocolon

Duodenojejunal junction

Paraduodenal fold (containing inferior mesenteric vein)

Left colic (splenic) flexure

Retroduodenal fossa

Descending colon

Sigmoid mesocolon

Sigmoid colon

Rectum

B. Marginal artery

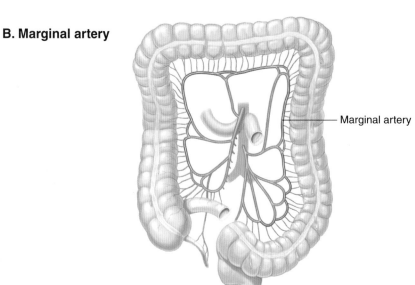

Marginal artery

A. Dissection

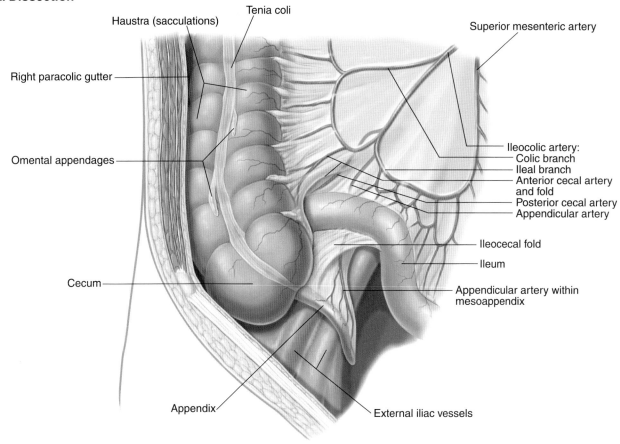

Haustra (sacculations)

Tenia coli

Superior mesenteric artery

Right paracolic gutter

Omental appendages

Ileocolic artery:
Colic branch
Ileal branch
Anterior cecal artery
and fold
Posterior cecal artery
Appendicular artery

Ileocecal fold

Ileum

Cecum

Appendicular artery within
mesoappendix

Appendix

External iliac vessels

C. Location of appendix

B. Ileocecal valve

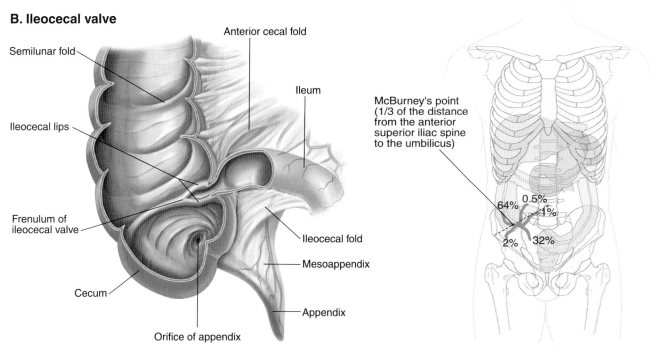

Anterior cecal fold

Semilunar fold

Ileum

Ileocecal lips

McBurney's point
(1/3 of the distance
from the anterior
superior iliac spine
to the umbilicus)

Frenulum of
ileocecal valve

Ileocecal fold

0.5%
64%
1%
2%
32%

Mesoappendix

Cecum

Appendix

Orifice of appendix

PLATE 5-16   Jejunum and Ileum

A. Orientation

Figure B

Figure C

B. Jejunum

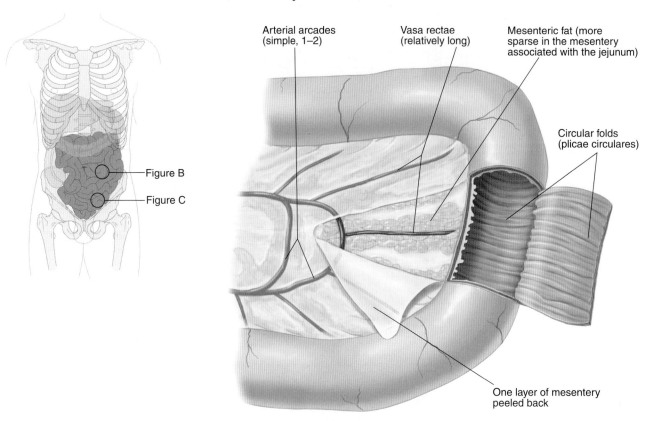

Arterial arcades (simple, 1–2)

Vasa rectae (relatively long)

Mesenteric fat (more sparse in the mesentery associated with the jejunum)

Circular folds (plicae circulares)

One layer of mesentery peeled back

C. Ileum

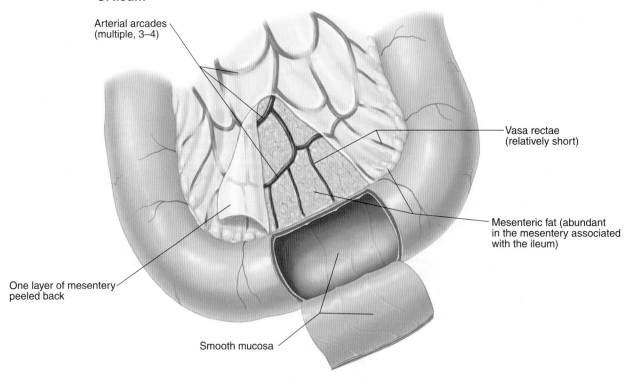

Arterial arcades (multiple, 3–4)

Vasa rectae (relatively short)

Mesenteric fat (abundant in the mesentery associated with the ileum)

One layer of mesentery peeled back

Smooth mucosa

A. Stomach and small intestine

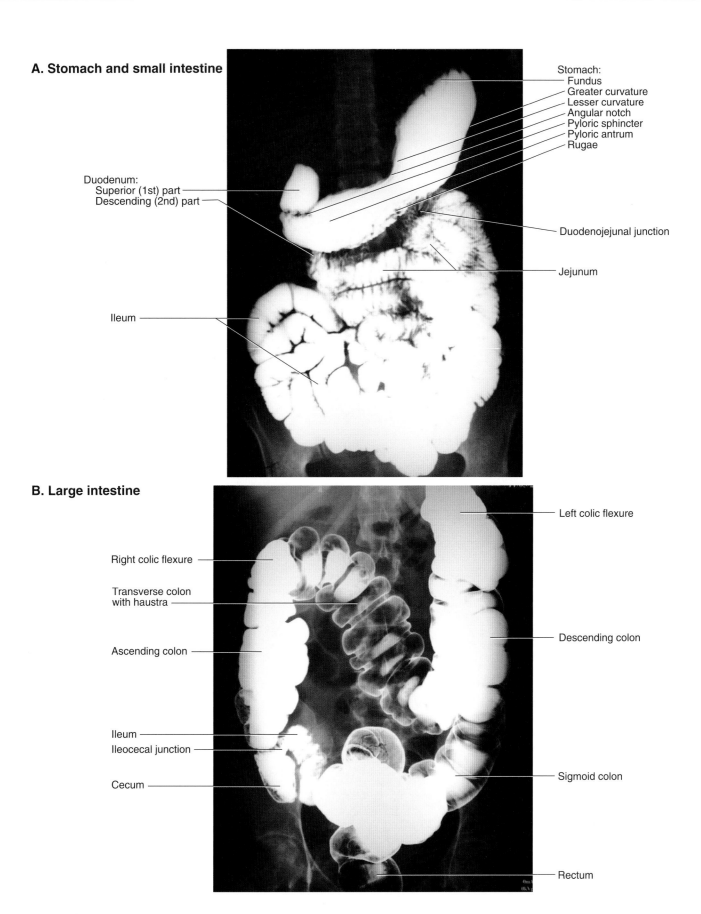

Stomach:
Fundus
Greater curvature
Lesser curvature
Angular notch
Pyloric sphincter
Pyloric antrum
Rugae

Duodenum:
Superior (1st) part
Descending (2nd) part

Duodenojejunal junction

Jejunum

Ileum

B. Large intestine

Left colic flexure

Right colic flexure

Transverse colon
with haustra

Ascending colon

Descending colon

Ileum
Ileocecal junction

Cecum

Sigmoid colon

Rectum

PLATE 5-18   Stomach and Lesser Omentum

A. Parts of stomach and lesser omentum

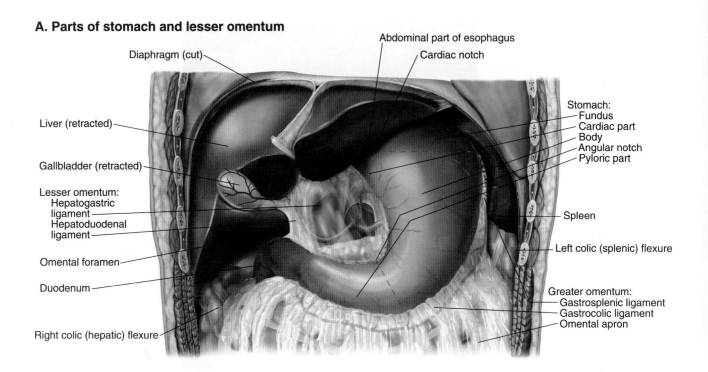

Diaphragm (cut)

Abdominal part of esophagus

Cardiac notch

Liver (retracted)

Stomach:
Fundus
Cardiac part
Body
Angular notch
Pyloric part

Gallbladder (retracted)

Lesser omentum:
Hepatogastric ligament
Hepatoduodenal ligament

Omental foramen

Duodenum

Right colic (hepatic) flexure

Spleen

Left colic (splenic) flexure

Greater omentum:
Gastrosplenic ligament
Gastrocolic ligament
Omental apron

B. Omental bursa (lesser peritoneal sac)

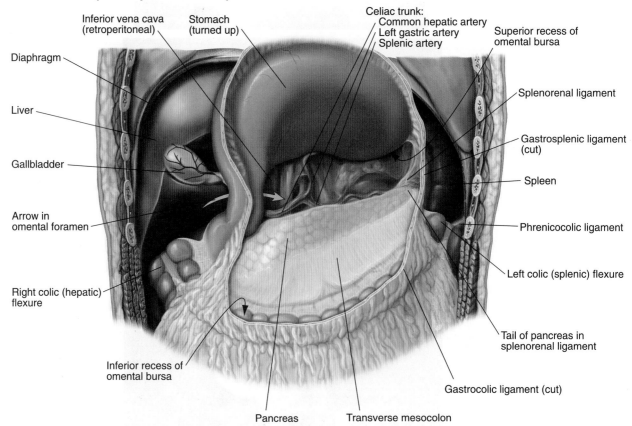

Inferior vena cava (retroperitoneal)

Stomach (turned up)

Celiac trunk:
Common hepatic artery
Left gastric artery
Splenic artery

Superior recess of omental bursa

Diaphragm

Liver

Splenorenal ligament

Gastrosplenic ligament (cut)

Gallbladder

Spleen

Arrow in omental foramen

Phrenicocolic ligament

Left colic (splenic) flexure

Right colic (hepatic) flexure

Tail of pancreas in splenorenal ligament

Inferior recess of omental bursa

Gastrocolic ligament (cut)

Pancreas

Transverse mesocolon

A. Celiac trunk

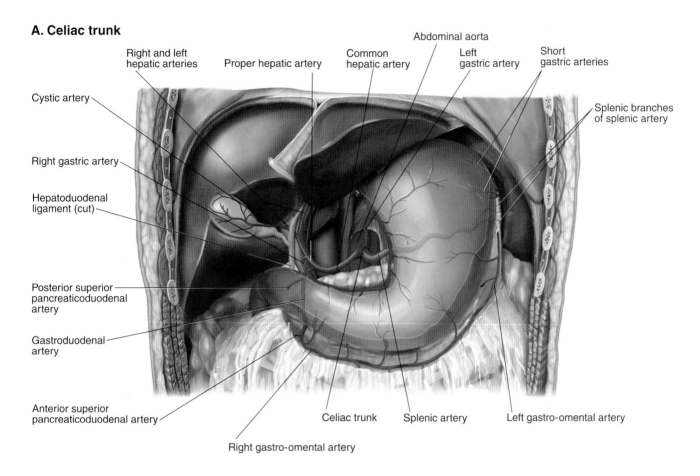

Right and left hepatic arteries

Proper hepatic artery

Common hepatic artery

Abdominal aorta

Left gastric artery

Short gastric arteries

Cystic artery

Splenic branches of splenic artery

Right gastric artery

Hepatoduodenal ligament (cut)

Posterior superior pancreaticoduodenal artery

Gastroduodenal artery

Anterior superior pancreaticoduodenal artery

Celiac trunk

Splenic artery

Left gastro-omental artery

Right gastro-omental artery

B. Stomach, internal view

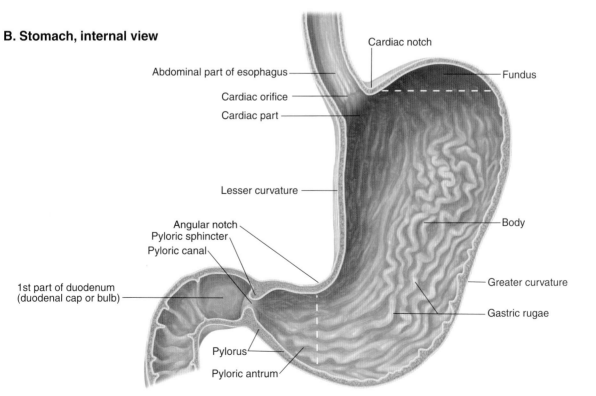

Cardiac notch

Abdominal part of esophagus

Fundus

Cardiac orifice

Cardiac part

Lesser curvature

Body

Angular notch

Pyloric sphincter

Pyloric canal

1st part of duodenum (duodenal cap or bulb)

Greater curvature

Gastric rugae

Pylorus

Pyloric antrum

PLATE 5-20 **Spleen**

A. Dissection

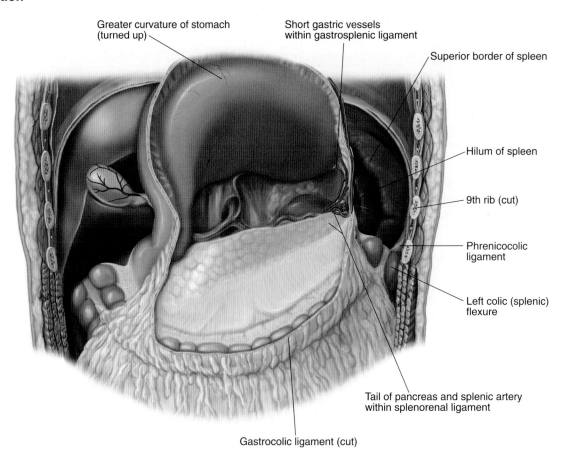

Greater curvature of stomach (turned up)

Short gastric vessels within gastrosplenic ligament

Superior border of spleen

Hilum of spleen

9th rib (cut)

Phrenicocolic ligament

Left colic (splenic) flexure

Tail of pancreas and splenic artery within splenorenal ligament

Gastrocolic ligament (cut)

B. Visceral surface

C. Diaphragmatic surface

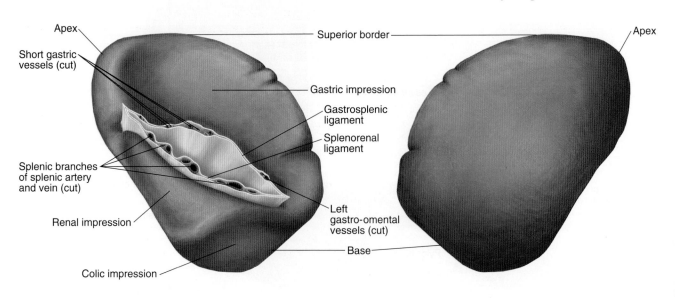

Apex

Short gastric vessels (cut)

Superior border

Apex

Gastric impression

Gastrosplenic ligament

Splenorenal ligament

Splenic branches of splenic artery and vein (cut)

Renal impression

Left gastro-omental vessels (cut)

Colic impression

Base

A. Orientation

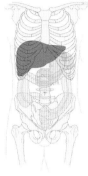

B. Anterior view

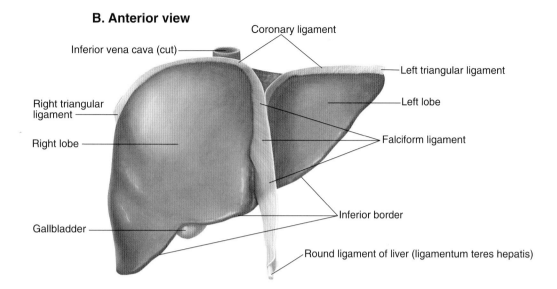

Coronary ligament

Inferior vena cava (cut)

Left triangular ligament

Right triangular ligament

Left lobe

Right lobe

Falciform ligament

Gallbladder

Inferior border

Round ligament of liver (ligamentum teres hepatis)

C. Inferior view

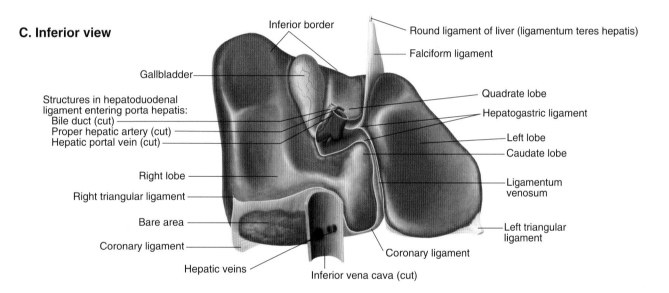

Inferior border

Round ligament of liver (ligamentum teres hepatis)

Falciform ligament

Gallbladder

Structures in hepatoduodenal ligament entering porta hepatis:
Bile duct (cut)
Proper hepatic artery (cut)
Hepatic portal vein (cut)

Quadrate lobe

Hepatogastric ligament

Left lobe

Caudate lobe

Right lobe

Right triangular ligament

Ligamentum venosum

Bare area

Coronary ligament

Left triangular ligament

Coronary ligament

Hepatic veins

Inferior vena cava (cut)

D. Superior view

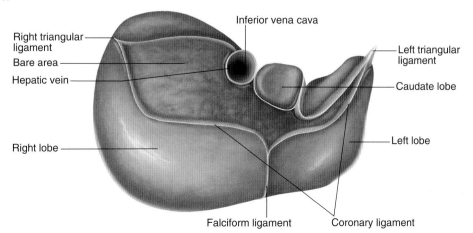

Inferior vena cava

Right triangular ligament

Bare area

Left triangular ligament

Hepatic vein

Caudate lobe

Right lobe

Left lobe

Falciform ligament

Coronary ligament

PLATE 5-22   Liver, Internal Features

A. Portal vein, hepatic artery, and biliary duct system

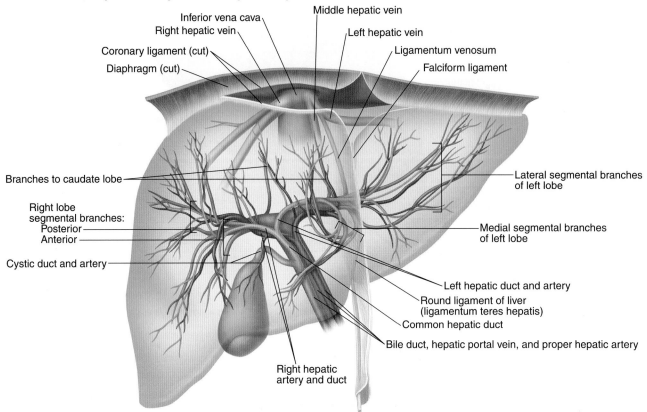

Inferior vena cava

Middle hepatic vein

Right hepatic vein

Left hepatic vein

Coronary ligament (cut)

Ligamentum venosum

Diaphragm (cut)

Falciform ligament

Branches to caudate lobe

Lateral segmental branches of left lobe

Right lobe segmental branches:
Posterior
Anterior

Medial segmental branches of left lobe

Cystic duct and artery

Left hepatic duct and artery

Round ligament of liver (ligamentum teres hepatis)

Common hepatic duct

Bile duct, hepatic portal vein, and proper hepatic artery

Right hepatic artery and duct

B. Portal vein and hepatic veins

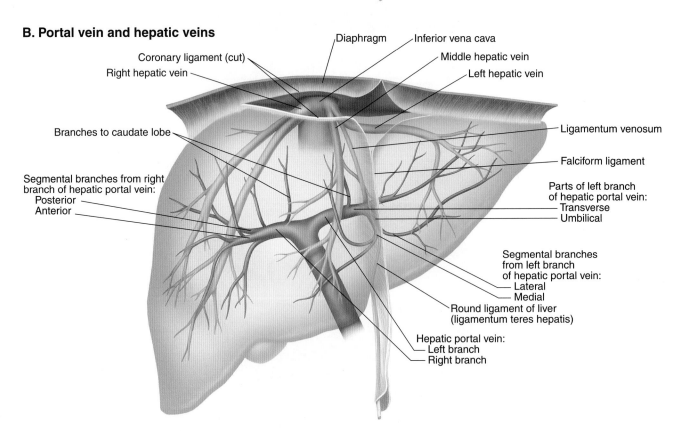

Diaphragm

Inferior vena cava

Coronary ligament (cut)

Middle hepatic vein

Right hepatic vein

Left hepatic vein

Branches to caudate lobe

Ligamentum venosum

Segmental branches from right branch of hepatic portal vein:
Posterior
Anterior

Falciform ligament

Parts of left branch of hepatic portal vein:
Transverse
Umbilical

Segmental branches from left branch of hepatic portal vein:
Lateral
Medial

Round ligament of liver (ligamentum teres hepatis)

Hepatic portal vein:
Left branch
Right branch

A. Anterior view

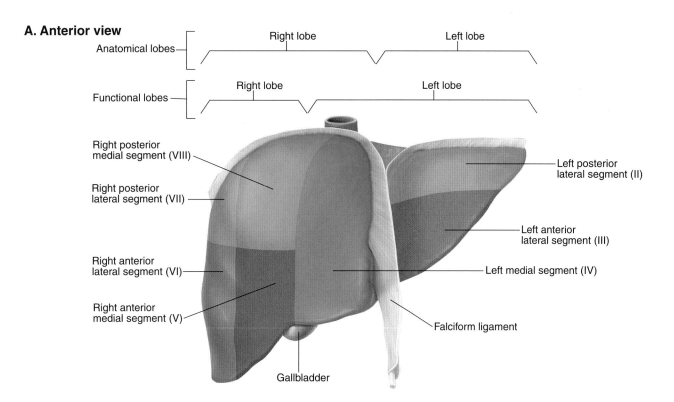

Anatomical lobes — Right lobe | Left lobe

Functional lobes — Right lobe | Left lobe

Right posterior medial segment (VIII)

Right posterior lateral segment (VII)

Right anterior lateral segment (VI)

Right anterior medial segment (V)

Left posterior lateral segment (II)

Left anterior lateral segment (III)

Left medial segment (IV)

Falciform ligament

Gallbladder

B. Visceral surface

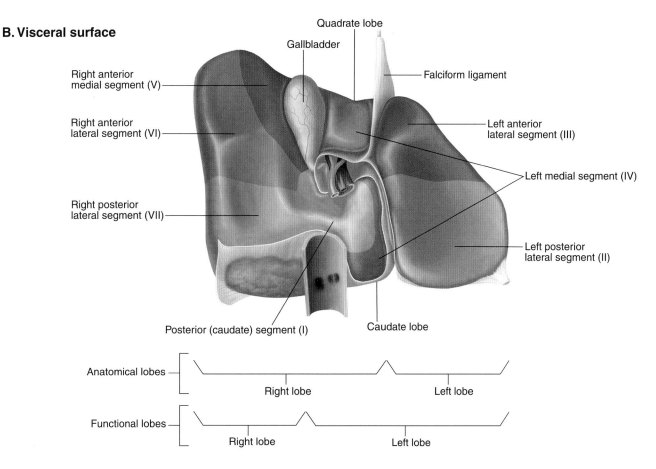

Quadrate lobe

Gallbladder

Right anterior medial segment (V)

Right anterior lateral segment (VI)

Right posterior lateral segment (VII)

Falciform ligament

Left anterior lateral segment (III)

Left medial segment (IV)

Left posterior lateral segment (II)

Posterior (caudate) segment (I)

Caudate lobe

Anatomical lobes — Right lobe | Left lobe

Functional lobes — Right lobe | Left lobe

PLATE 5-24   Gallbladder

A. Orientation

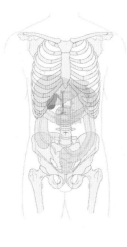

B. Dissection

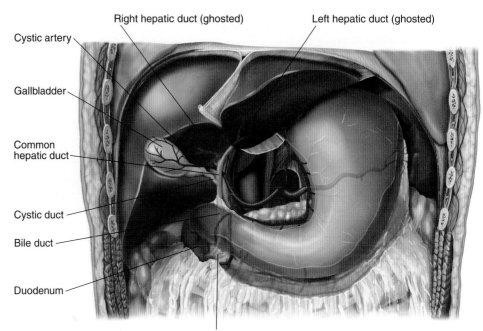

Cystic artery

Gallbladder

Common hepatic duct

Cystic duct

Bile duct

Duodenum

Right hepatic duct (ghosted)

Left hepatic duct (ghosted)

Main pancreatic duct

C. Internal view

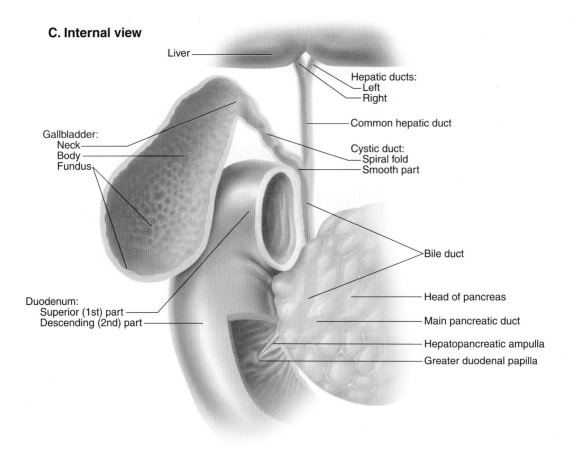

Liver

Hepatic ducts:
Left
Right

Common hepatic duct

Cystic duct:
Spiral fold
Smooth part

Gallbladder:
Neck
Body
Fundus

Bile duct

Head of pancreas

Main pancreatic duct

Hepatopancreatic ampulla

Greater duodenal papilla

Duodenum:
Superior (1st) part
Descending (2nd) part

A. Variations in the hepatic arteries

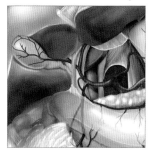 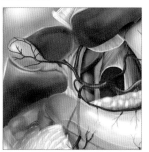 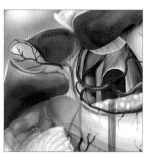 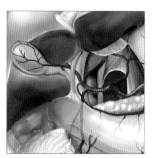

Right and left hepatic arteries arising from proper hepatic artery; right hepatic artery passing posterior to common hepatic duct (64%)

Right hepatic artery passing anterior to common hepatic duct (24%)

Right hepatic artery arising from superior mesenteric artery (12%)

Left hepatic artery arising from left gastric artery (11%)

B. Variations in the cystic artery

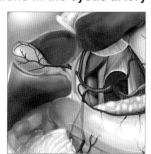 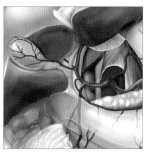 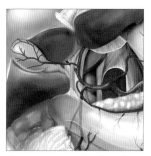

Cystic artery arising from right hepatic artery and passing posterior to common hepatic duct (76%)

Cystic artery arising from right hepatic artery and passing anterior to common hepatic duct (13%)

Cystic artery arising from left hepatic artery and passing anterior to common hepatic duct (6%)

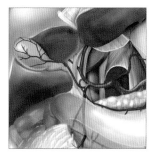 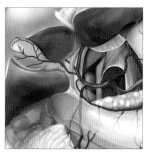

Cystic artery arising from gastroduodenal artery and passing anterior to common hepatic duct (3%)

Cystic artery arising from proper hepatic artery and passing anterior to common hepatic duct (2%)

PLATE 5-26   Duodenum and Pancreas I

A. Orientation

B. Surface features

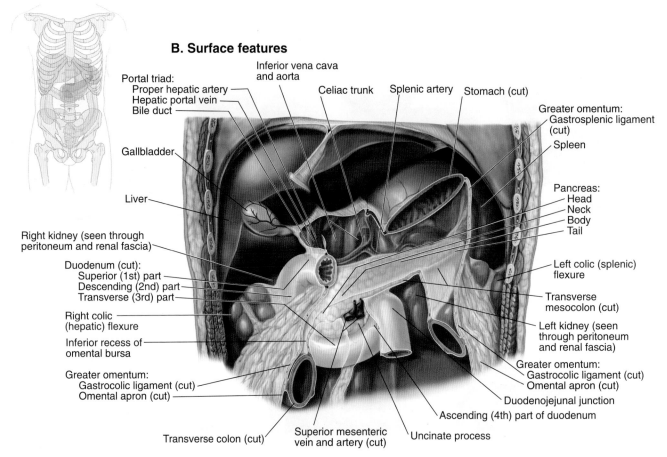

Portal triad:
Proper hepatic artery
Hepatic portal vein
Bile duct

Inferior vena cava and aorta

Celiac trunk

Splenic artery

Stomach (cut)

Greater omentum:
Gastrosplenic ligament (cut)

Spleen

Gallbladder

Liver

Pancreas:
Head
Neck
Body
Tail

Right kidney (seen through peritoneum and renal fascia)

Duodenum (cut):
Superior (1st) part
Descending (2nd) part
Transverse (3rd) part

Left colic (splenic) flexure

Transverse mesocolon (cut)

Right colic (hepatic) flexure

Inferior recess of omental bursa

Left kidney (seen through peritoneum and renal fascia)

Greater omentum:
Gastrocolic ligament (cut)
Omental apron (cut)

Greater omentum:
Gastrocolic ligament (cut)
Omental apron (cut)

Duodenojejunal junction

Ascending (4th) part of duodenum

Transverse colon (cut)

Superior mesenteric vein and artery (cut)

Uncinate process

C. Dissection

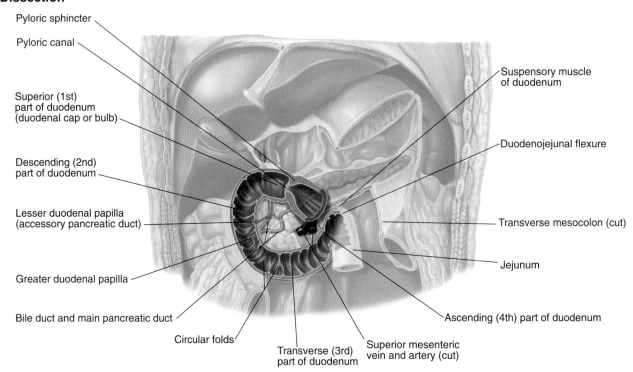

Pyloric sphincter

Pyloric canal

Suspensory muscle of duodenum

Superior (1st) part of duodenum (duodenal cap or bulb)

Descending (2nd) part of duodenum

Duodenojejunal flexure

Lesser duodenal papilla (accessory pancreatic duct)

Transverse mesocolon (cut)

Greater duodenal papilla

Jejunum

Bile duct and main pancreatic duct

Circular folds

Transverse (3rd) part of duodenum

Superior mesenteric vein and artery (cut)

Ascending (4th) part of duodenum

A. Parts

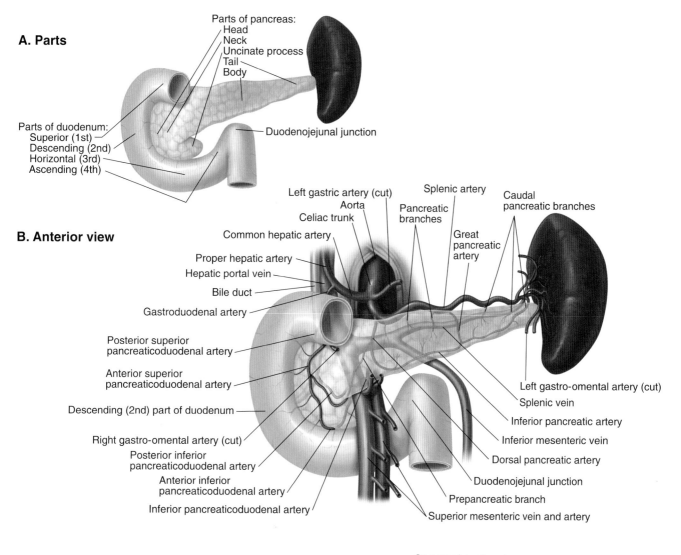

Parts of pancreas:
Head
Neck
Uncinate process
Tail
Body

Parts of duodenum:
Superior (1st)
Descending (2nd)
Horizontal (3rd)
Ascending (4th)

Duodenojejunal junction

B. Anterior view

Left gastric artery (cut)
Aorta
Celiac trunk
Common hepatic artery
Proper hepatic artery
Hepatic portal vein
Bile duct
Gastroduodenal artery
Posterior superior pancreaticoduodenal artery
Anterior superior pancreaticoduodenal artery
Descending (2nd) part of duodenum
Right gastro-omental artery (cut)
Posterior inferior pancreaticoduodenal artery
Anterior inferior pancreaticoduodenal artery
Inferior pancreaticoduodenal artery

Splenic artery
Pancreatic branches
Great pancreatic artery
Caudal pancreatic branches
Left gastro-omental artery (cut)
Splenic vein
Inferior pancreatic artery
Inferior mesenteric vein
Dorsal pancreatic artery
Duodenojejunal junction
Prepancreatic branch
Superior mesenteric vein and artery

C. Posterior view

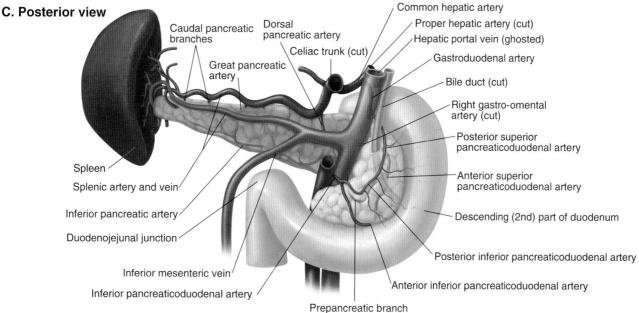

Caudal pancreatic branches
Dorsal pancreatic artery
Great pancreatic artery
Celiac trunk (cut)
Common hepatic artery
Proper hepatic artery (cut)
Hepatic portal vein (ghosted)
Gastroduodenal artery
Bile duct (cut)
Right gastro-omental artery (cut)
Posterior superior pancreaticoduodenal artery
Anterior superior pancreaticoduodenal artery
Descending (2nd) part of duodenum
Posterior inferior pancreaticoduodenal artery
Anterior inferior pancreaticoduodenal artery

Spleen
Splenic artery and vein
Inferior pancreatic artery
Duodenojejunal junction
Inferior mesenteric vein
Inferior pancreaticoduodenal artery
Prepancreatic branch

PLATE 5-28   **Hepatic Portal Vein**

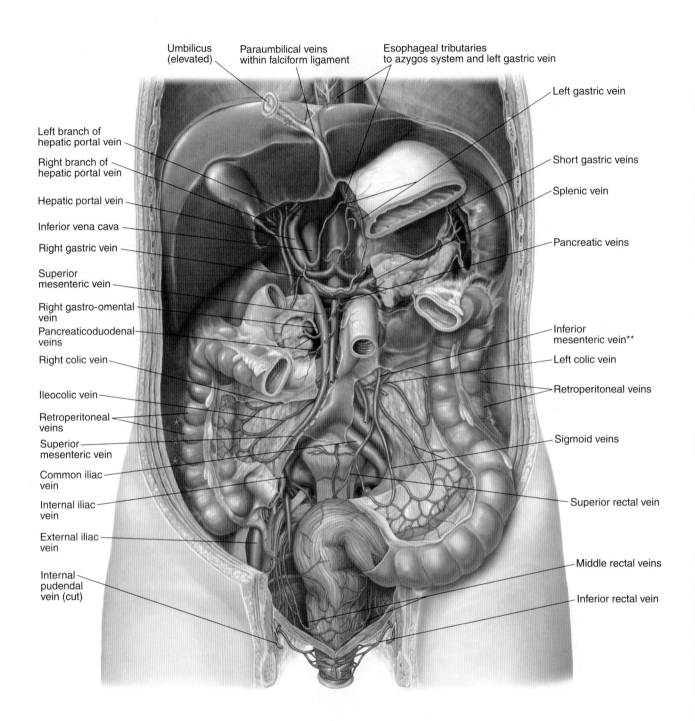

Umbilicus (elevated)

Paraumbilical veins within falciform ligament

Esophageal tributaries to azygos system and left gastric vein

Left gastric vein

Left branch of hepatic portal vein

Right branch of hepatic portal vein

Hepatic portal vein

Inferior vena cava

Right gastric vein

Superior mesenteric vein

Right gastro-omental vein

Pancreaticoduodenal veins

Right colic vein

Ileocolic vein

Retroperitoneal veins

Superior mesenteric vein

Common iliac vein

Internal iliac vein

External iliac vein

Internal pudendal vein (cut)

Short gastric veins

Splenic vein

Pancreatic veins

Inferior mesenteric vein**

Left colic vein

Retroperitoneal veins

Sigmoid veins

Superior rectal vein

Middle rectal veins

Inferior rectal vein

★Denotes sites of portal–caval anastomosis in cases of portal hypertension:
  1. Esophageal tributaries of left gastric vein to esophageal tributaries of azygos system of veins
  2. Superior rectal vein to middle and inferior rectal veins
  3. Paraumbilical tributaries of left hepatic portal vein to superficial veins of anterior body wall
  4. Retroperitoneal veins to veins of posterior body wall

**Inferior mesenteric vein can join the splenic vein (34%), the superior mesenteric vein (33%), or the junction of the splenic and superior mesenteric veins (32%)

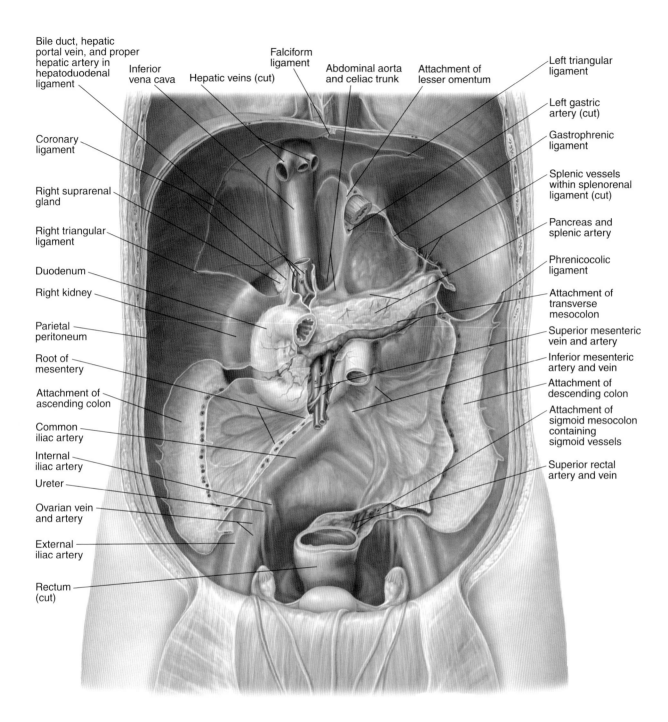

Bile duct, hepatic portal vein, and proper hepatic artery in hepatoduodenal ligament

Inferior vena cava

Hepatic veins (cut)

Falciform ligament

Abdominal aorta and celiac trunk

Attachment of lesser omentum

Left triangular ligament

Left gastric artery (cut)

Gastrophrenic ligament

Splenic vessels within splenorenal ligament (cut)

Pancreas and splenic artery

Phrenicocolic ligament

Attachment of transverse mesocolon

Superior mesenteric vein and artery

Inferior mesenteric artery and vein

Attachment of descending colon

Attachment of sigmoid mesocolon containing sigmoid vessels

Superior rectal artery and vein

Coronary ligament

Right suprarenal gland

Right triangular ligament

Duodenum

Right kidney

Parietal peritoneum

Root of mesentery

Attachment of ascending colon

Common iliac artery

Internal iliac artery

Ureter

Ovarian vein and artery

External iliac artery

Rectum (cut)

PLATE 5-30   Kidneys and Retroperitoneum

A. Orientation

B. Anterior view

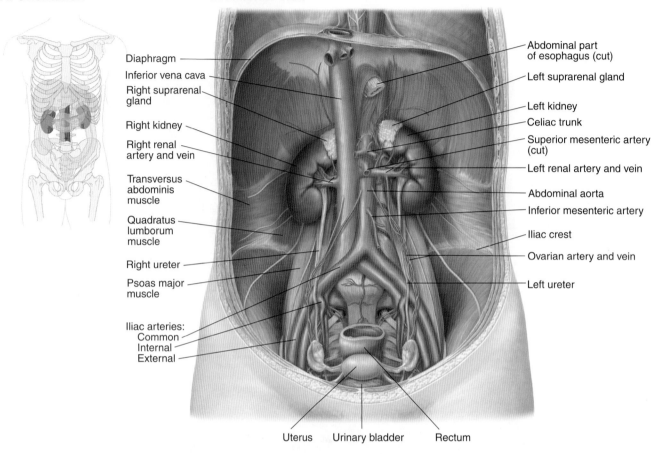

Diaphragm

Inferior vena cava

Right suprarenal gland

Right kidney

Right renal artery and vein

Transversus abdominis muscle

Quadratus lumborum muscle

Right ureter

Psoas major muscle

Iliac arteries:
Common
Internal
External

Abdominal part of esophagus (cut)

Left suprarenal gland

Left kidney

Celiac trunk

Superior mesenteric artery (cut)

Left renal artery and vein

Abdominal aorta

Inferior mesenteric artery

Iliac crest

Ovarian artery and vein

Left ureter

Uterus   Urinary bladder   Rectum

C. Posterior view

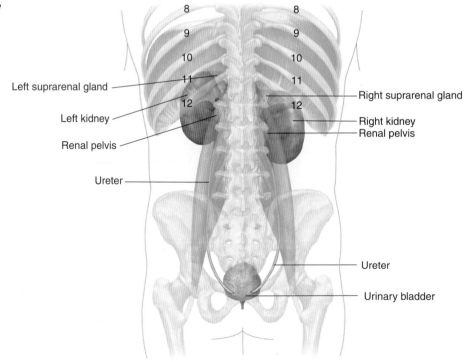

8   8
9   9
10   10
11   11
12   12

Left suprarenal gland

Left kidney

Renal pelvis

Ureter

Right suprarenal gland

Right kidney
Renal pelvis

Ureter

Urinary bladder

A. Orientation

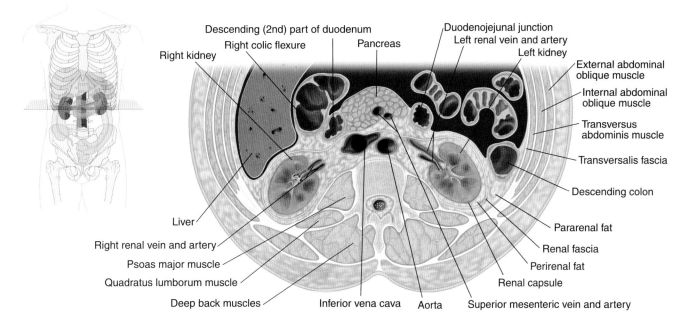

B. Cross section through the L2 vertebra

Descending (2nd) part of duodenum
Right colic flexure
Right kidney
Pancreas
Duodenojejunal junction
Left renal vein and artery
Left kidney
External abdominal oblique muscle
Internal abdominal oblique muscle
Transversus abdominis muscle
Transversalis fascia
Descending colon
Pararenal fat
Renal fascia
Perirenal fat
Renal capsule
Superior mesenteric vein and artery
Aorta
Inferior vena cava
Deep back muscles
Quadratus lumborum muscle
Psoas major muscle
Right renal vein and artery
Liver

C. Dissection

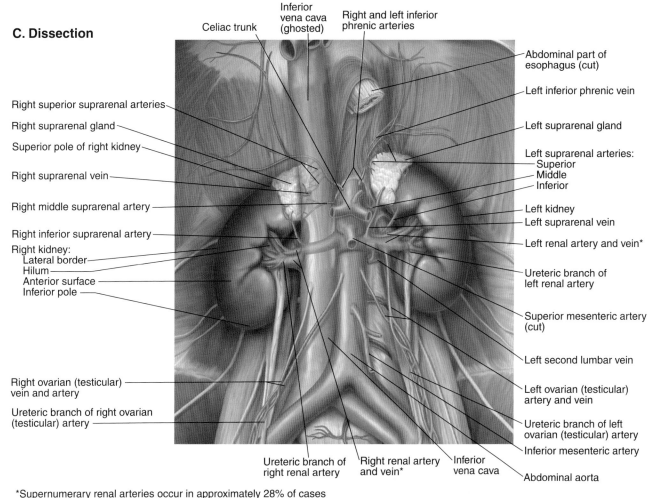

Celiac trunk
Inferior vena cava (ghosted)
Right and left inferior phrenic arteries
Abdominal part of esophagus (cut)
Left inferior phrenic vein
Left suprarenal gland
Left suprarenal arteries:
— Superior
— Middle
— Inferior
Left kidney
Left suprarenal vein
Left renal artery and vein*
Ureteric branch of left renal artery
Superior mesenteric artery (cut)
Left second lumbar vein
Left ovarian (testicular) artery and vein
Ureteric branch of left ovarian (testicular) artery
Inferior mesenteric artery
Abdominal aorta

Right superior suprarenal arteries
Right suprarenal gland
Superior pole of right kidney
Right suprarenal vein
Right middle suprarenal artery
Right inferior suprarenal artery
Right kidney:
  Lateral border
  Hilum
  Anterior surface
  Inferior pole
Right ovarian (testicular) vein and artery
Ureteric branch of right ovarian (testicular) artery

Ureteric branch of right renal artery
Right renal artery and vein*
Inferior vena cava

*Supernumerary renal arteries occur in approximately 28% of cases

PLATE 5-32   **Kidney and Suprarenal Gland, Internal Features**

A. Arteries

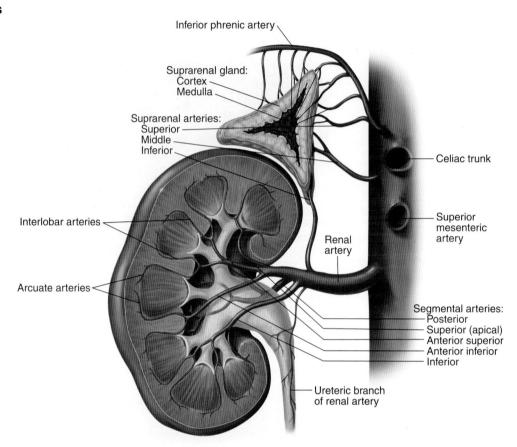

Inferior phrenic artery

Suprarenal gland:
Cortex
Medulla

Suprarenal arteries:
Superior
Middle
Inferior

Celiac trunk

Superior mesenteric artery

Interlobar arteries

Renal artery

Arcuate arteries

Segmental arteries:
Posterior
Superior (apical)
Anterior superior
Anterior inferior
Inferior

Ureteric branch
of renal artery

B. Renal collecting system

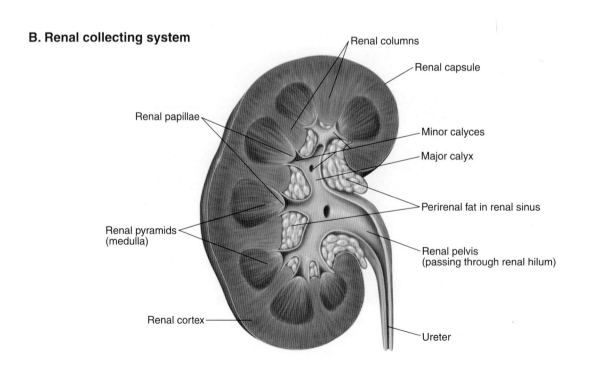

Renal columns

Renal capsule

Renal papillae

Minor calyces

Major calyx

Perirenal fat in renal sinus

Renal pyramids
(medulla)

Renal pelvis
(passing through renal hilum)

Renal cortex

Ureter

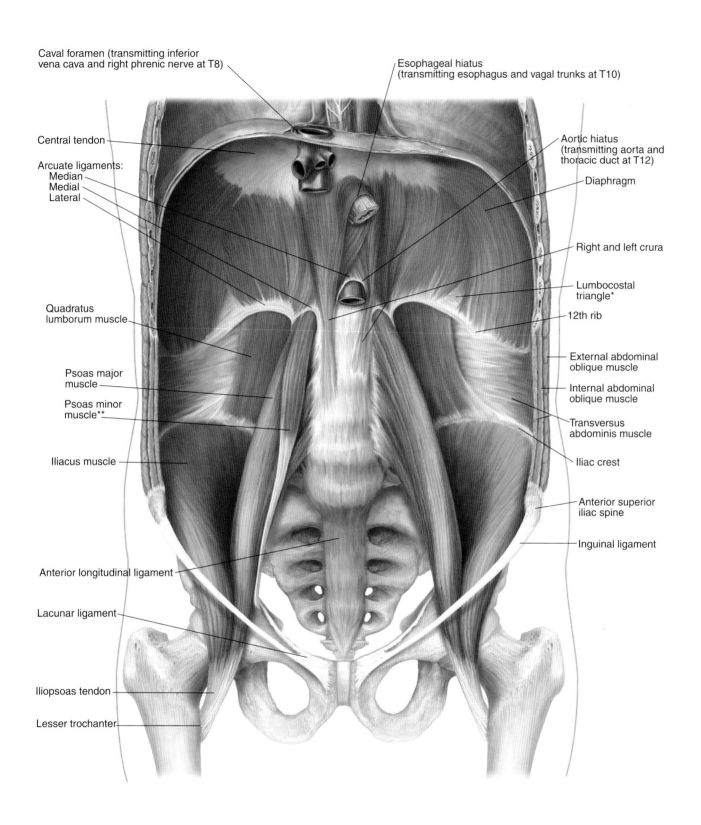

Caval foramen (transmitting inferior vena cava and right phrenic nerve at T8)

Esophageal hiatus (transmitting esophagus and vagal trunks at T10)

Central tendon

Arcuate ligaments:
Median
Medial
Lateral

Aortic hiatus (transmitting aorta and thoracic duct at T12)

Diaphragm

Right and left crura

Lumbocostal triangle*

Quadratus lumborum muscle

12th rib

External abdominal oblique muscle

Psoas major muscle

Internal abdominal oblique muscle

Psoas minor muscle**

Transversus abdominis muscle

Iliacus muscle

Iliac crest

Anterior superior iliac spine

Inguinal ligament

Anterior longitudinal ligament

Lacunar ligament

Iliopsoas tendon

Lesser trochanter

* Lumbocostal triangle is present in 80% of cases
** Psoas minor muscle is present in 50% of cases

PLATE 5-34   **Vessels of the Posterior Abdominal Wall**

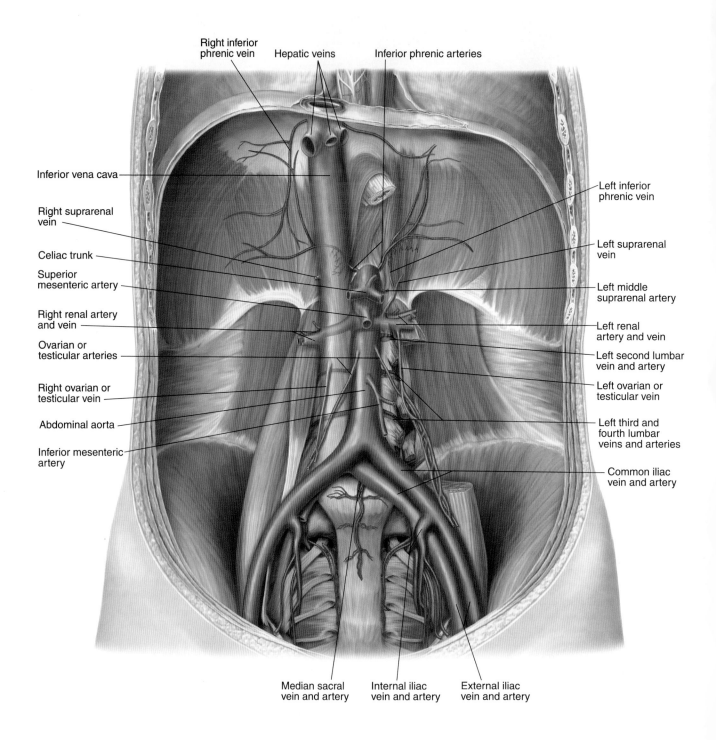

Right inferior phrenic vein

Hepatic veins

Inferior phrenic arteries

Inferior vena cava

Right suprarenal vein

Celiac trunk

Superior mesenteric artery

Right renal artery and vein

Ovarian or testicular arteries

Right ovarian or testicular vein

Abdominal aorta

Inferior mesenteric artery

Left inferior phrenic vein

Left suprarenal vein

Left middle suprarenal artery

Left renal artery and vein

Left second lumbar vein and artery

Left ovarian or testicular vein

Left third and fourth lumbar veins and arteries

Common iliac vein and artery

Median sacral vein and artery

Internal iliac vein and artery

External iliac vein and artery

A. Superficial dissection

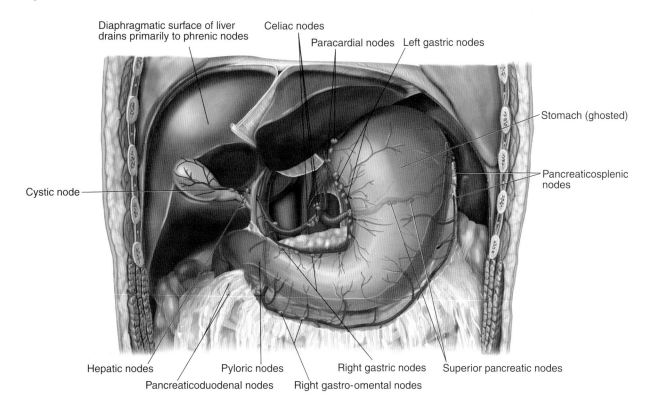

Diaphragmatic surface of liver drains primarily to phrenic nodes

Celiac nodes

Paracardial nodes

Left gastric nodes

Stomach (ghosted)

Pancreaticosplenic nodes

Cystic node

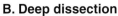

Hepatic nodes

Pancreaticoduodenal nodes

Pyloric nodes

Right gastro-omental nodes

Right gastric nodes

Superior pancreatic nodes

B. Deep dissection

Hepatic nodes

Celiac nodes

Left gastric nodes

Splenic nodes

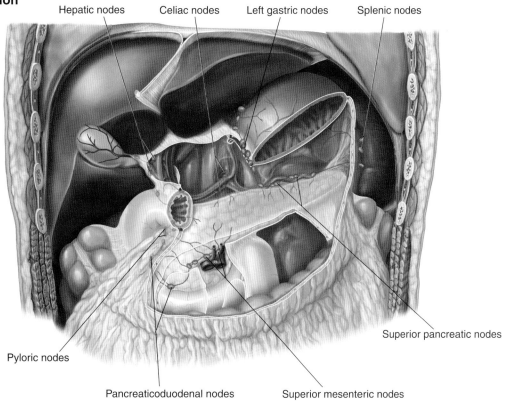

Superior pancreatic nodes

Pyloric nodes

Pancreaticoduodenal nodes

Superior mesenteric nodes

PLATE 5-36   **Lymphatic Drainage of the Small and Large Intestines**

A. Small intestine, cecum, ascending colon, and transverse colon

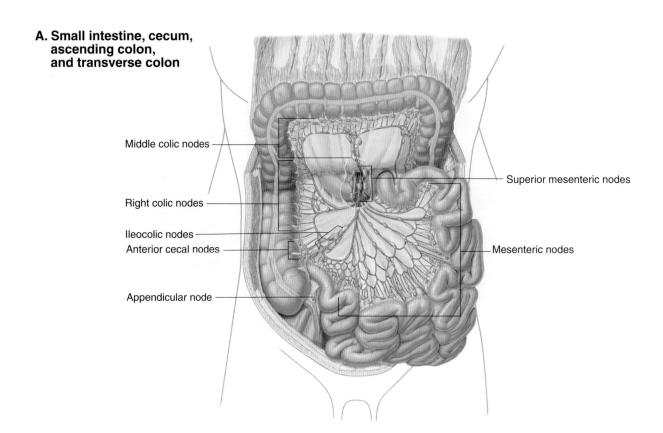

Middle colic nodes

Right colic nodes

Ileocolic nodes

Anterior cecal nodes

Appendicular node

Superior mesenteric nodes

Mesenteric nodes

B. Descending colon, sigmoid colon, and rectum

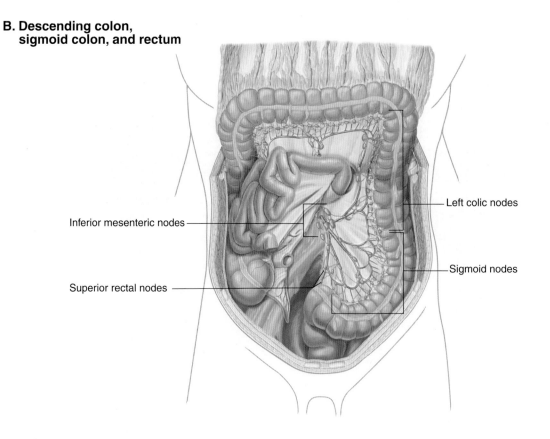

Inferior mesenteric nodes

Superior rectal nodes

Left colic nodes

Sigmoid nodes

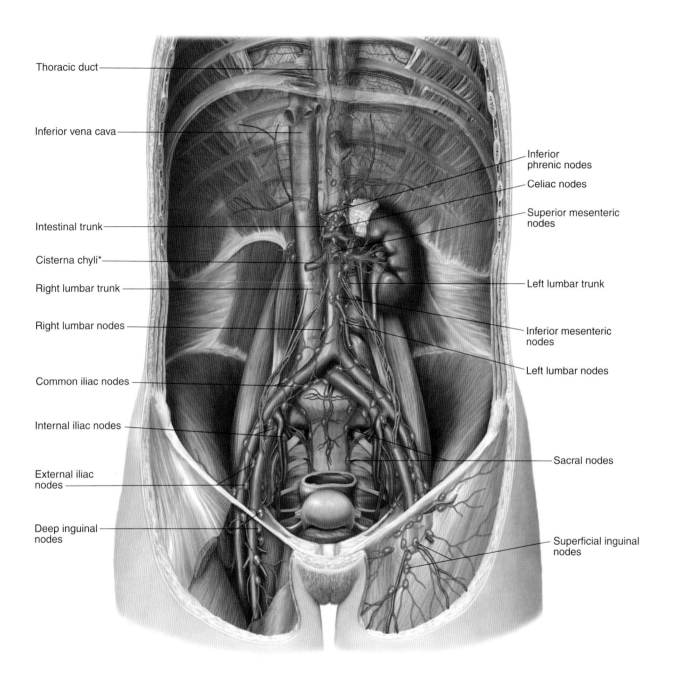

Thoracic duct

Inferior vena cava

Intestinal trunk

Cisterna chyli*

Right lumbar trunk

Right lumbar nodes

Common iliac nodes

Internal iliac nodes

External iliac nodes

Deep inguinal nodes

Inferior phrenic nodes

Celiac nodes

Superior mesenteric nodes

Left lumbar trunk

Inferior mesenteric nodes

Left lumbar nodes

Sacral nodes

Superficial inguinal nodes

*Cisterna chyli is present in approximately 25% of cases

PLATE 5-38 | **Nerves of the Posterior Abdominal Wall**

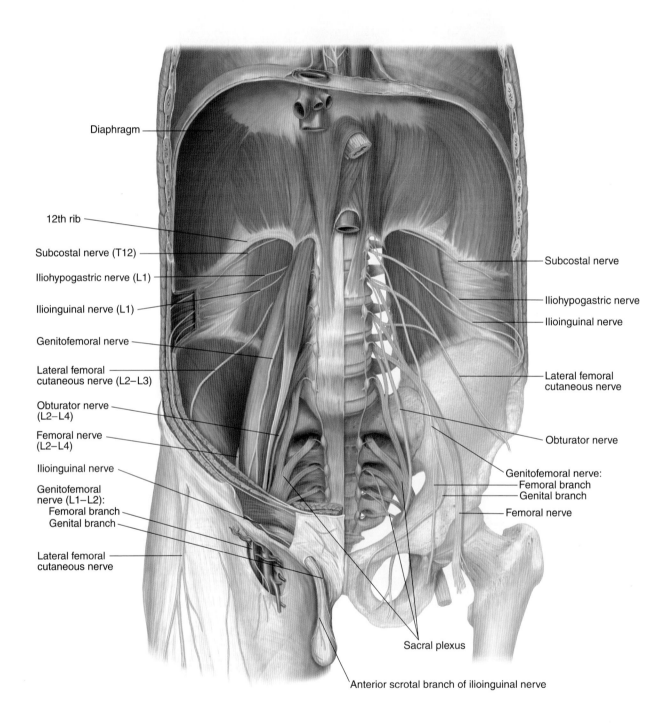

Diaphragm

12th rib

Subcostal nerve (T12)

Iliohypogastric nerve (L1)

Ilioinguinal nerve (L1)

Genitofemoral nerve

Lateral femoral
cutaneous nerve (L2–L3)

Obturator nerve
(L2–L4)

Femoral nerve
(L2–L4)

Ilioinguinal nerve

Genitofemoral
nerve (L1–L2):
  Femoral branch
  Genital branch

Lateral femoral
cutaneous nerve

Subcostal nerve

Iliohypogastric nerve

Ilioinguinal nerve

Lateral femoral
cutaneous nerve

Obturator nerve

Genitofemoral nerve:
  Femoral branch
  Genital branch

Femoral nerve

Sacral plexus

Anterior scrotal branch of ilioinguinal nerve

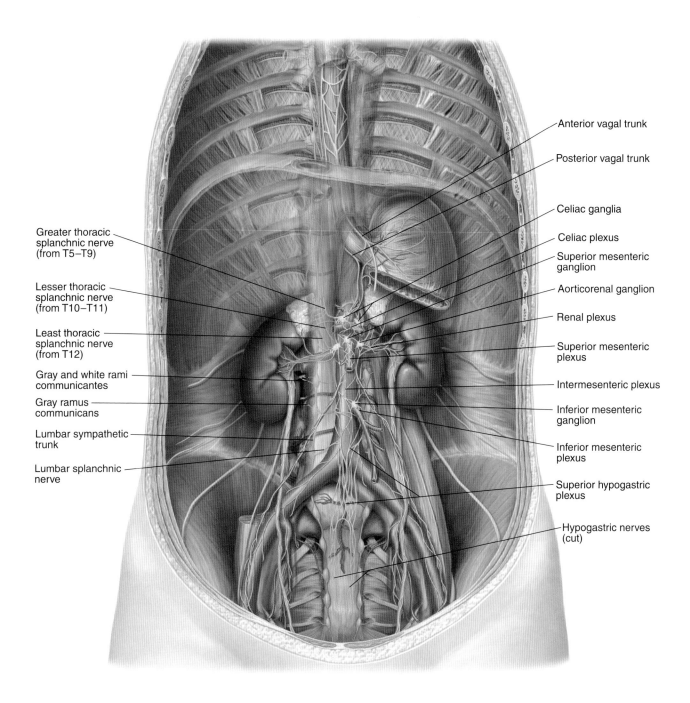

Greater thoracic
splanchnic nerve
(from T5–T9)

Lesser thoracic
splanchnic nerve
(from T10–T11)

Least thoracic
splanchnic nerve
(from T12)

Gray and white rami
communicantes

Gray ramus
communicans

Lumbar sympathetic
trunk

Lumbar splanchnic
nerve

Anterior vagal trunk

Posterior vagal trunk

Celiac ganglia

Celiac plexus

Superior mesenteric
ganglion

Aorticorenal ganglion

Renal plexus

Superior mesenteric
plexus

Intermesenteric plexus

Inferior mesenteric
ganglion

Inferior mesenteric
plexus

Superior hypogastric
plexus

Hypogastric nerves
(cut)

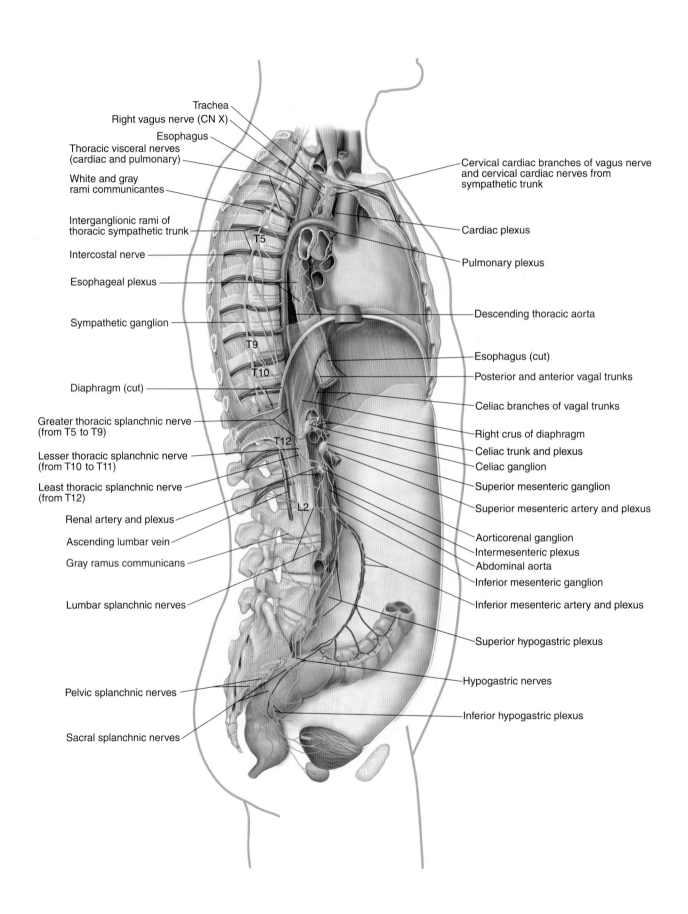

Trachea

Right vagus nerve (CN X)

Esophagus

Thoracic visceral nerves
(cardiac and pulmonary)

White and gray
rami communicantes

Interganglionic rami of
thoracic sympathetic trunk

Intercostal nerve

Esophageal plexus

Sympathetic ganglion

Diaphragm (cut)

Greater thoracic splanchnic nerve
(from T5 to T9)

Lesser thoracic splanchnic nerve
(from T10 to T11)

Least thoracic splanchnic nerve
(from T12)

Renal artery and plexus

Ascending lumbar vein

Gray ramus communicans

Lumbar splanchnic nerves

Pelvic splanchnic nerves

Sacral splanchnic nerves

T5

T9

T10

T12

L2

Cervical cardiac branches of vagus nerve
and cervical cardiac nerves from
sympathetic trunk

Cardiac plexus

Pulmonary plexus

Descending thoracic aorta

Esophagus (cut)

Posterior and anterior vagal trunks

Celiac branches of vagal trunks

Right crus of diaphragm

Celiac trunk and plexus

Celiac ganglion

Superior mesenteric ganglion

Superior mesenteric artery and plexus

Aorticorenal ganglion

Intermesenteric plexus

Abdominal aorta

Inferior mesenteric ganglion

Inferior mesenteric artery and plexus

Superior hypogastric plexus

Hypogastric nerves

Inferior hypogastric plexus

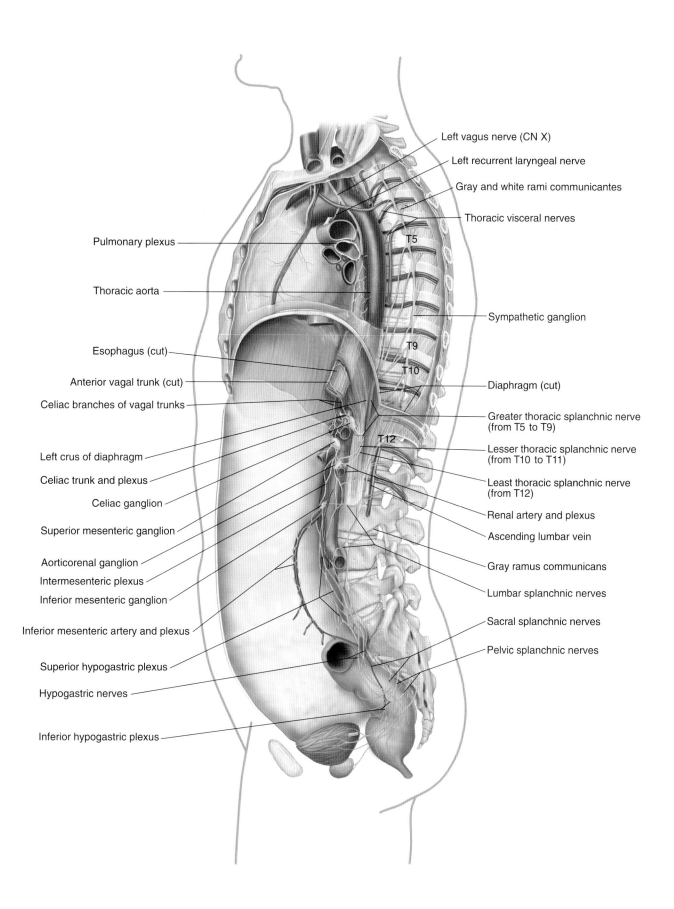

Left vagus nerve (CN X)

Left recurrent laryngeal nerve

Gray and white rami communicantes

Thoracic visceral nerves

Pulmonary plexus

T5

Thoracic aorta

Sympathetic ganglion

T9

T10

Esophagus (cut)

Anterior vagal trunk (cut)

Diaphragm (cut)

Celiac branches of vagal trunks

Greater thoracic splanchnic nerve (from T5 to T9)

T12

Lesser thoracic splanchnic nerve (from T10 to T11)

Left crus of diaphragm

Least thoracic splanchnic nerve (from T12)

Celiac trunk and plexus

Celiac ganglion

Renal artery and plexus

Superior mesenteric ganglion

Ascending lumbar vein

Aorticorenal ganglion

Gray ramus communicans

Intermesenteric plexus

Inferior mesenteric ganglion

Lumbar splanchnic nerves

Inferior mesenteric artery and plexus

Sacral splanchnic nerves

Superior hypogastric plexus

Pelvic splanchnic nerves

Hypogastric nerves

Inferior hypogastric plexus

PLATE 5-42 **Cross Sections Through Vertebral Levels T10 and L1**

A. T10 vertebral level

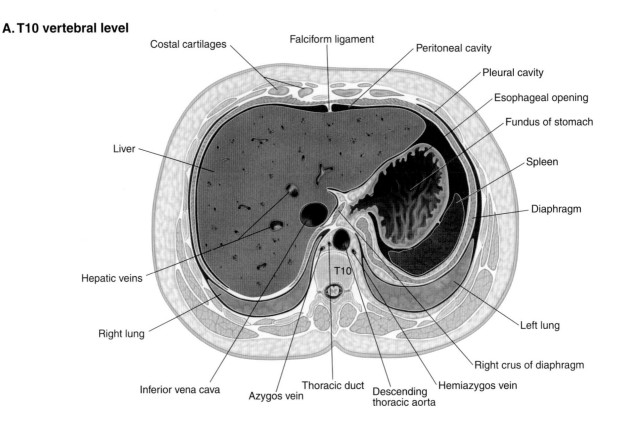

Costal cartilages — Falciform ligament — Peritoneal cavity — Pleural cavity — Esophageal opening — Fundus of stomach — Liver — Spleen — Diaphragm — Hepatic veins — T10 — Left lung — Right lung — Right crus of diaphragm — Inferior vena cava — Azygos vein — Thoracic duct — Descending thoracic aorta — Hemiazygos vein

B. L1 vertebral level

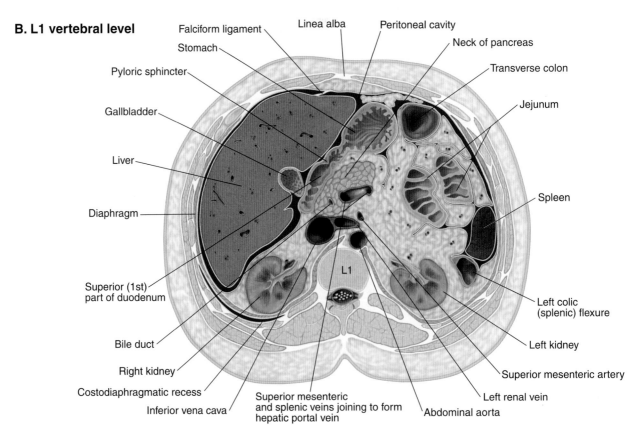

Falciform ligament — Linea alba — Peritoneal cavity — Neck of pancreas — Stomach — Transverse colon — Pyloric sphincter — Jejunum — Gallbladder — Liver — Spleen — Diaphragm — L1 — Superior (1st) part of duodenum — Left colic (splenic) flexure — Bile duct — Left kidney — Right kidney — Superior mesenteric artery — Costodiaphragmatic recess — Left renal vein — Inferior vena cava — Superior mesenteric and splenic veins joining to form hepatic portal vein — Abdominal aorta

A. L3 vertebral level

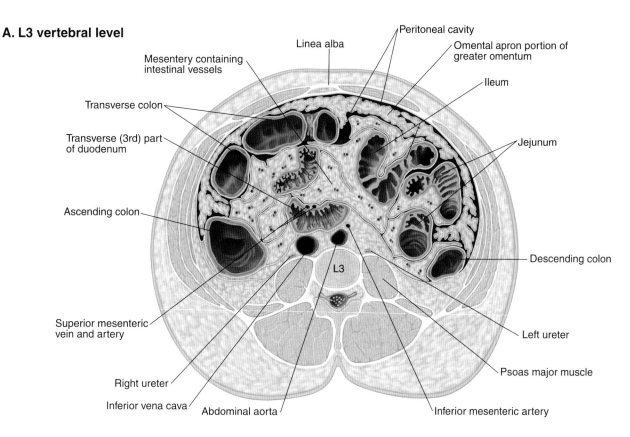

Peritoneal cavity

Linea alba

Omental apron portion of
greater omentum

Mesentery containing
intestinal vessels

Ileum

Transverse colon

Jejunum

Transverse (3rd) part
of duodenum

Ascending colon

Descending colon

L3

Superior mesenteric
vein and artery

Left ureter

Psoas major muscle

Right ureter

Inferior vena cava   Abdominal aorta   Inferior mesenteric artery

B. L5/S1 vertebral level

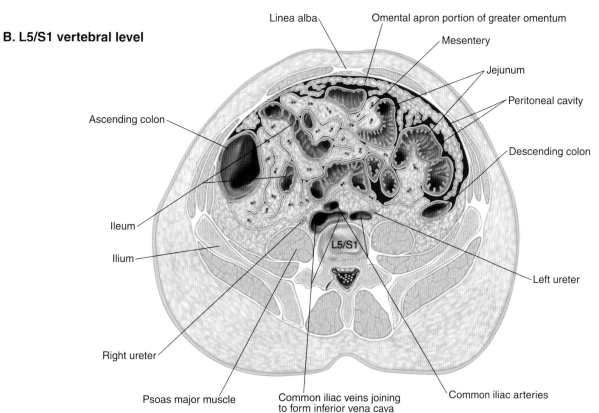

Linea alba   Omental apron portion of greater omentum

Mesentery

Jejunum

Ascending colon

Peritoneal cavity

Descending colon

L5/S1

Ileum

Ilium

Left ureter

Right ureter

Psoas major muscle   Common iliac veins joining
to form inferior vena cava   Common iliac arteries

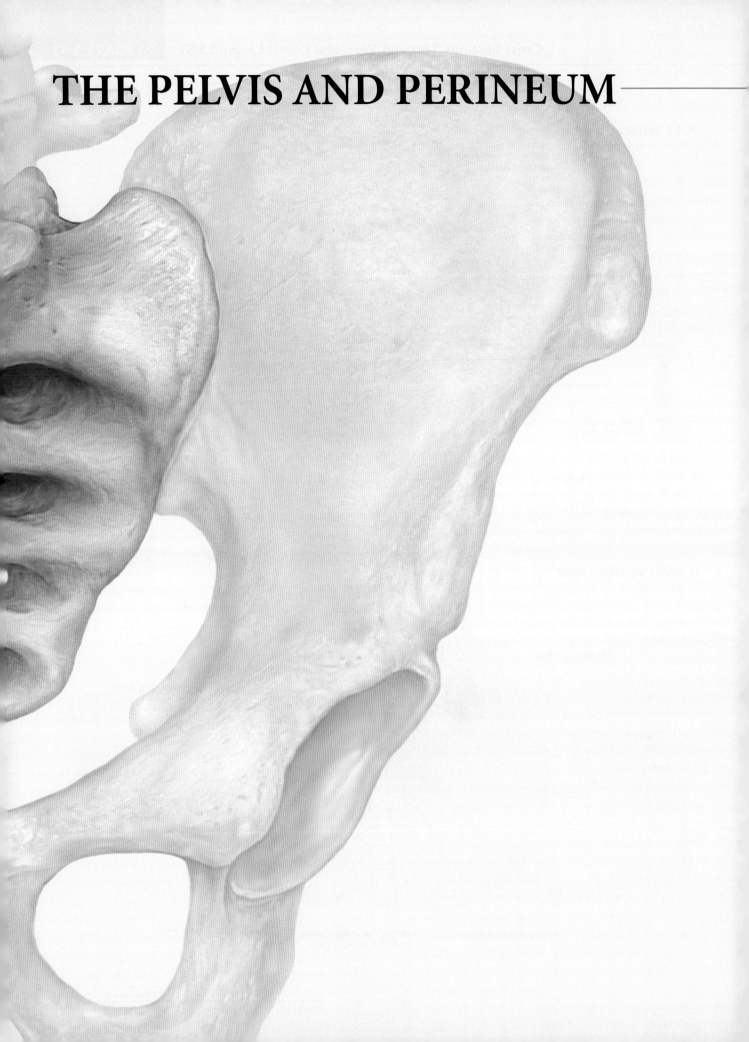

THE PELVIS AND PERINEUM

A. Anterior view

Palpable bony structures

Iliac crest

Anterior superior
iliac spine

Inguinal ligament

Pubic:
Crest
Tubercle
Symphysis

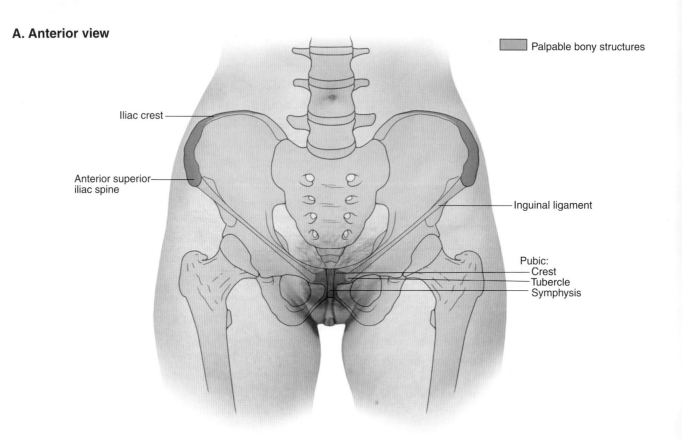

B. Posterior view

Iliac crest

Posterior superior
iliac spine

Sacrum

Coccyx

Ischial tuberosity

Greater sciatic notch

Ischial spine
Lesser sciatic notch

A. Anterior view

Palpable bony structures

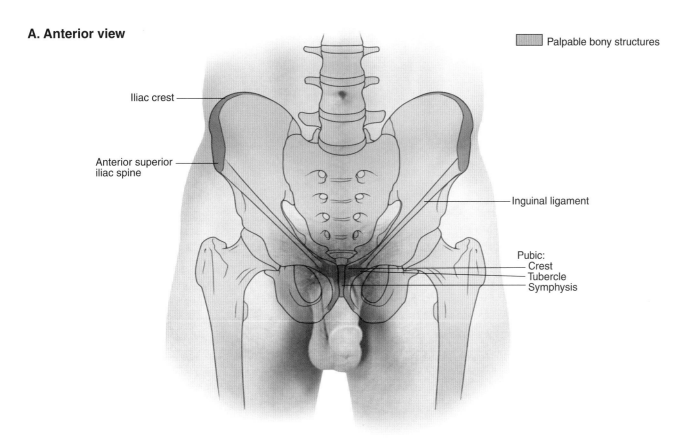

Iliac crest

Anterior superior
iliac spine

Inguinal ligament

Pubic:
Crest
Tubercle
Symphysis

B. Posterior view

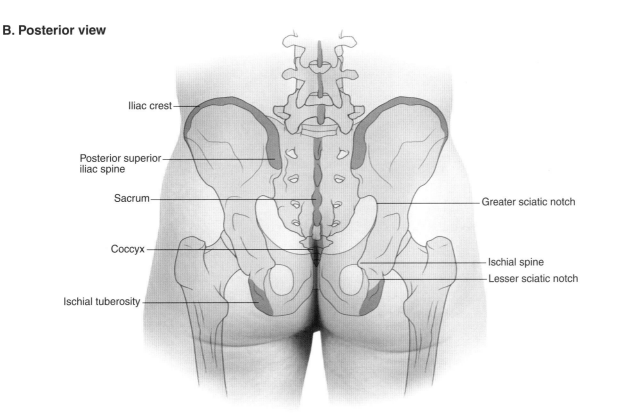

Iliac crest

Posterior superior
iliac spine

Sacrum

Greater sciatic notch

Coccyx

Ischial spine
Lesser sciatic notch

Ischial tuberosity

PLATE 6-03   **Skeleton of the Hip (Os Coxae)**

A. Medial view

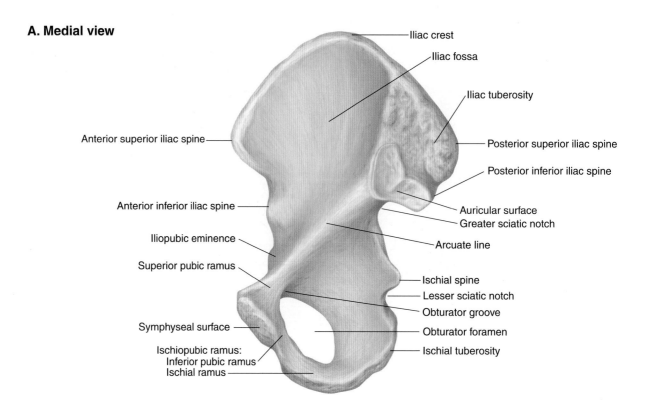

Iliac crest

Iliac fossa

Iliac tuberosity

Anterior superior iliac spine

Posterior superior iliac spine

Posterior inferior iliac spine

Anterior inferior iliac spine

Auricular surface

Greater sciatic notch

Iliopubic eminence

Arcuate line

Superior pubic ramus

Ischial spine

Lesser sciatic notch

Obturator groove

Symphyseal surface

Obturator foramen

Ischiopubic ramus:
  Inferior pubic ramus
  Ischial ramus

Ischial tuberosity

B. Lateral view

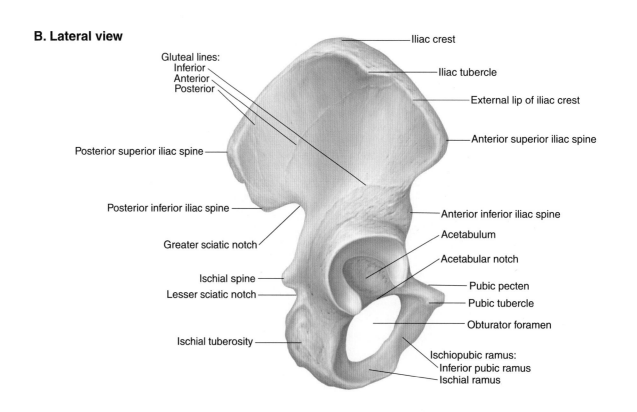

Gluteal lines:
  Inferior
  Anterior
  Posterior

Iliac crest

Iliac tubercle

External lip of iliac crest

Posterior superior iliac spine

Anterior superior iliac spine

Posterior inferior iliac spine

Anterior inferior iliac spine

Greater sciatic notch

Acetabulum

Acetabular notch

Ischial spine

Pubic pecten

Lesser sciatic notch

Pubic tubercle

Obturator foramen

Ischial tuberosity

Ischiopubic ramus:
  Inferior pubic ramus
  Ischial ramus

A. Anterior view

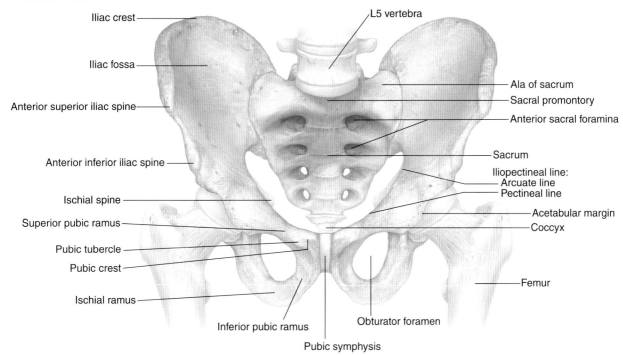

Iliac crest

Iliac fossa

Anterior superior iliac spine

Anterior inferior iliac spine

Ischial spine

Superior pubic ramus

Pubic tubercle

Pubic crest

Ischial ramus

Inferior pubic ramus

Pubic symphysis

L5 vertebra

Ala of sacrum

Sacral promontory

Anterior sacral foramina

Sacrum

Iliopectineal line:
Arcuate line
Pectineal line

Acetabular margin

Coccyx

Femur

Obturator foramen

B. Posterior view

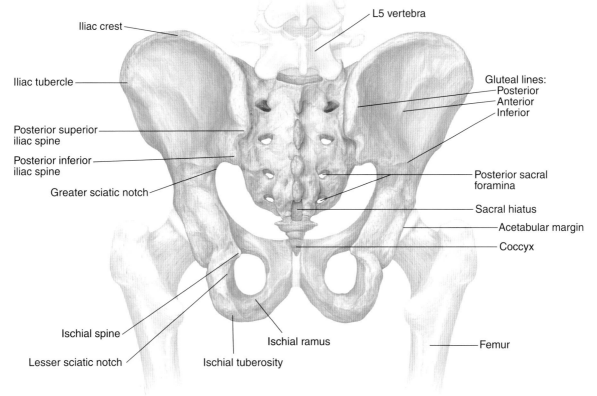

Iliac crest

Iliac tubercle

Posterior superior iliac spine

Posterior inferior iliac spine

Greater sciatic notch

Ischial spine

Lesser sciatic notch

Ischial tuberosity

Ischial ramus

L5 vertebra

Gluteal lines:
Posterior
Anterior
Inferior

Posterior sacral foramina

Sacral hiatus

Acetabular margin

Coccyx

Femur

PLATE 6-05   Comparison of Female and Male Pelves

A. Female, anterior view

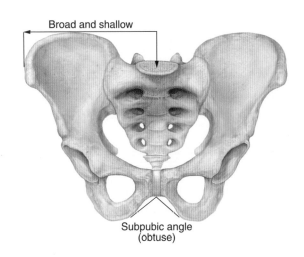

Broad and shallow

Subpubic angle
(obtuse)

B. Male, anterior view

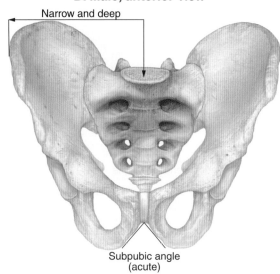

Narrow and deep

Subpubic angle
(acute)

C. Female, superior view

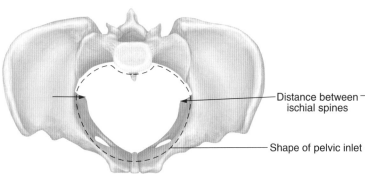

D. Male, superior view

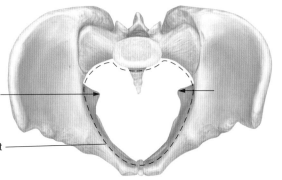

Distance between
ischial spines

Shape of pelvic inlet

E. Female, medial view

F. Male, medial view

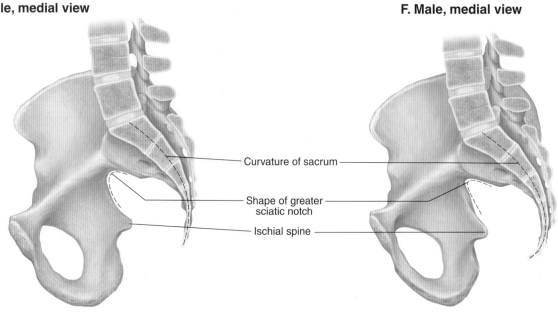

Curvature of sacrum

Shape of greater
sciatic notch

Ischial spine

A. Anterior view

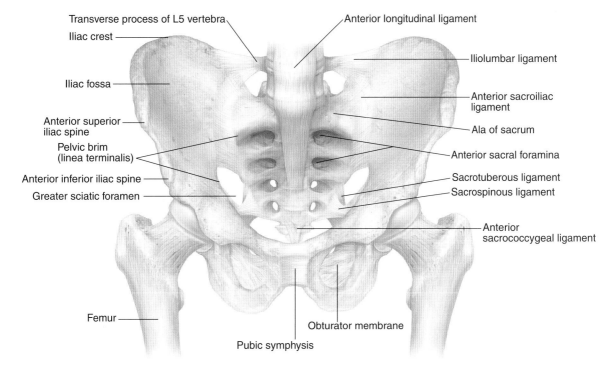

Transverse process of L5 vertebra

Iliac crest

Iliac fossa

Anterior superior iliac spine

Pelvic brim (linea terminalis)

Anterior inferior iliac spine

Greater sciatic foramen

Femur

Pubic symphysis

Anterior longitudinal ligament

Iliolumbar ligament

Anterior sacroiliac ligament

Ala of sacrum

Anterior sacral foramina

Sacrotuberous ligament

Sacrospinous ligament

Anterior sacrococcygeal ligament

Obturator membrane

B. Posterior view

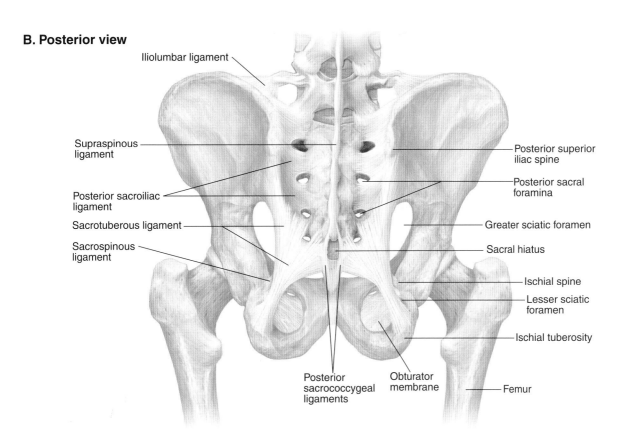

Iliolumbar ligament

Supraspinous ligament

Posterior sacroiliac ligament

Sacrotuberous ligament

Sacrospinous ligament

Posterior sacrococcygeal ligaments

Obturator membrane

Posterior superior iliac spine

Posterior sacral foramina

Greater sciatic foramen

Sacral hiatus

Ischial spine

Lesser sciatic foramen

Ischial tuberosity

Femur

PLATE 6-07   Pelvic Peritoneum, Superior View

A. Female

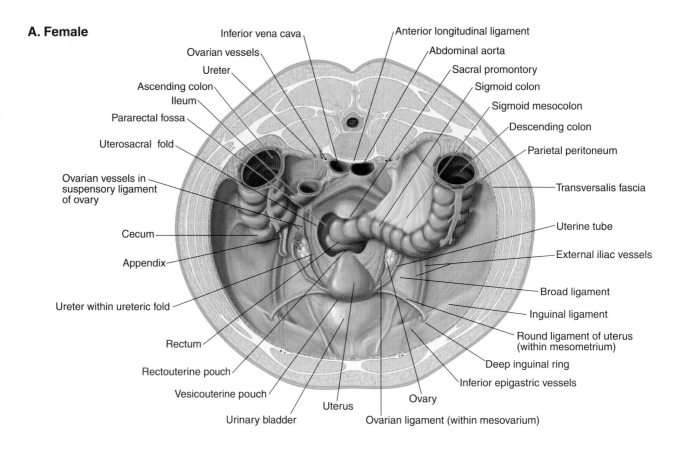

Inferior vena cava
Ovarian vessels
Ureter
Ascending colon
Ileum
Pararectal fossa
Uterosacral fold
Ovarian vessels in suspensory ligament of ovary
Cecum
Appendix
Ureter within ureteric fold
Rectum
Rectouterine pouch
Vesicouterine pouch
Urinary bladder
Uterus
Ovary
Ovarian ligament (within mesovarium)
Inferior epigastric vessels
Deep inguinal ring
Round ligament of uterus (within mesometrium)
Inguinal ligament
Broad ligament
External iliac vessels
Uterine tube
Transversalis fascia
Parietal peritoneum
Descending colon
Sigmoid mesocolon
Sigmoid colon
Sacral promontory
Abdominal aorta
Anterior longitudinal ligament

B. Male

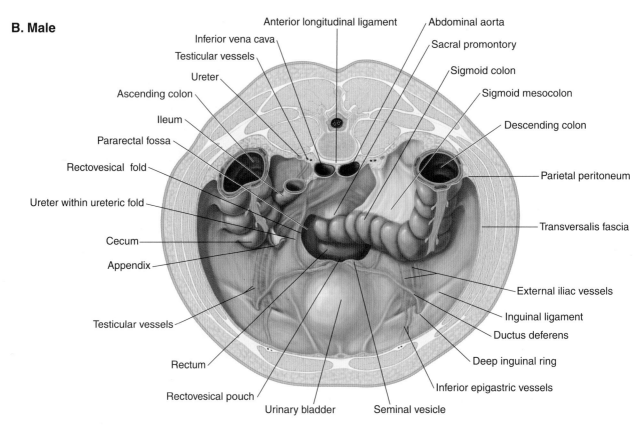

Anterior longitudinal ligament
Inferior vena cava
Testicular vessels
Ureter
Ascending colon
Ileum
Pararectal fossa
Rectovesical fold
Ureter within ureteric fold
Cecum
Appendix
Testicular vessels
Rectum
Rectovesical pouch
Urinary bladder
Seminal vesicle
Inferior epigastric vessels
Deep inguinal ring
Ductus deferens
Inguinal ligament
External iliac vessels
Transversalis fascia
Parietal peritoneum
Descending colon
Sigmoid mesocolon
Sigmoid colon
Sacral promontory
Abdominal aorta

A. Female

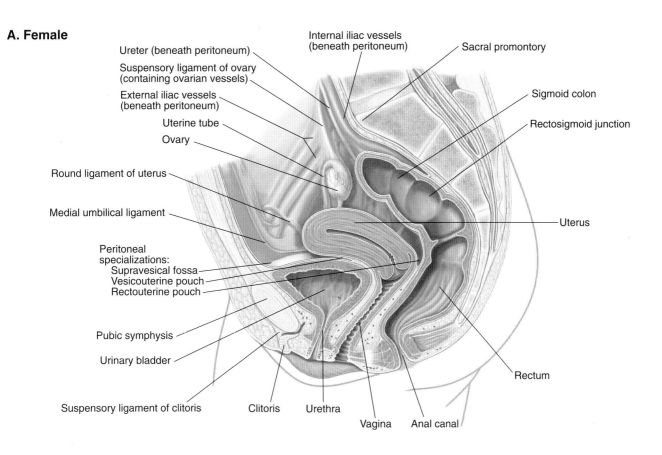

Ureter (beneath peritoneum)
Suspensory ligament of ovary (containing ovarian vessels)
External iliac vessels (beneath peritoneum)
Uterine tube
Ovary
Round ligament of uterus
Medial umbilical ligament
Peritoneal specializations:
Supravesical fossa
Vesicouterine pouch
Rectouterine pouch
Pubic symphysis
Urinary bladder
Suspensory ligament of clitoris
Clitoris
Urethra
Vagina
Anal canal
Internal iliac vessels (beneath peritoneum)
Sacral promontory
Sigmoid colon
Rectosigmoid junction
Uterus
Rectum

B. Male

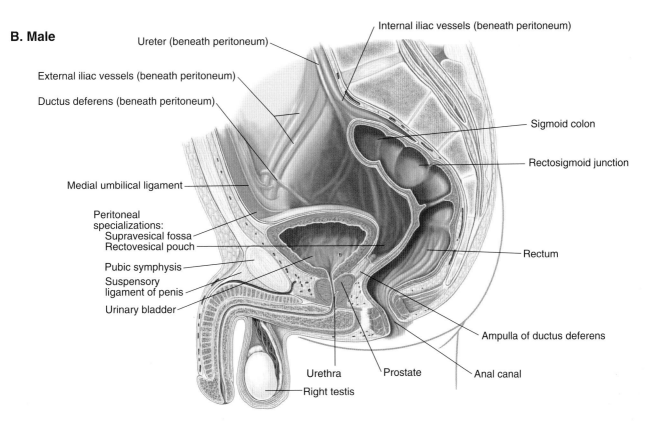

Ureter (beneath peritoneum)
External iliac vessels (beneath peritoneum)
Ductus deferens (beneath peritoneum)
Medial umbilical ligament
Peritoneal specializations:
Supravesical fossa
Rectovesical pouch
Pubic symphysis
Suspensory ligament of penis
Urinary bladder
Right testis
Urethra
Prostate
Internal iliac vessels (beneath peritoneum)
Sigmoid colon
Rectosigmoid junction
Rectum
Ampulla of ductus deferens
Anal canal

PLATE 6-09 **Urinary Bladder, Lateral View**

A. Female

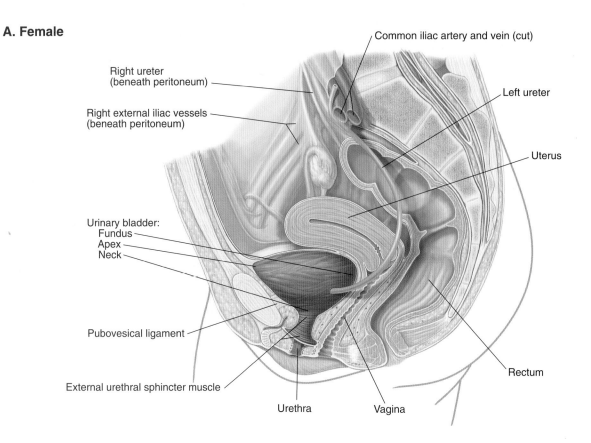

Common iliac artery and vein (cut)

Right ureter
(beneath peritoneum)

Right external iliac vessels
(beneath peritoneum)

Left ureter

Uterus

Urinary bladder:
Fundus
Apex
Neck

Pubovesical ligament

Rectum

External urethral sphincter muscle

Urethra

Vagina

B. Male

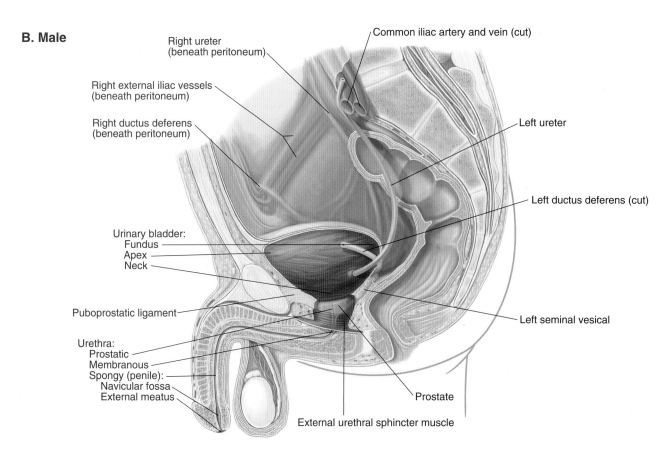

Common iliac artery and vein (cut)

Right ureter
(beneath peritoneum)

Right external iliac vessels
(beneath peritoneum)

Right ductus deferens
(beneath peritoneum)

Left ureter

Left ductus deferens (cut)

Urinary bladder:
Fundus
Apex
Neck

Puboprostatic ligament

Left seminal vesical

Urethra:
Prostatic
Membranous
Spongy (penile):
Navicular fossa
External meatus

Prostate

External urethral sphincter muscle

A. Female

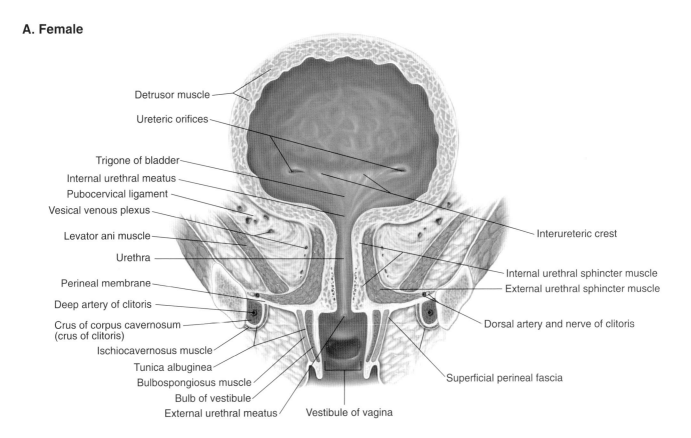

Detrusor muscle

Ureteric orifices

Trigone of bladder

Internal urethral meatus

Pubocervical ligament

Vesical venous plexus

Levator ani muscle

Urethra

Perineal membrane

Deep artery of clitoris

Crus of corpus cavernosum (crus of clitoris)

Ischiocavernosus muscle

Tunica albuginea

Bulbospongiosus muscle

Bulb of vestibule

External urethral meatus

Interureteric crest

Internal urethral sphincter muscle

External urethral sphincter muscle

Dorsal artery and nerve of clitoris

Superficial perineal fascia

Vestibule of vagina

B. Male

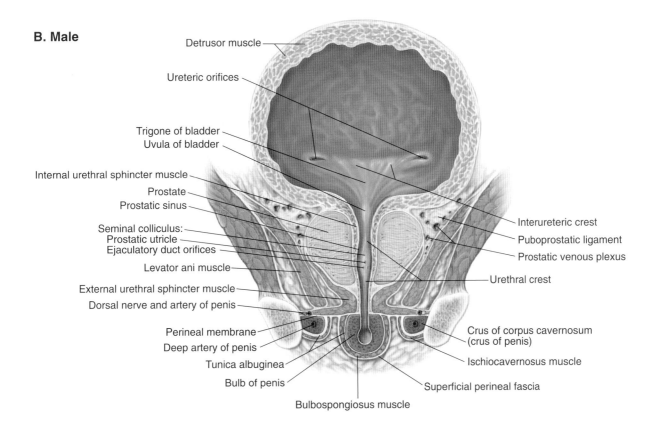

Detrusor muscle

Ureteric orifices

Trigone of bladder

Uvula of bladder

Internal urethral sphincter muscle

Prostate

Prostatic sinus

Seminal colliculus:
Prostatic utricle
Ejaculatory duct orifices

Levator ani muscle

External urethral sphincter muscle

Dorsal nerve and artery of penis

Perineal membrane

Deep artery of penis

Tunica albuginea

Bulb of penis

Bulbospongiosus muscle

Interureteric crest

Puboprostatic ligament

Prostatic venous plexus

Urethral crest

Crus of corpus cavernosum (crus of penis)

Ischiocavernosus muscle

Superficial perineal fascia

PLATE 6-11 **Uterus and Vagina I**

A. Lateral view

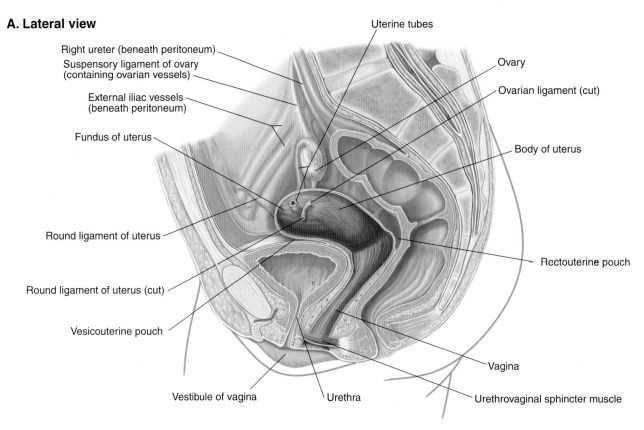

Right ureter (beneath peritoneum)

Suspensory ligament of ovary (containing ovarian vessels)

External iliac vessels (beneath peritoneum)

Fundus of uterus

Round ligament of uterus

Round ligament of uterus (cut)

Vesicouterine pouch

Vestibule of vagina

Urethra

Uterine tubes

Ovary

Ovarian ligament (cut)

Body of uterus

Rectouterine pouch

Vagina

Urethrovaginal sphincter muscle

B. Posterior view

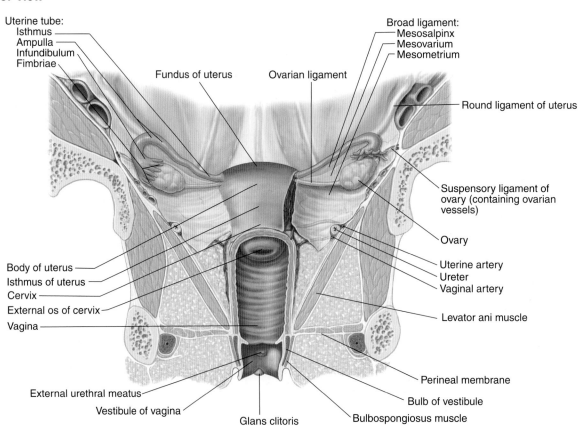

Uterine tube:
Isthmus
Ampulla
Infundibulum
Fimbriae

Fundus of uterus

Ovarian ligament

Broad ligament:
Mesosalpinx
Mesovarium
Mesometrium

Round ligament of uterus

Suspensory ligament of ovary (containing ovarian vessels)

Ovary

Uterine artery
Ureter
Vaginal artery

Levator ani muscle

Body of uterus

Isthmus of uterus

Cervix

External os of cervix

Vagina

Perineal membrane

External urethral meatus

Vestibule of vagina

Glans clitoris

Bulbospongiosus muscle

Bulb of vestibule

A. Posterior view

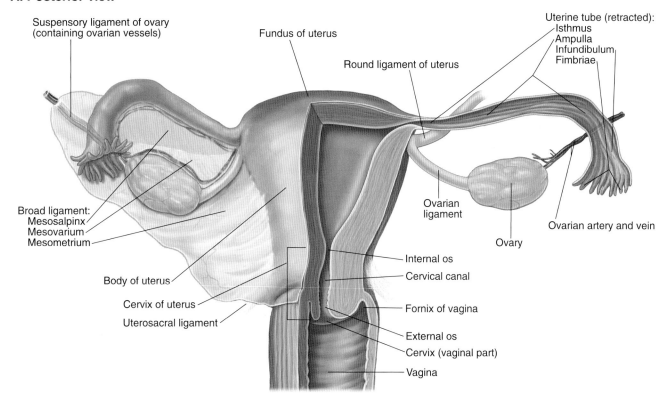

Suspensory ligament of ovary
(containing ovarian vessels)

Fundus of uterus

Round ligament of uterus

Uterine tube (retracted):
Isthmus
Ampulla
Infundibulum
Fimbriae

Broad ligament:
Mesosalpinx
Mesovarium
Mesometrium

Ovarian
ligament

Ovarian artery and vein

Ovary

Body of uterus

Internal os

Cervical canal

Cervix of uterus

Fornix of vagina

Uterosacral ligament

External os

Cervix (vaginal part)

Vagina

B. Hysterosalpingogram

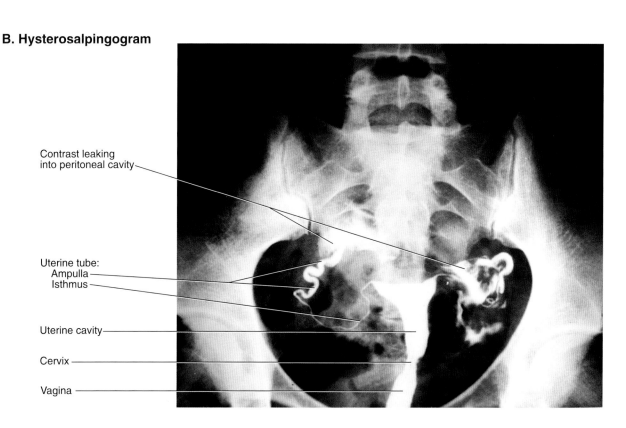

Contrast leaking
into peritoneal cavity

Uterine tube:
Ampulla
Isthmus

Uterine cavity

Cervix

Vagina

A. Normal positions

Anteflexed

Anteverted

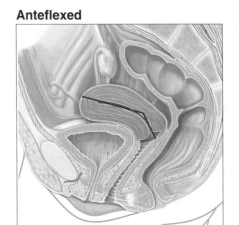
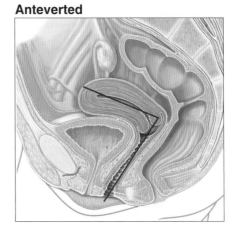

B. Retroflexed

C. Retroverted

D. Prolapsed

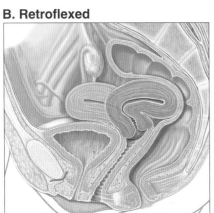
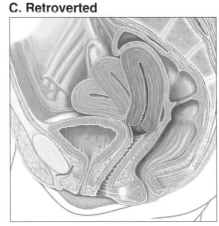
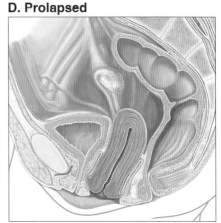

E. Supporting structures of the uterus, superior view

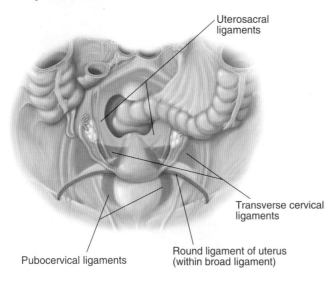

Uterosacral ligaments

Transverse cervical ligaments

Pubocervical ligaments

Round ligament of uterus (within broad ligament)

F. Supporting structures of the uterus, lateral view

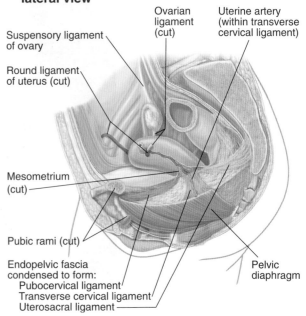

Ovarian ligament (cut)

Uterine artery (within transverse cervical ligament)

Suspensory ligament of ovary

Round ligament of uterus (cut)

Mesometrium (cut)

Pubic rami (cut)

Endopelvic fascia condensed to form:
  Pubocervical ligament
  Transverse cervical ligament
  Uterosacral ligament

Pelvic diaphragm

A. Posterior view

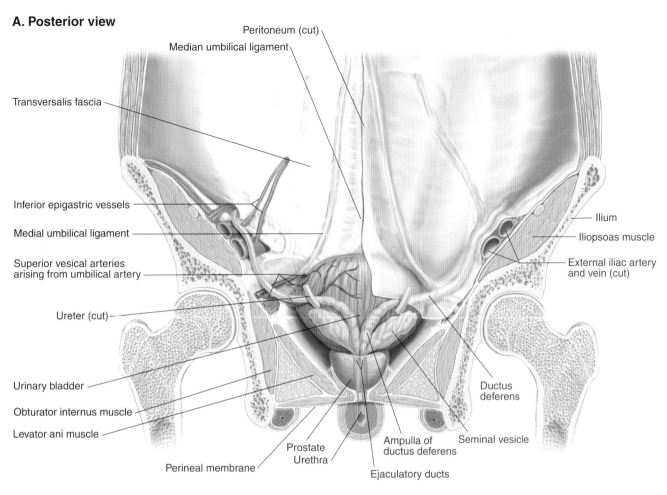

Peritoneum (cut)
Median umbilical ligament
Transversalis fascia
Inferior epigastric vessels
Medial umbilical ligament
Superior vesical arteries arising from umbilical artery
Ureter (cut)
Urinary bladder
Obturator internus muscle
Levator ani muscle
Perineal membrane
Prostate
Urethra
Ejaculatory ducts
Ampulla of ductus deferens
Seminal vesicle
Ductus deferens
External iliac artery and vein (cut)
Iliopsoas muscle
Ilium

B. Vasogram

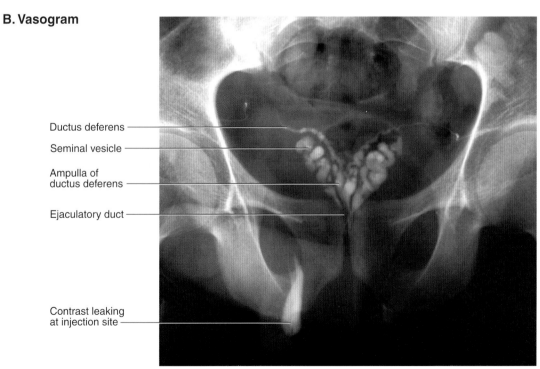

Ductus deferens
Seminal vesicle
Ampulla of ductus deferens
Ejaculatory duct
Contrast leaking at injection site

PLATE 6-15   Rectum and Anal Canal, Relationships

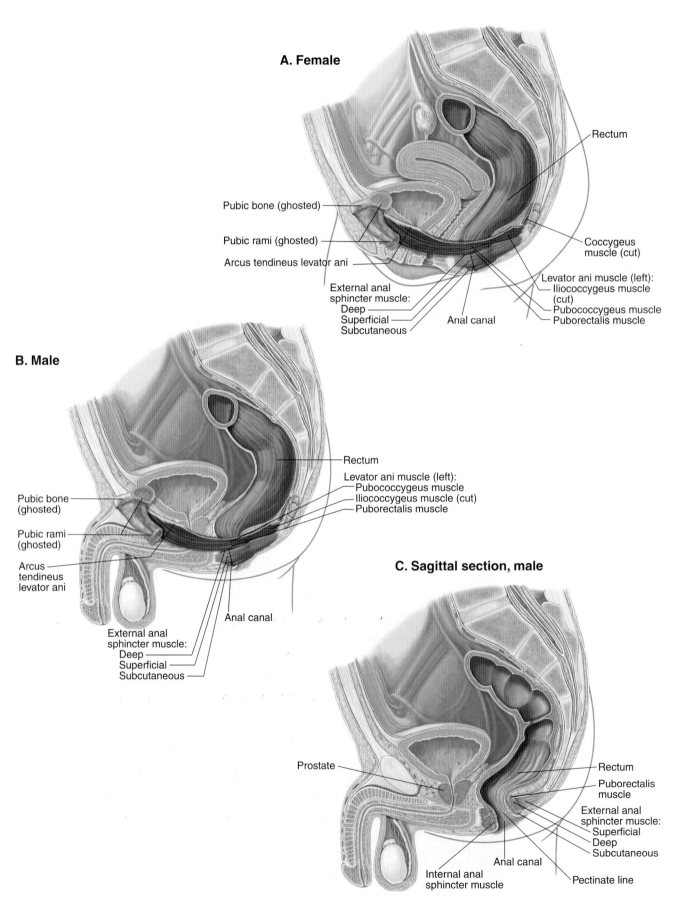

A. Female

Rectum

Pubic bone (ghosted)

Pubic rami (ghosted)

Arcus tendineus levator ani

External anal
sphincter muscle:
Deep
Superficial
Subcutaneous

Anal canal

Coccygeus
muscle (cut)

Levator ani muscle (left):
Iliococcygeus muscle
(cut)
Pubococcygeus muscle
Puborectalis muscle

B. Male

Rectum

Levator ani muscle (left):
Pubococcygeus muscle
Iliococcygeus muscle (cut)
Puborectalis muscle

Pubic bone
(ghosted)

Pubic rami
(ghosted)

Arcus
tendineus
levator ani

External anal
sphincter muscle:
Deep
Superficial
Subcutaneous

Anal canal

C. Sagittal section, male

Prostate

Rectum

Puborectalis
muscle

External anal
sphincter muscle:
Superficial
Deep
Subcutaneous

Anal canal

Internal anal
sphincter muscle

Pectinate line

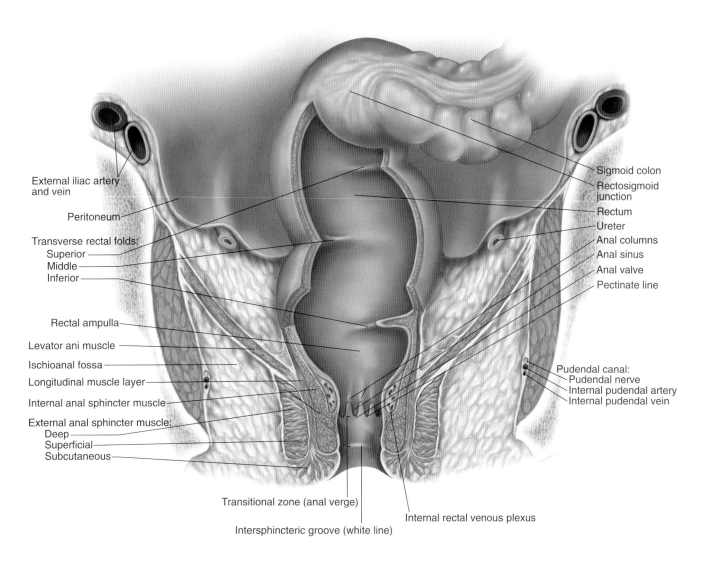

External iliac artery and vein

Peritoneum

Transverse rectal folds:
Superior
Middle
Inferior

Rectal ampulla

Levator ani muscle

Ischioanal fossa

Longitudinal muscle layer

Internal anal sphincter muscle

External anal sphincter muscle:
Deep
Superficial
Subcutaneous

Transitional zone (anal verge)

Intersphincteric groove (white line)

Sigmoid colon

Rectosigmoid junction

Rectum

Ureter

Anal columns

Anal sinus

Anal valve

Pectinate line

Pudendal canal:
Pudendal nerve
Internal pudendal artery
Internal pudendal vein

Internal rectal venous plexus

PLATE 6-17   **Blood Supply of the Pelvis**

A. Female

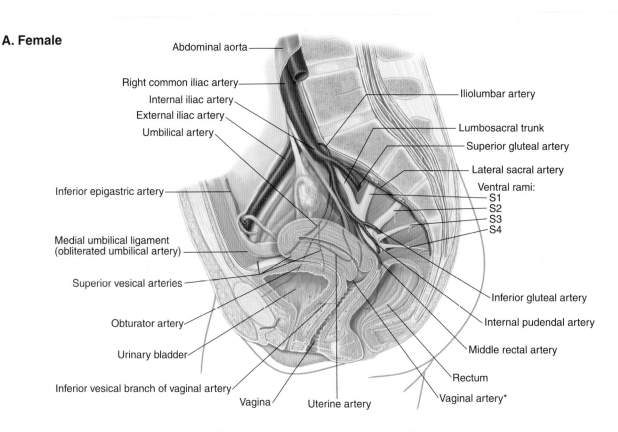

Abdominal aorta

Right common iliac artery

Internal iliac artery

External iliac artery

Umbilical artery

Iliolumbar artery

Lumbosacral trunk

Superior gluteal artery

Lateral sacral artery

Ventral rami:
S1
S2
S3
S4

Inferior epigastric artery

Medial umbilical ligament
(obliterated umbilical artery)

Superior vesical arteries

Obturator artery

Urinary bladder

Inferior vesical branch of vaginal artery

Vagina

Uterine artery

Inferior gluteal artery

Internal pudendal artery

Middle rectal artery

Rectum

Vaginal artery*

*Vaginal artery arises from uterine artery in 11% of cases

B. Male

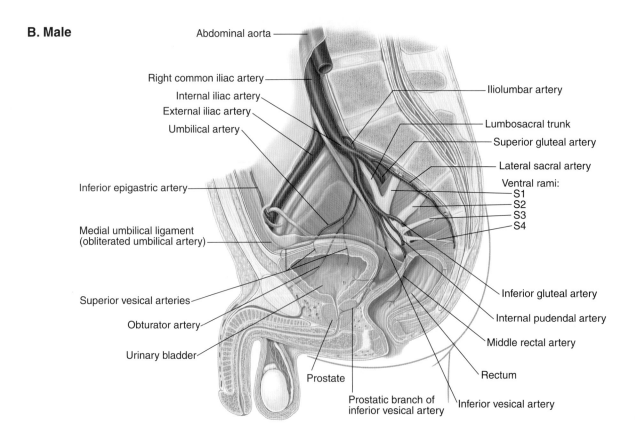

Abdominal aorta

Right common iliac artery

Internal iliac artery

External iliac artery

Umbilical artery

Iliolumbar artery

Lumbosacral trunk

Superior gluteal artery

Lateral sacral artery

Ventral rami:
S1
S2
S3
S4

Inferior epigastric artery

Medial umbilical ligament
(obliterated umbilical artery)

Superior vesical arteries

Obturator artery

Urinary bladder

Prostate

Prostatic branch of
inferior vesical artery

Inferior gluteal artery

Internal pudendal artery

Middle rectal artery

Rectum

Inferior vesical artery

A. Medial view

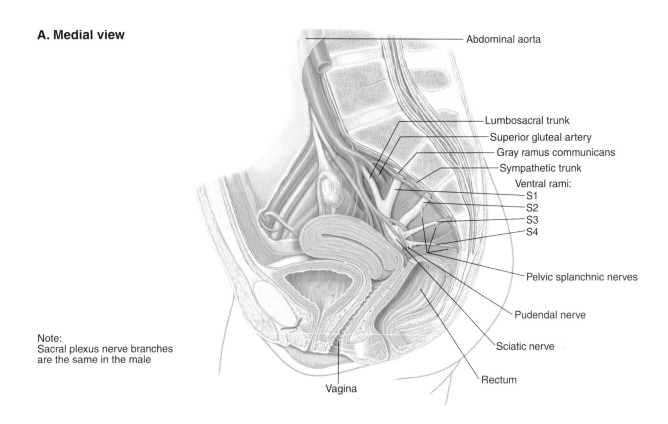

Abdominal aorta

Lumbosacral trunk
Superior gluteal artery
Gray ramus communicans
Sympathetic trunk
Ventral rami:
S1
S2
S3
S4

Pelvic splanchnic nerves

Pudendal nerve

Sciatic nerve

Rectum

Vagina

Note:
Sacral plexus nerve branches
are the same in the male

B. Anterior view

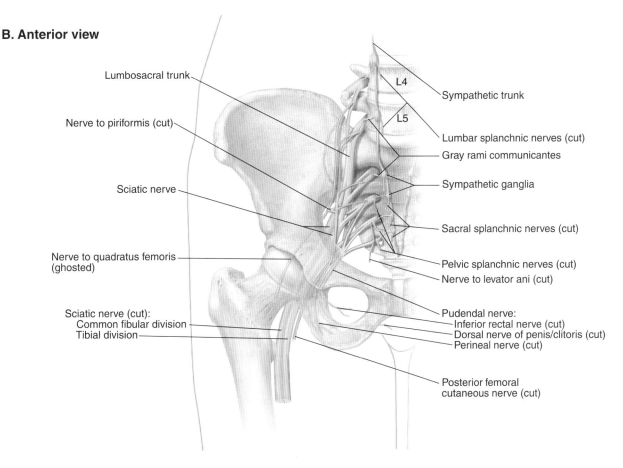

Lumbosacral trunk

Nerve to piriformis (cut)

Sciatic nerve

Nerve to quadratus femoris
(ghosted)

Sciatic nerve (cut):
Common fibular division
Tibial division

L4

L5

Sympathetic trunk

Lumbar splanchnic nerves (cut)
Gray rami communicantes

Sympathetic ganglia

Sacral splanchnic nerves (cut)

Pelvic splanchnic nerves (cut)
Nerve to levator ani (cut)

Pudendal nerve:
Inferior rectal nerve (cut)
Dorsal nerve of penis/clitoris (cut)
Perineal nerve (cut)

Posterior femoral
cutaneous nerve (cut)

PLATE 6-19 **Autonomic Nerves of the Pelvis**

A. Female

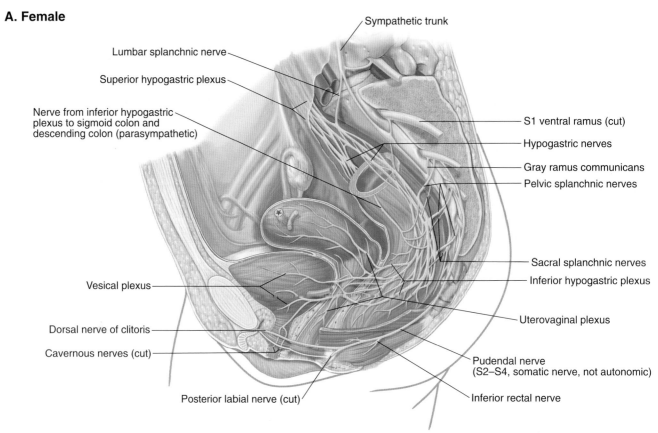

Lumbar splanchnic nerve

Superior hypogastric plexus

Nerve from inferior hypogastric plexus to sigmoid colon and descending colon (parasympathetic)

Vesical plexus

Dorsal nerve of clitoris

Cavernous nerves (cut)

Posterior labial nerve (cut)

Sympathetic trunk

S1 ventral ramus (cut)

Hypogastric nerves

Gray ramus communicans

Pelvic splanchnic nerves

Sacral splanchnic nerves

Inferior hypogastric plexus

Uterovaginal plexus

Pudendal nerve (S2–S4, somatic nerve, not autonomic)

Inferior rectal nerve

B. Male

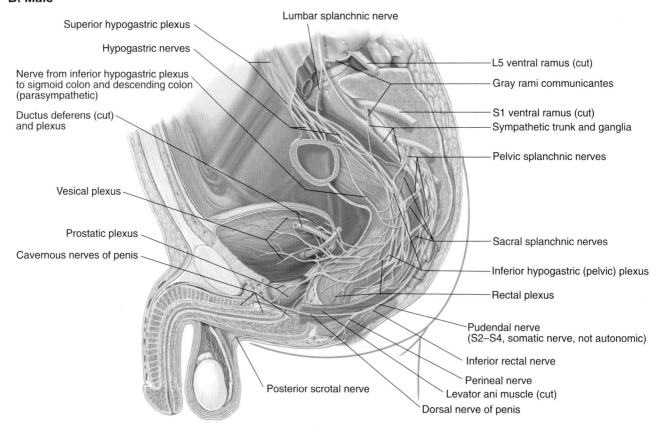

Superior hypogastric plexus

Hypogastric nerves

Nerve from inferior hypogastric plexus to sigmoid colon and descending colon (parasympathetic)

Ductus deferens (cut) and plexus

Vesical plexus

Prostatic plexus

Cavernous nerves of penis

Posterior scrotal nerve

Lumbar splanchnic nerve

L5 ventral ramus (cut)

Gray rami communicantes

S1 ventral ramus (cut)

Sympathetic trunk and ganglia

Pelvic splanchnic nerves

Sacral splanchnic nerves

Inferior hypogastric (pelvic) plexus

Rectal plexus

Pudendal nerve (S2–S4, somatic nerve, not autonomic)

Inferior rectal nerve

Perineal nerve

Levator ani muscle (cut)

Dorsal nerve of penis

A. Female

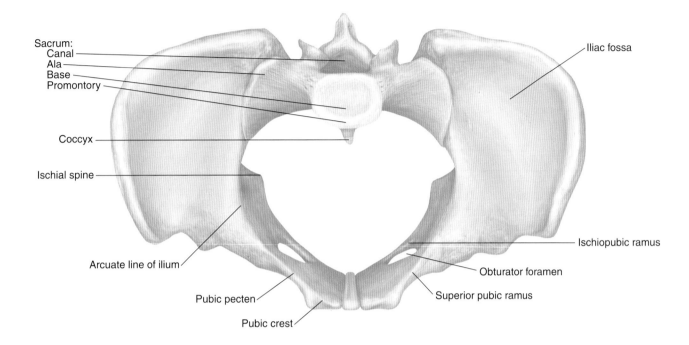

Sacrum:
Canal
Ala
Base
Promontory

Coccyx

Ischial spine

Arcuate line of ilium

Pubic pecten

Pubic crest

Iliac fossa

Ischiopubic ramus

Obturator foramen

Superior pubic ramus

B. Male

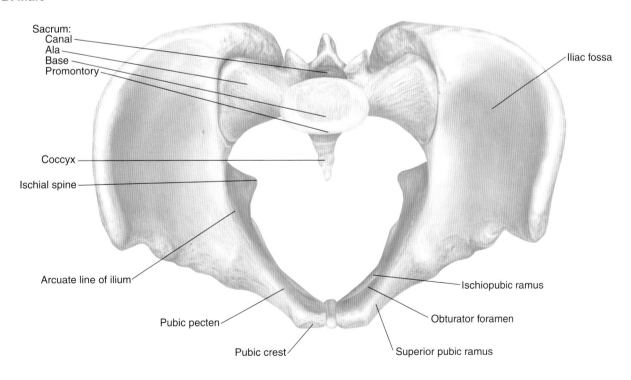

Sacrum:
Canal
Ala
Base
Promontory

Coccyx

Ischial spine

Arcuate line of ilium

Pubic pecten

Pubic crest

Iliac fossa

Ischiopubic ramus

Obturator foramen

Superior pubic ramus

PLATE 6-21   Pelvic Diaphragm, Superior View

A. Female

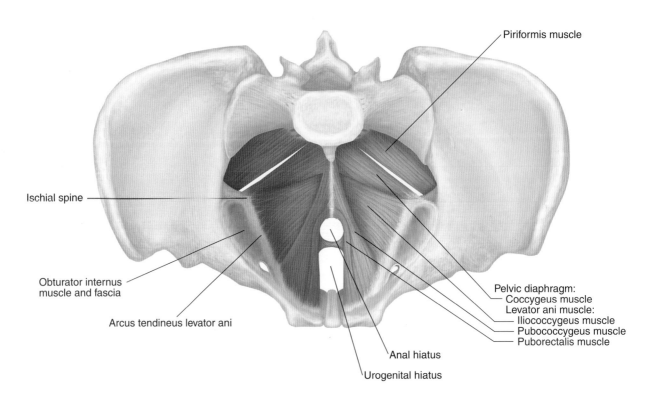

Piriformis muscle

Ischial spine

Obturator internus
muscle and fascia

Arcus tendineus levator ani

Pelvic diaphragm:
   Coccygeus muscle
Levator ani muscle:
   Iliococcygeus muscle
   Pubococcygeus muscle
   Puborectalis muscle

Anal hiatus

Urogenital hiatus

B. Male

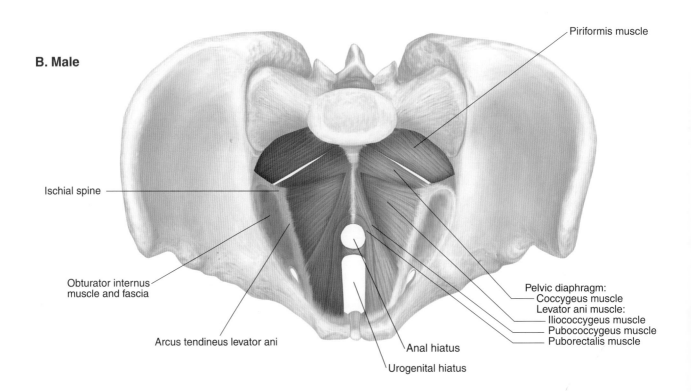

Piriformis muscle

Ischial spine

Obturator internus
muscle and fascia

Arcus tendineus levator ani

Pelvic diaphragm:
   Coccygeus muscle
Levator ani muscle:
   Iliococcygeus muscle
   Pubococcygeus muscle
   Puborectalis muscle

Anal hiatus

Urogenital hiatus

A. Medial view

Obturator internus muscle and fascia

Arcus tendineus levator ani

Obturator canal

Piriformis muscle

Ischial spine

Coccygeus muscle

Levator ani muscle:
— Iliococcygeus muscle
— Pubococcygeus muscle
— Puborectalis muscle

B. Relationships to nerves and vessels, medial view

Iliac arteries:
Common
Internal
External

Sacral plexus

C. Lateral view

Piriformis muscle

Sacrospinous ligament (ghosted)

Coccygeus muscle (seen through sacrospinous ligament)

Sacrotuberous ligament (cut)

Arcus tendineus levator ani

Levator ani muscle

D. Relationships to nerves and vessels, lateral view

Superior gluteal artery and nerve

Inferior gluteal artery and nerve

Sciatic nerve (cut)

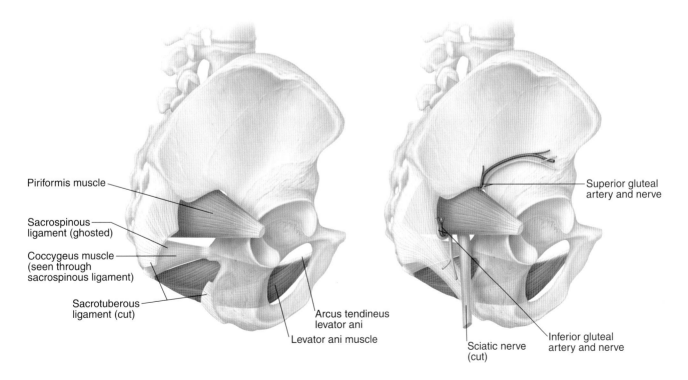

PLATE 6-23 Pelvic Diaphragm, Inferior View

A. Female

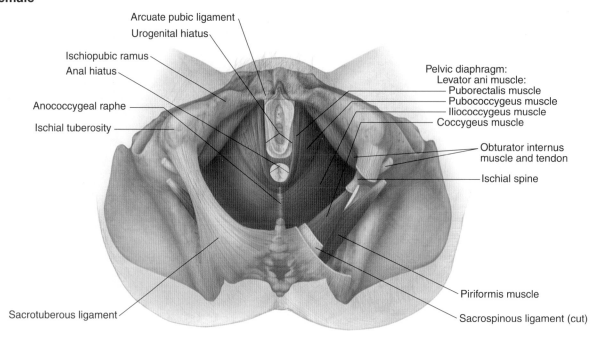

Arcuate pubic ligament
Urogenital hiatus
Ischiopubic ramus
Anal hiatus
Anococcygeal raphe
Ischial tuberosity

Pelvic diaphragm:
Levator ani muscle:
Puborectalis muscle
Pubococcygeus muscle
Iliococcygeus muscle
Coccygeus muscle

Obturator internus
muscle and tendon

Ischial spine

Piriformis muscle

Sacrotuberous ligament

Sacrospinous ligament (cut)

B. Male

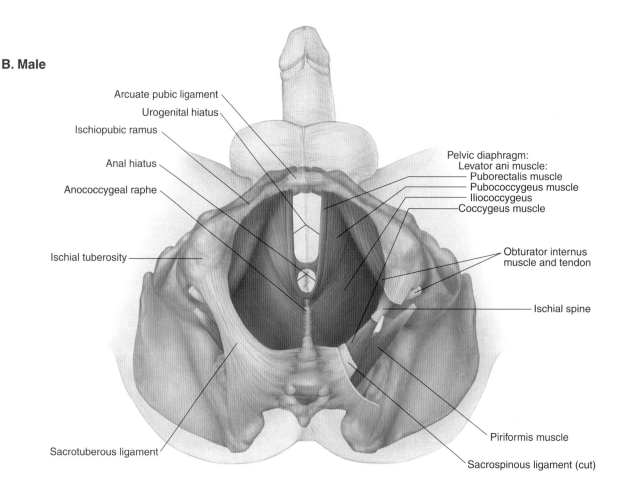

Arcuate pubic ligament
Urogenital hiatus
Ischiopubic ramus
Anal hiatus
Anococcygeal raphe

Ischial tuberosity

Pelvic diaphragm:
Levator ani muscle:
Puborectalis muscle
Pubococcygeus muscle
Iliococcygeus
Coccygeus muscle

Obturator internus
muscle and tendon

Ischial spine

Piriformis muscle

Sacrotuberous ligament

Sacrospinous ligament (cut)

A. Female

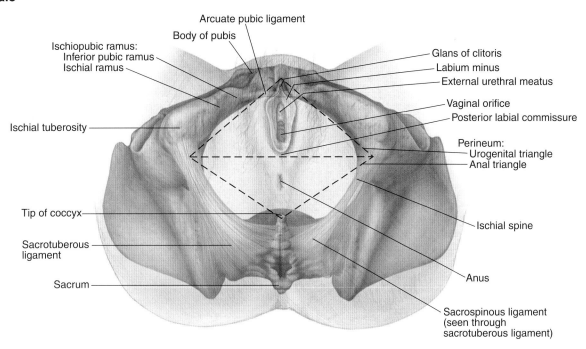

Arcuate pubic ligament

Body of pubis

Ischiopubic ramus:
Inferior pubic ramus
Ischial ramus

Glans of clitoris

Labium minus

External urethral meatus

Vaginal orifice

Posterior labial commissure

Ischial tuberosity

Perineum:
Urogenital triangle
Anal triangle

Tip of coccyx

Ischial spine

Sacrotuberous
ligament

Anus

Sacrum

Sacrospinous ligament
(seen through
sacrotuberous ligament)

B. Male

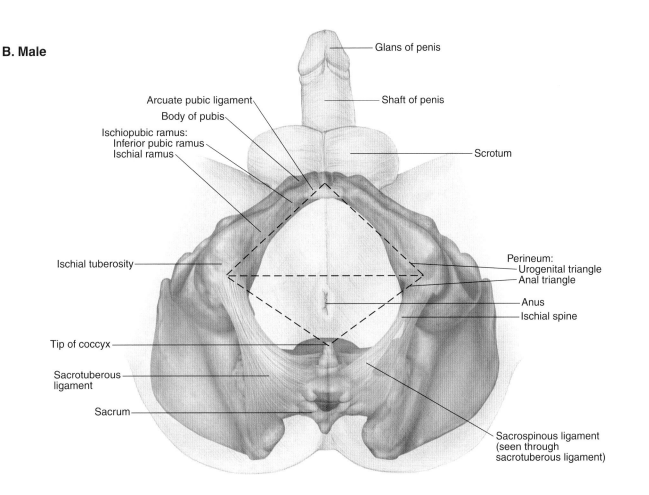

Glans of penis

Arcuate pubic ligament

Body of pubis

Ischiopubic ramus:
Inferior pubic ramus
Ischial ramus

Shaft of penis

Scrotum

Ischial tuberosity

Perineum:
Urogenital triangle
Anal triangle

Anus

Ischial spine

Tip of coccyx

Sacrotuberous
ligament

Sacrum

Sacrospinous ligament
(seen through
sacrotuberous ligament)

PLATE 6-25   Perineum, Surface Anatomy

A. Female

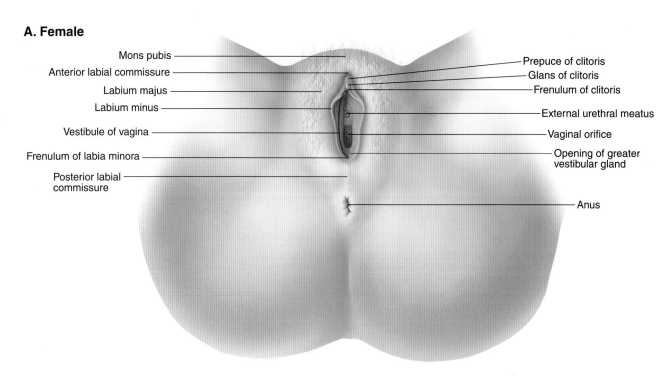

Mons pubis

Anterior labial commissure

Labium majus

Labium minus

Vestibule of vagina

Frenulum of labia minora

Posterior labial
commissure

Prepuce of clitoris

Glans of clitoris

Frenulum of clitoris

External urethral meatus

Vaginal orifice

Opening of greater
vestibular gland

Anus

B. Male

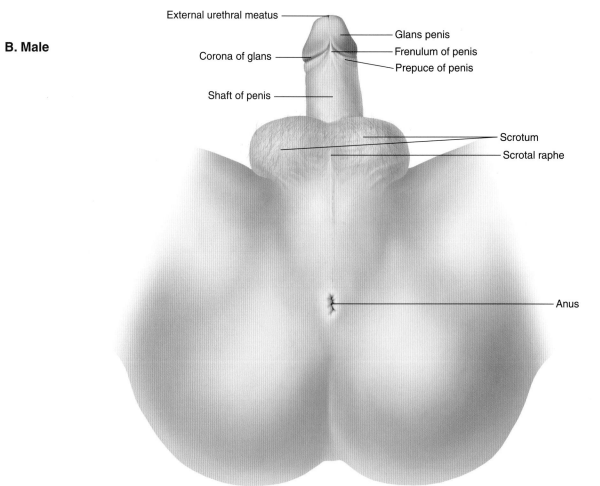

External urethral meatus

Glans penis

Corona of glans

Frenulum of penis

Prepuce of penis

Shaft of penis

Scrotum

Scrotal raphe

Anus

A. Female

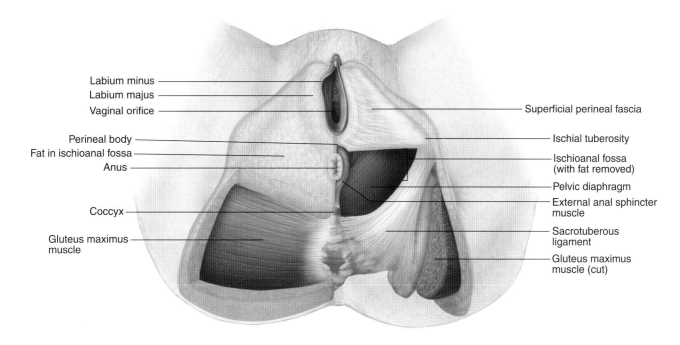

Labium minus
Labium majus
Vaginal orifice
Perineal body
Fat in ischioanal fossa
Anus
Coccyx
Gluteus maximus muscle

Superficial perineal fascia
Ischial tuberosity
Ischioanal fossa (with fat removed)
Pelvic diaphragm
External anal sphincter muscle
Sacrotuberous ligament
Gluteus maximus muscle (cut)

B. Male

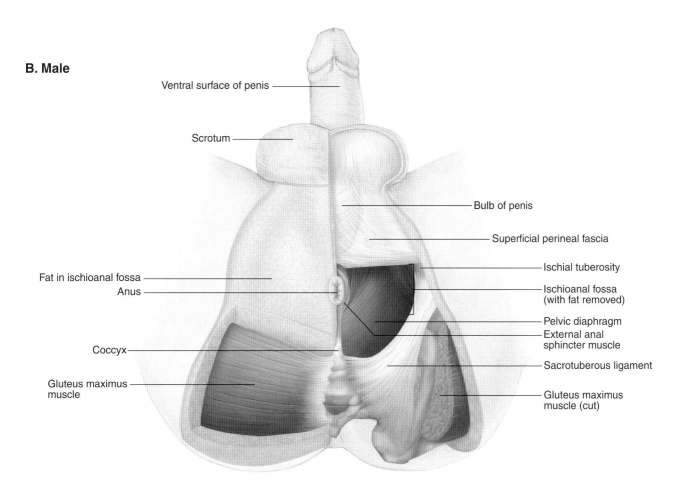

Ventral surface of penis
Scrotum
Fat in ischioanal fossa
Anus
Coccyx
Gluteus maximus muscle

Bulb of penis
Superficial perineal fascia
Ischial tuberosity
Ischioanal fossa (with fat removed)
Pelvic diaphragm
External anal sphincter muscle
Sacrotuberous ligament
Gluteus maximus muscle (cut)

PLATE 6-27   Perineum, Intermediate Dissection

A. Female

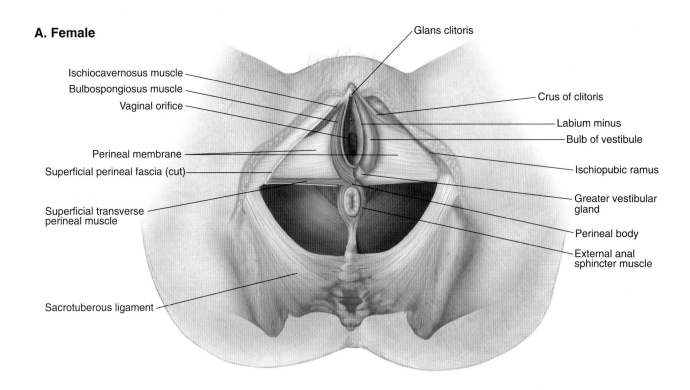

Ischiocavernosus muscle

Bulbospongiosus muscle

Vaginal orifice

Perineal membrane

Superficial perineal fascia (cut)

Superficial transverse perineal muscle

Sacrotuberous ligament

Glans clitoris

Crus of clitoris

Labium minus

Bulb of vestibule

Ischiopubic ramus

Greater vestibular gland

Perineal body

External anal sphincter muscle

B. Male

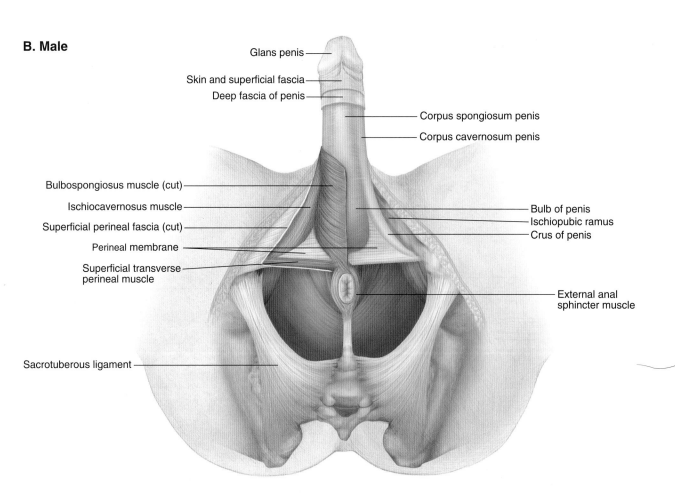

Glans penis

Skin and superficial fascia

Deep fascia of penis

Corpus spongiosum penis

Corpus cavernosum penis

Bulbospongiosus muscle (cut)

Ischiocavernosus muscle

Superficial perineal fascia (cut)

Perineal membrane

Superficial transverse perineal muscle

Sacrotuberous ligament

Bulb of penis

Ischiopubic ramus

Crus of penis

External anal sphincter muscle

A. Female

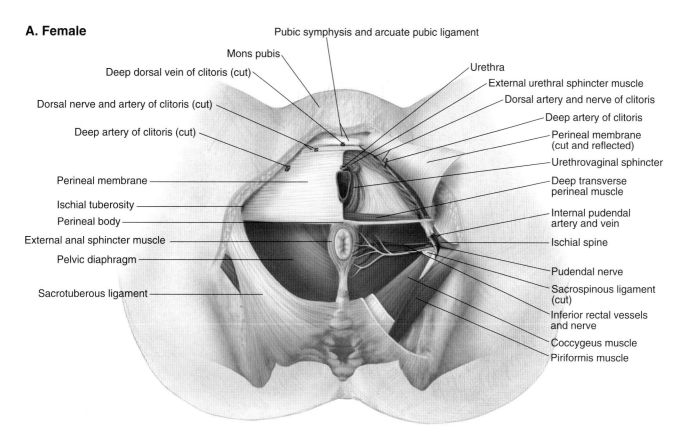

Pubic symphysis and arcuate pubic ligament

Mons pubis

Deep dorsal vein of clitoris (cut)

Dorsal nerve and artery of clitoris (cut)

Deep artery of clitoris (cut)

Perineal membrane

Ischial tuberosity

Perineal body

External anal sphincter muscle

Pelvic diaphragm

Sacrotuberous ligament

Urethra

External urethral sphincter muscle

Dorsal artery and nerve of clitoris

Deep artery of clitoris

Perineal membrane (cut and reflected)

Urethrovaginal sphincter

Deep transverse perineal muscle

Internal pudendal artery and vein

Ischial spine

Pudendal nerve

Sacrospinous ligament (cut)

Inferior rectal vessels and nerve

Coccygeus muscle

Piriformis muscle

B. Male

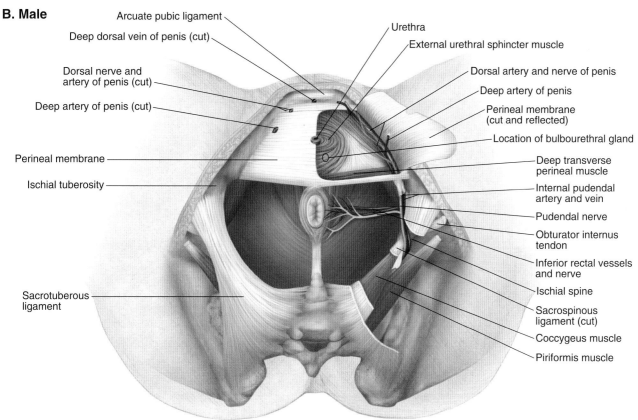

Arcuate pubic ligament

Deep dorsal vein of penis (cut)

Dorsal nerve and artery of penis (cut)

Deep artery of penis (cut)

Perineal membrane

Ischial tuberosity

Sacrotuberous ligament

Urethra

External urethral sphincter muscle

Dorsal artery and nerve of penis

Deep artery of penis

Perineal membrane (cut and reflected)

Location of bulbourethral gland

Deep transverse perineal muscle

Internal pudendal artery and vein

Pudendal nerve

Obturator internus tendon

Inferior rectal vessels and nerve

Ischial spine

Sacrospinous ligament (cut)

Coccygeus muscle

Piriformis muscle

PLATE 6-29   **Arteries of the Perineum**

A. Female

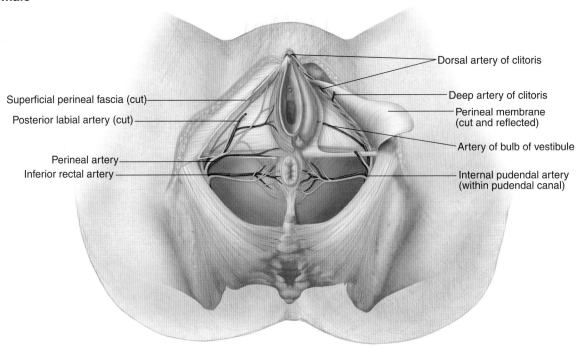

Dorsal artery of clitoris

Deep artery of clitoris

Superficial perineal fascia (cut)

Posterior labial artery (cut)

Perineal membrane
(cut and reflected)

Artery of bulb of vestibule

Perineal artery

Inferior rectal artery

Internal pudendal artery
(within pudendal canal)

B. Male

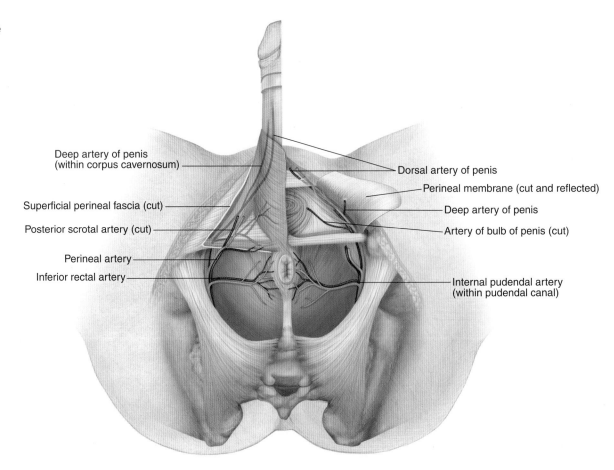

Deep artery of penis
(within corpus cavernosum)

Dorsal artery of penis

Perineal membrane (cut and reflected)

Superficial perineal fascia (cut)

Deep artery of penis

Posterior scrotal artery (cut)

Artery of bulb of penis (cut)

Perineal artery

Inferior rectal artery

Internal pudendal artery
(within pudendal canal)

A. Female

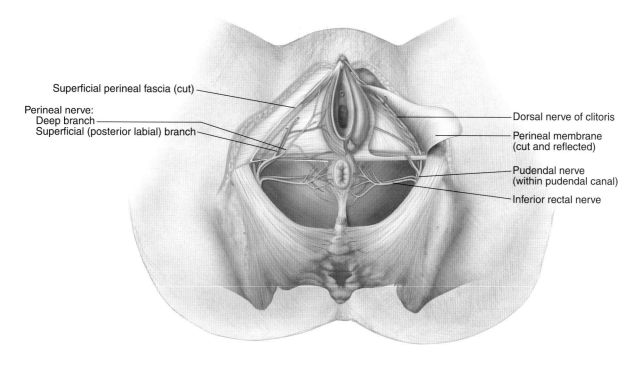

Superficial perineal fascia (cut)

Perineal nerve:
Deep branch
Superficial (posterior labial) branch

Dorsal nerve of clitoris

Perineal membrane
(cut and reflected)

Pudendal nerve
(within pudendal canal)

Inferior rectal nerve

B. Male

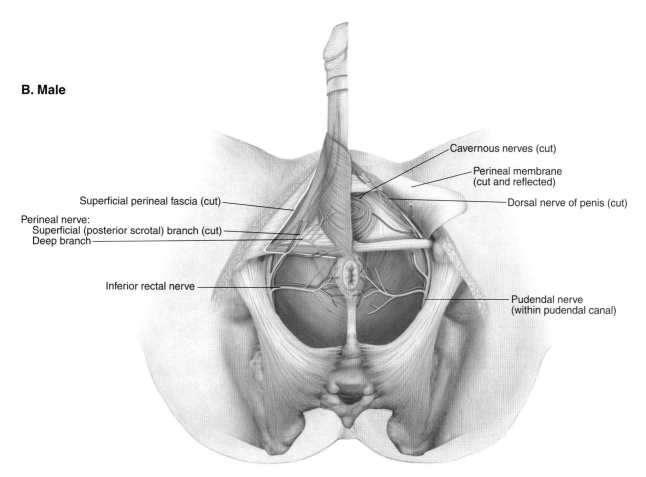

Cavernous nerves (cut)

Perineal membrane
(cut and reflected)

Dorsal nerve of penis (cut)

Superficial perineal fascia (cut)

Perineal nerve:
Superficial (posterior scrotal) branch (cut)
Deep branch

Inferior rectal nerve

Pudendal nerve
(within pudendal canal)

PLATE 6-31   Penis and Testes

A. Anterior view

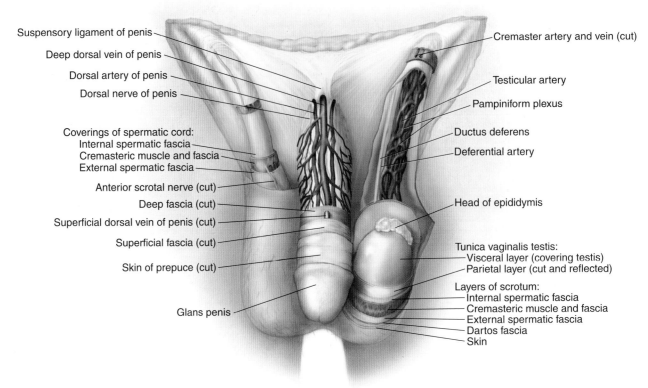

Suspensory ligament of penis

Deep dorsal vein of penis

Dorsal artery of penis

Dorsal nerve of penis

Coverings of spermatic cord:
Internal spermatic fascia
Cremasteric muscle and fascia
External spermatic fascia

Anterior scrotal nerve (cut)

Deep fascia (cut)

Superficial dorsal vein of penis (cut)

Superficial fascia (cut)

Skin of prepuce (cut)

Glans penis

Cremaster artery and vein (cut)

Testicular artery

Pampiniform plexus

Ductus deferens

Deferential artery

Head of epididymis

Tunica vaginalis testis:
Visceral layer (covering testis)
Parietal layer (cut and reflected)

Layers of scrotum:
Internal spermatic fascia
Cremasteric muscle and fascia
External spermatic fascia
Dartos fascia
Skin

B. Lateral view

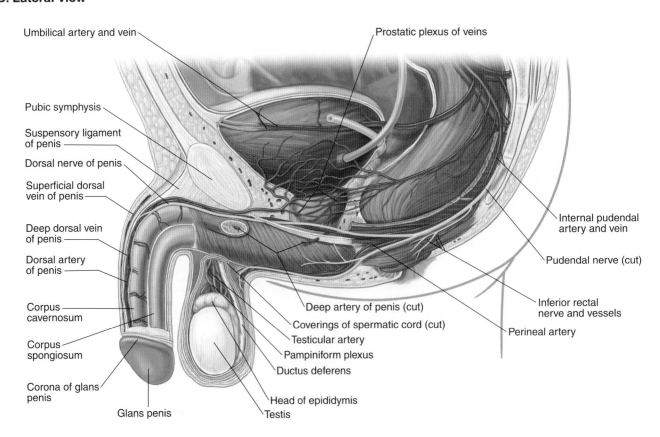

Umbilical artery and vein

Pubic symphysis

Suspensory ligament
of penis

Dorsal nerve of penis

Superficial dorsal
vein of penis

Deep dorsal vein
of penis

Dorsal artery
of penis

Corpus
cavernosum

Corpus
spongiosum

Corona of glans
penis

Glans penis

Prostatic plexus of veins

Internal pudendal
artery and vein

Pudendal nerve (cut)

Inferior rectal
nerve and vessels

Perineal artery

Deep artery of penis (cut)

Coverings of spermatic cord (cut)

Testicular artery

Pampiniform plexus

Ductus deferens

Head of epididymis

Testis

A. Orientation

Plane of section B

B. Section through penis

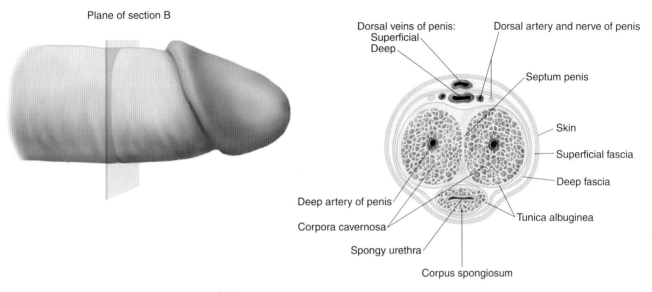

Dorsal veins of penis:
Superficial
Deep

Dorsal artery and nerve of penis

Septum penis

Skin

Superficial fascia

Deep fascia

Deep artery of penis

Tunica albuginea

Corpora cavernosa

Spongy urethra

Corpus spongiosum

C. Section through testis

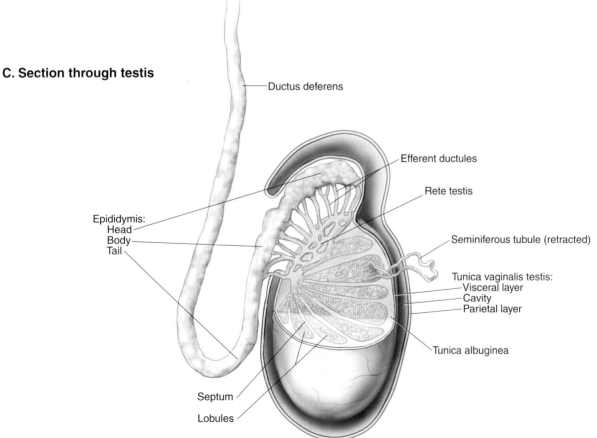

Ductus deferens

Efferent ductules

Rete testis

Epididymis:
Head
Body
Tail

Seminiferous tubule (retracted)

Tunica vaginalis testis:
Visceral layer
Cavity
Parietal layer

Tunica albuginea

Septum

Lobules

PLATE 6-33   **Lymphatics of the Pelvis and Perineum, Female**

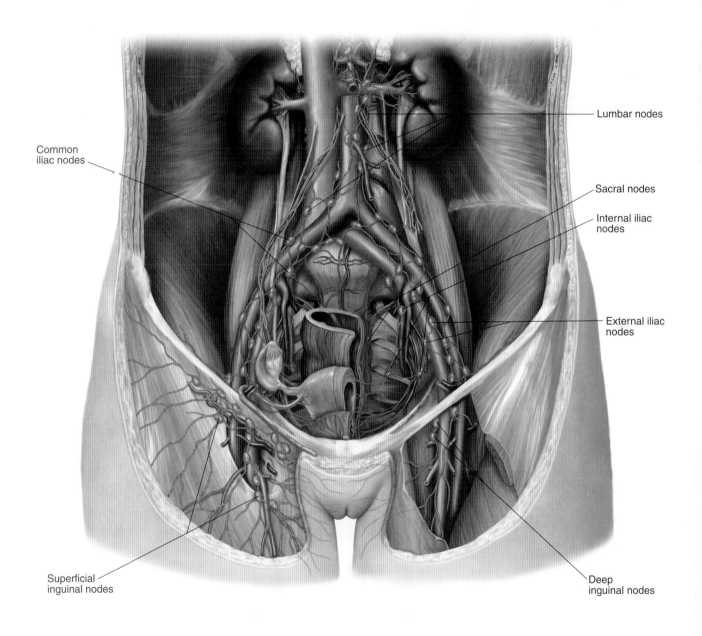

Common
iliac nodes

Lumbar nodes

Sacral nodes

Internal iliac
nodes

External iliac
nodes

Deep
inguinal nodes

Superficial
inguinal nodes

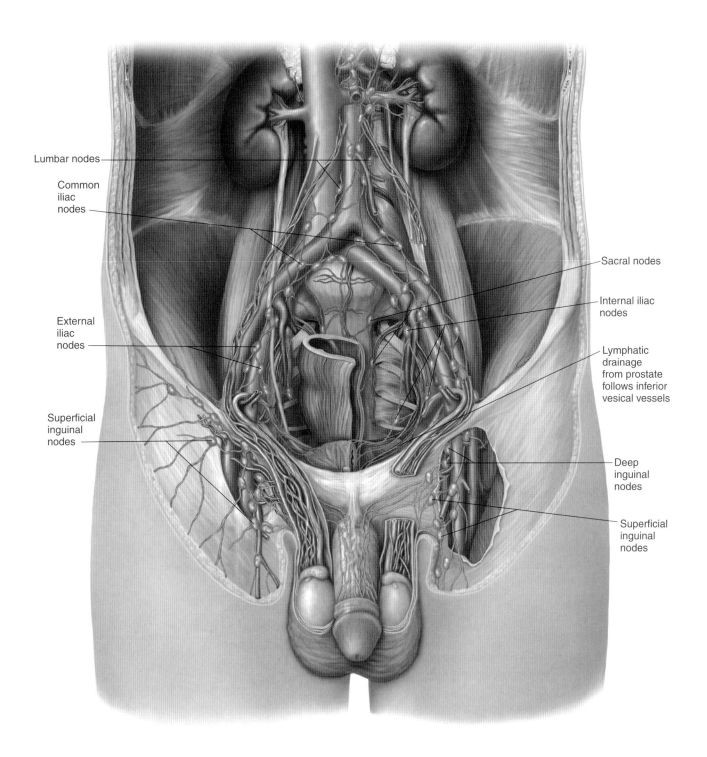

Lumbar nodes

Common
iliac
nodes

External
iliac
nodes

Superficial
inguinal
nodes

Sacral nodes

Internal iliac
nodes

Lymphatic
drainage
from prostate
follows inferior
vesical vessels

Deep
inguinal
nodes

Superficial
inguinal
nodes

PLATE 6-35   Cross Section of the Female Pelvis

A. Orientation

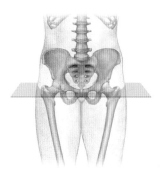

B. Cross section

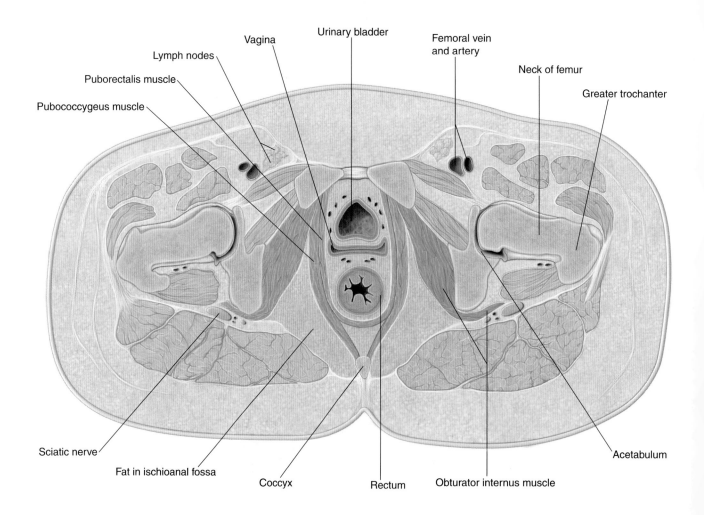

Lymph nodes

Vagina

Urinary bladder

Femoral vein
and artery

Neck of femur

Greater trochanter

Puborectalis muscle

Pubococcygeus muscle

Sciatic nerve

Fat in ischioanal fossa

Coccyx

Rectum

Obturator internus muscle

Acetabulum

A. Orientation

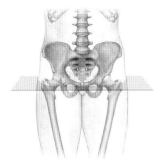

B. Cross section

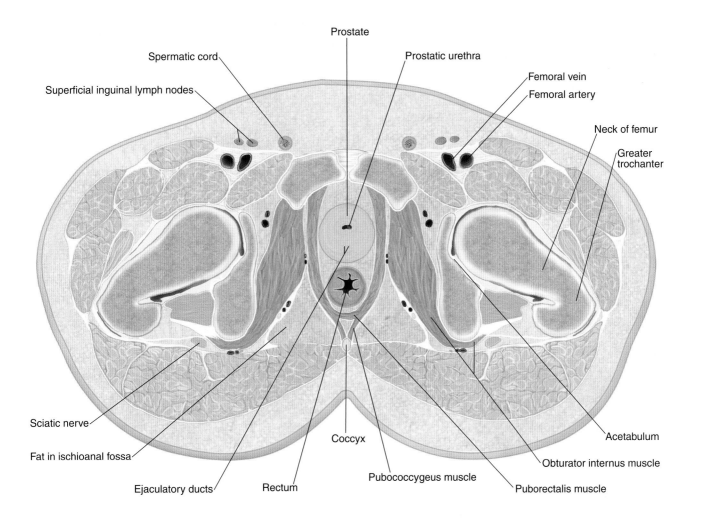

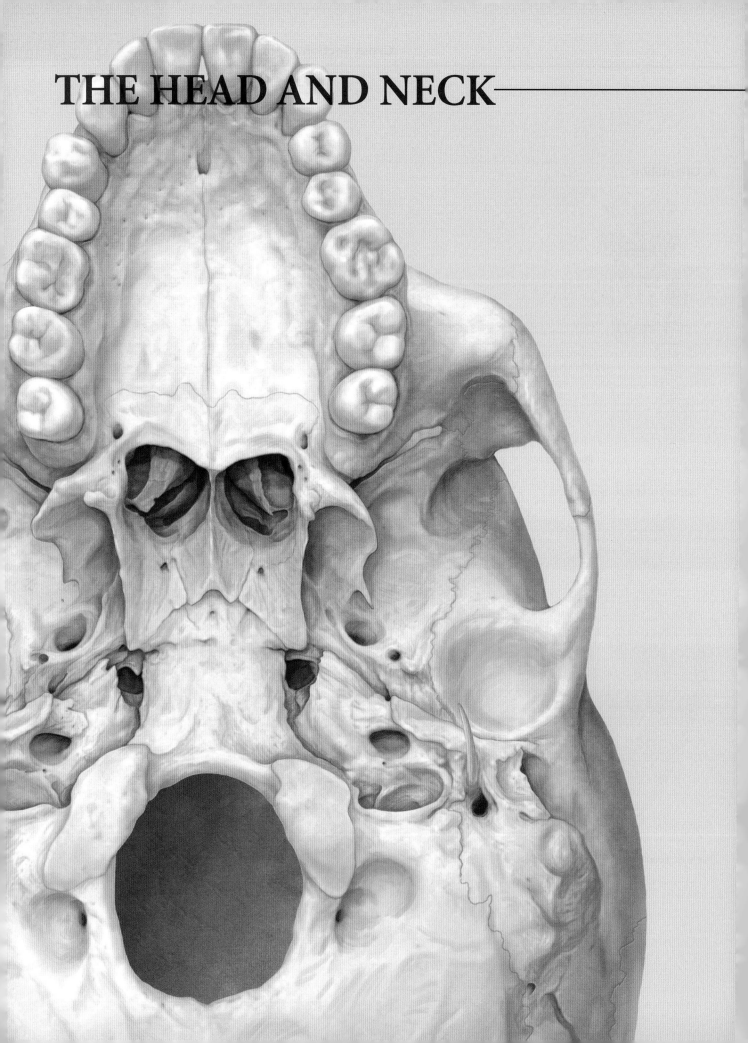

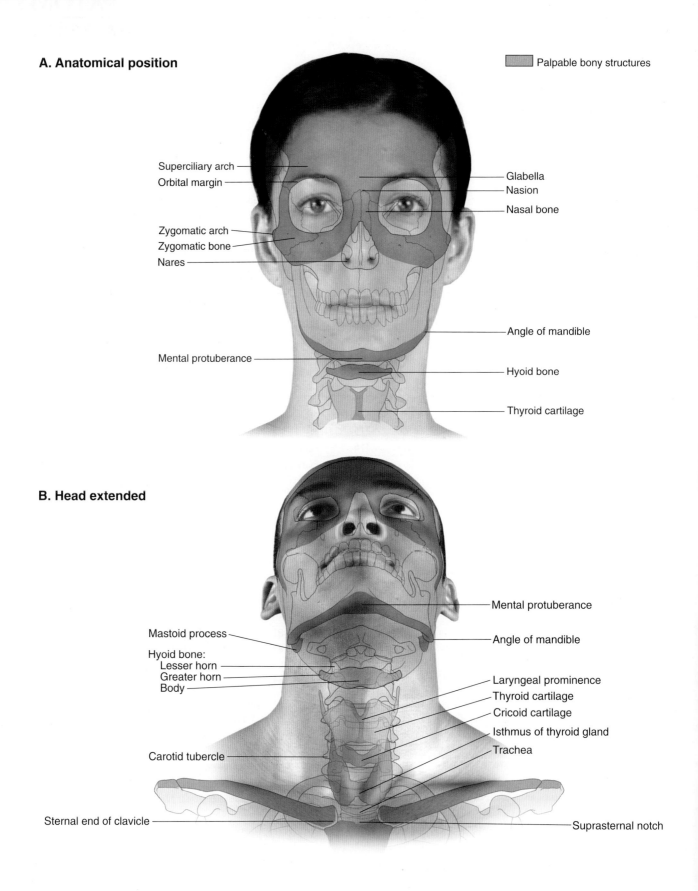

A. Anatomical position

Palpable bony structures

Superciliary arch
Orbital margin
Zygomatic arch
Zygomatic bone
Nares
Mental protuberance

Glabella
Nasion
Nasal bone
Angle of mandible
Hyoid bone
Thyroid cartilage

B. Head extended

Mastoid process
Hyoid bone:
  Lesser horn
  Greater horn
  Body
Carotid tubercle
Sternal end of clavicle

Mental protuberance
Angle of mandible
Laryngeal prominence
Thyroid cartilage
Cricoid cartilage
Isthmus of thyroid gland
Trachea
Suprasternal notch

A. Anterior view

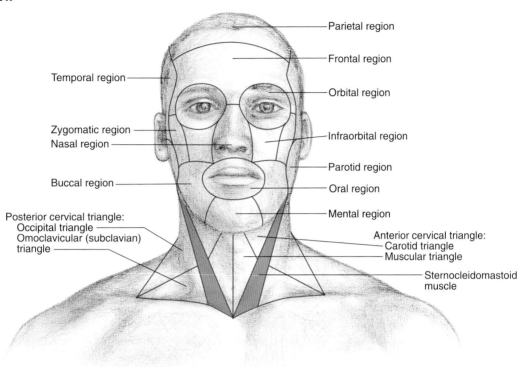

Parietal region
Frontal region
Temporal region
Orbital region
Zygomatic region
Nasal region
Infraorbital region
Parotid region
Buccal region
Oral region
Posterior cervical triangle:
Occipital triangle
Omoclavicular (subclavian) triangle
Mental region
Anterior cervical triangle:
Carotid triangle
Muscular triangle
Sternocleidomastoid muscle

B. Lateral view

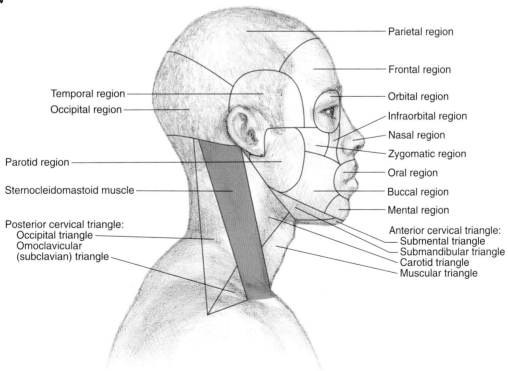

Parietal region
Frontal region
Temporal region
Occipital region
Orbital region
Infraorbital region
Nasal region
Zygomatic region
Parotid region
Oral region
Sternocleidomastoid muscle
Buccal region
Mental region
Posterior cervical triangle:
Occipital triangle
Omoclavicular (subclavian) triangle
Anterior cervical triangle:
Submental triangle
Submandibular triangle
Carotid triangle
Muscular triangle

PLATE 7-03   **Skull, Anterior View**

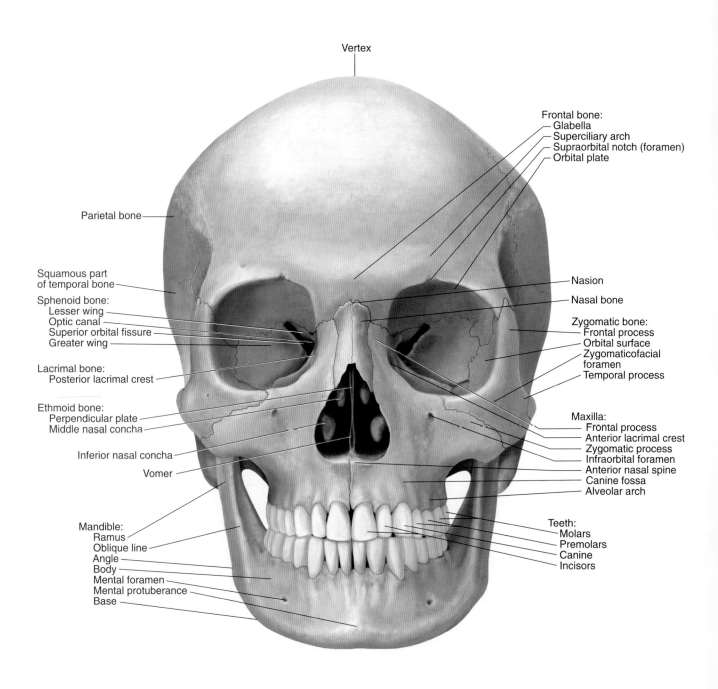

Vertex

Frontal bone:
Glabella
Superciliary arch
Supraorbital notch (foramen)
Orbital plate

Parietal bone

Squamous part
of temporal bone

Sphenoid bone:
Lesser wing
Optic canal
Superior orbital fissure
Greater wing

Lacrimal bone:
Posterior lacrimal crest

Ethmoid bone:
Perpendicular plate
Middle nasal concha

Inferior nasal concha

Vomer

Mandible:
Ramus
Oblique line
Angle
Body
Mental foramen
Mental protuberance
Base

Nasion

Nasal bone

Zygomatic bone:
Frontal process
Orbital surface
Zygomaticofacial
foramen
Temporal process

Maxilla:
Frontal process
Anterior lacrimal crest
Zygomatic process
Infraorbital foramen
Anterior nasal spine
Canine fossa
Alveolar arch

Teeth:
Molars
Premolars
Canine
Incisors

A. Bones

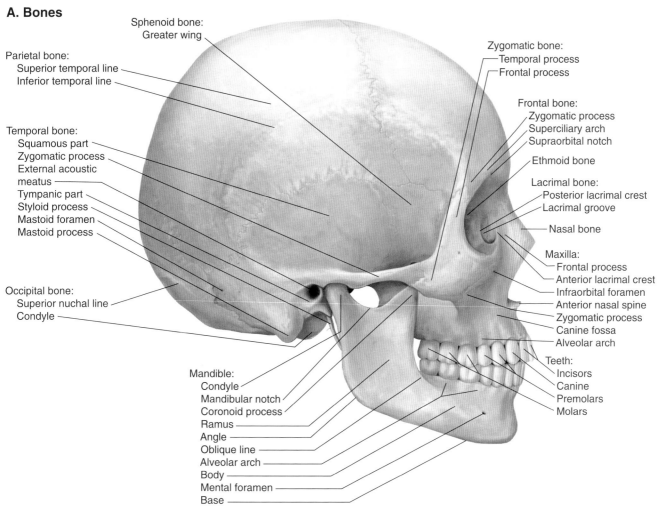

Sphenoid bone:
  Greater wing

Parietal bone:
  Superior temporal line
  Inferior temporal line

Temporal bone:
  Squamous part
  Zygomatic process
  External acoustic
  meatus
  Tympanic part
  Styloid process
  Mastoid foramen
  Mastoid process

Occipital bone:
  Superior nuchal line
  Condyle

Mandible:
  Condyle
  Mandibular notch
  Coronoid process
  Ramus
  Angle
  Oblique line
  Alveolar arch
  Body
  Mental foramen
  Base

Zygomatic bone:
  Temporal process
  Frontal process

Frontal bone:
  Zygomatic process
  Superciliary arch
  Supraorbital notch

Ethmoid bone

Lacrimal bone:
  Posterior lacrimal crest
  Lacrimal groove

Nasal bone

Maxilla:
  Frontal process
  Anterior lacrimal crest
  Infraorbital foramen
  Anterior nasal spine
  Zygomatic process
  Canine fossa
  Alveolar arch

Teeth:
  Incisors
  Canine
  Premolars
  Molars

B. Sutures and landmarks

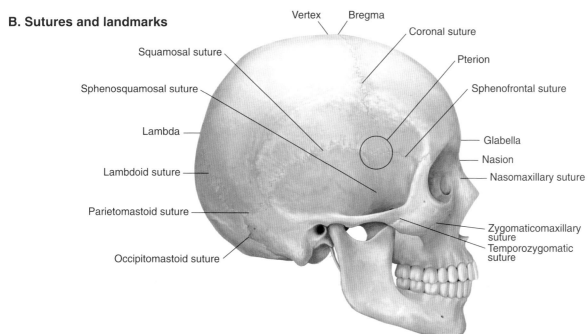

Vertex   Bregma

Coronal suture

Squamosal suture

Pterion

Sphenosquamosal suture

Sphenofrontal suture

Lambda

Glabella

Lambdoid suture

Nasion

Nasomaxillary suture

Parietomastoid suture

Zygomaticomaxillary
suture
Temporozygomatic
suture

Occipitomastoid suture

PLATE 7-05   Skull and Calvaria

A. Posterior view

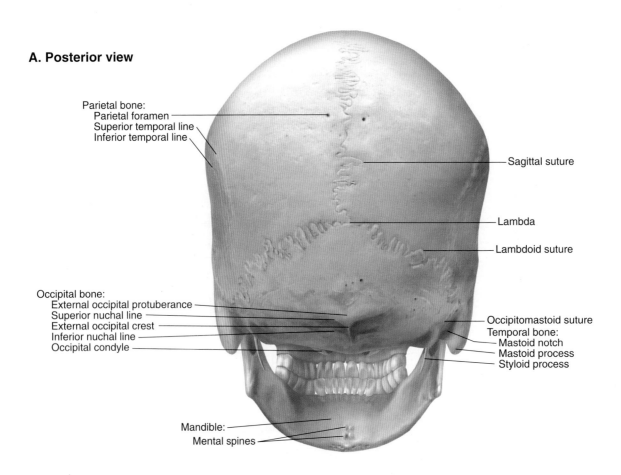

Parietal bone:
Parietal foramen
Superior temporal line
Inferior temporal line

Sagittal suture

Lambda

Lambdoid suture

Occipital bone:
External occipital protuberance
Superior nuchal line
External occipital crest
Inferior nuchal line
Occipital condyle

Occipitomastoid suture
Temporal bone:
Mastoid notch
Mastoid process
Styloid process

Mandible:
Mental spines

B. Calvaria, superior view

C. Calvaria, internal surface

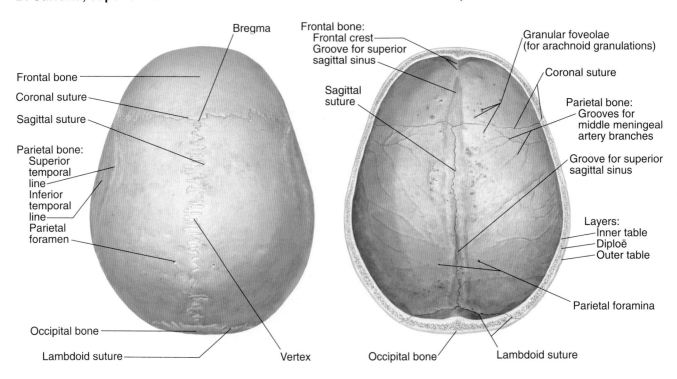

Bregma

Frontal bone

Coronal suture

Sagittal suture

Parietal bone:
Superior
temporal
line
Inferior
temporal
line
Parietal
foramen

Occipital bone

Lambdoid suture

Vertex

Frontal bone:
Frontal crest
Groove for superior
sagittal sinus

Sagittal
suture

Granular foveolae
(for arachnoid granulations)

Coronal suture

Parietal bone:
Grooves for
middle meningeal
artery branches

Groove for superior
sagittal sinus

Layers:
Inner table
Diploë
Outer table

Parietal foramina

Occipital bone

Lambdoid suture

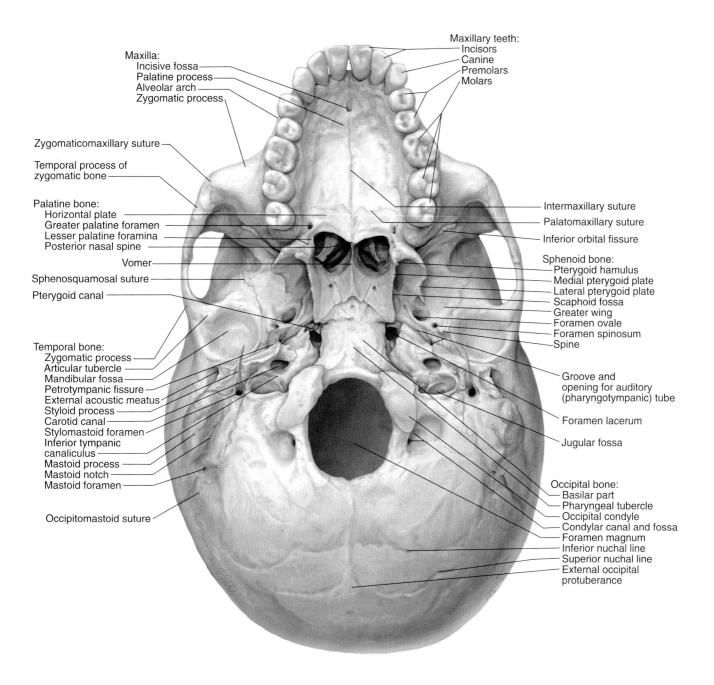

Maxilla:
Incisive fossa
Palatine process
Alveolar arch
Zygomatic process

Maxillary teeth:
Incisors
Canine
Premolars
Molars

Zygomaticomaxillary suture

Temporal process of
zygomatic bone

Palatine bone:
Horizontal plate
Greater palatine foramen
Lesser palatine foramina
Posterior nasal spine

Vomer

Sphenosquamosal suture

Pterygoid canal

Temporal bone:
Zygomatic process
Articular tubercle
Mandibular fossa
Petrotympanic fissure
External acoustic meatus
Styloid process
Carotid canal
Stylomastoid foramen
Inferior tympanic
canaliculus
Mastoid process
Mastoid notch
Mastoid foramen

Occipitomastoid suture

Intermaxillary suture
Palatomaxillary suture
Inferior orbital fissure

Sphenoid bone:
Pterygoid hamulus
Medial pterygoid plate
Lateral pterygoid plate
Scaphoid fossa
Greater wing
Foramen ovale
Foramen spinosum
Spine

Groove and
opening for auditory
(pharyngotympanic) tube

Foramen lacerum

Jugular fossa

Occipital bone:
Basilar part
Pharyngeal tubercle
Occipital condyle
Condylar canal and fossa
Foramen magnum
Inferior nuchal line
Superior nuchal line
External occipital
protuberance

PLATE 7-07 **Base of Skull, Interior**

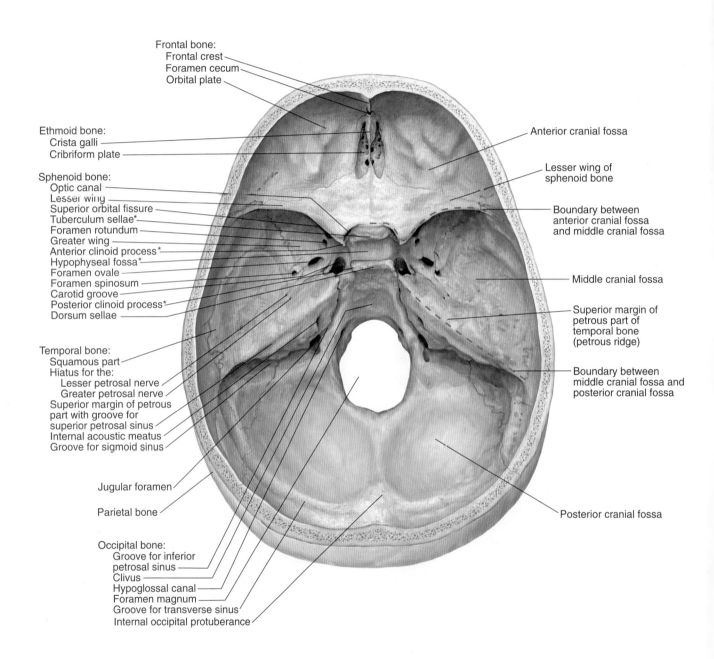

Frontal bone:
Frontal crest
Foramen cecum
Orbital plate

Anterior cranial fossa

Ethmoid bone:
Crista galli
Cribriform plate

Lesser wing of
sphenoid bone

Sphenoid bone:
Optic canal
Lesser wing
Superior orbital fissure
Tuberculum sellae*
Foramen rotundum
Greater wing
Anterior clinoid process*
Hypophyseal fossa*
Foramen ovale
Foramen spinosum
Carotid groove
Posterior clinoid process*
Dorsum sellae

Boundary between
anterior cranial fossa
and middle cranial fossa

Middle cranial fossa

Superior margin of
petrous part of
temporal bone
(petrous ridge)

Temporal bone:
Squamous part
Hiatus for the:
Lesser petrosal nerve
Greater petrosal nerve
Superior margin of petrous
part with groove for
superior petrosal sinus
Internal acoustic meatus
Groove for sigmoid sinus

Boundary between
middle cranial fossa and
posterior cranial fossa

Jugular foramen

Parietal bone

Posterior cranial fossa

Occipital bone:
Groove for inferior
petrosal sinus
Clivus
Hypoglossal canal
Foramen magnum
Groove for transverse sinus
Internal occipital protuberance

*These four structures make up the sella turcica

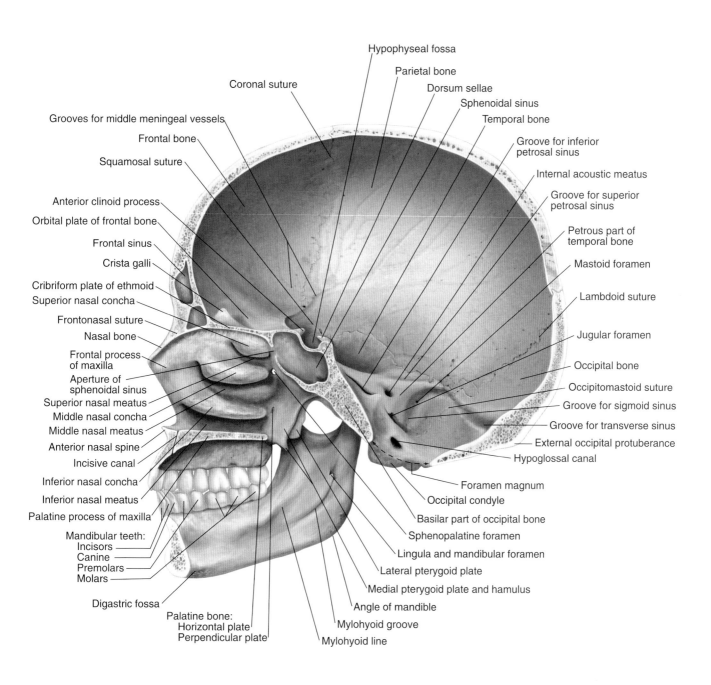

Hypophyseal fossa
Parietal bone
Coronal suture
Dorsum sellae
Sphenoidal sinus
Temporal bone
Grooves for middle meningeal vessels
Groove for inferior petrosal sinus
Frontal bone
Squamosal suture
Internal acoustic meatus
Groove for superior petrosal sinus
Anterior clinoid process
Orbital plate of frontal bone
Petrous part of temporal bone
Frontal sinus
Crista galli
Mastoid foramen
Cribriform plate of ethmoid
Superior nasal concha
Lambdoid suture
Frontonasal suture
Nasal bone
Jugular foramen
Frontal process of maxilla
Occipital bone
Aperture of sphenoidal sinus
Occipitomastoid suture
Superior nasal meatus
Groove for sigmoid sinus
Middle nasal concha
Groove for transverse sinus
Middle nasal meatus
External occipital protuberance
Anterior nasal spine
Hypoglossal canal
Incisive canal
Inferior nasal concha
Foramen magnum
Inferior nasal meatus
Occipital condyle
Palatine process of maxilla
Basilar part of occipital bone
Mandibular teeth:
Sphenopalatine foramen
Incisors
Canine
Lingula and mandibular foramen
Premolars
Lateral pterygoid plate
Molars
Medial pterygoid plate and hamulus
Digastric fossa
Angle of mandible
Palatine bone:
Mylohyoid groove
Horizontal plate
Perpendicular plate
Mylohyoid line

PLATE 7-09   **Skeleton of the Neck, Lateral View**

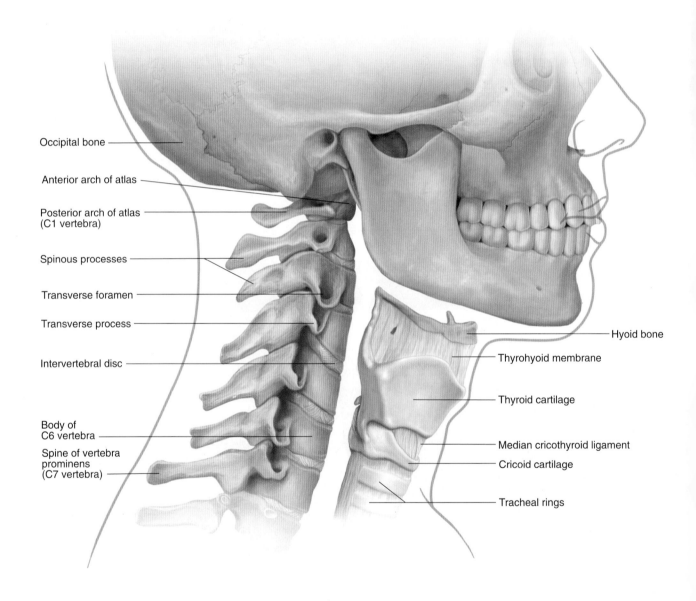

Occipital bone

Anterior arch of atlas

Posterior arch of atlas
(C1 vertebra)

Spinous processes

Transverse foramen

Transverse process

Intervertebral disc

Body of
C6 vertebra

Spine of vertebra
prominens
(C7 vertebra)

Hyoid bone

Thyrohyoid membrane

Thyroid cartilage

Median cricothyroid ligament

Cricoid cartilage

Tracheal rings

A. Sagittal section

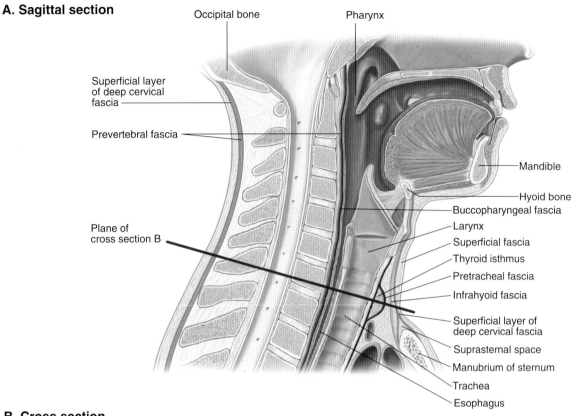

Occipital bone

Pharynx

Superficial layer
of deep cervical
fascia

Prevertebral fascia

Plane of
cross section B

Mandible

Hyoid bone

Buccopharyngeal fascia

Larynx

Superficial fascia

Thyroid isthmus

Pretracheal fascia

Infrahyoid fascia

Superficial layer of
deep cervical fascia

Suprasternal space

Manubrium of sternum

Trachea

Esophagus

B. Cross section

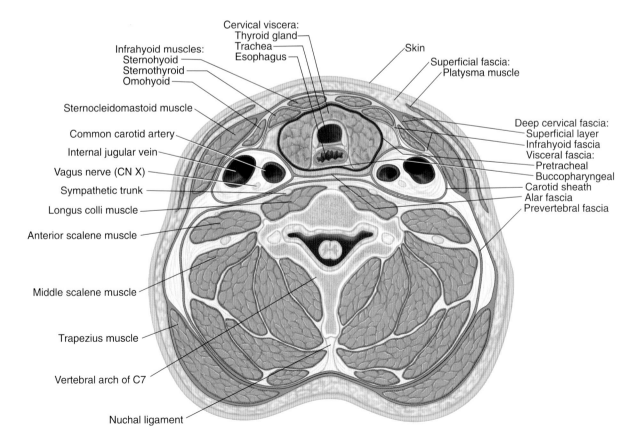

Cervical viscera:
Thyroid gland
Trachea
Esophagus

Infrahyoid muscles:
Sternohyoid
Sternothyroid
Omohyoid

Skin

Superficial fascia:
Platysma muscle

Sternocleidomastoid muscle

Common carotid artery

Internal jugular vein

Vagus nerve (CN X)

Sympathetic trunk

Longus colli muscle

Anterior scalene muscle

Deep cervical fascia:
Superficial layer
Infrahyoid fascia
Visceral fascia:
Pretracheal
Buccopharyngeal
Carotid sheath
Alar fascia
Prevertebral fascia

Middle scalene muscle

Trapezius muscle

Vertebral arch of C7

Nuchal ligament

PLATE 7-11   **Neck, Superficial Dissection**

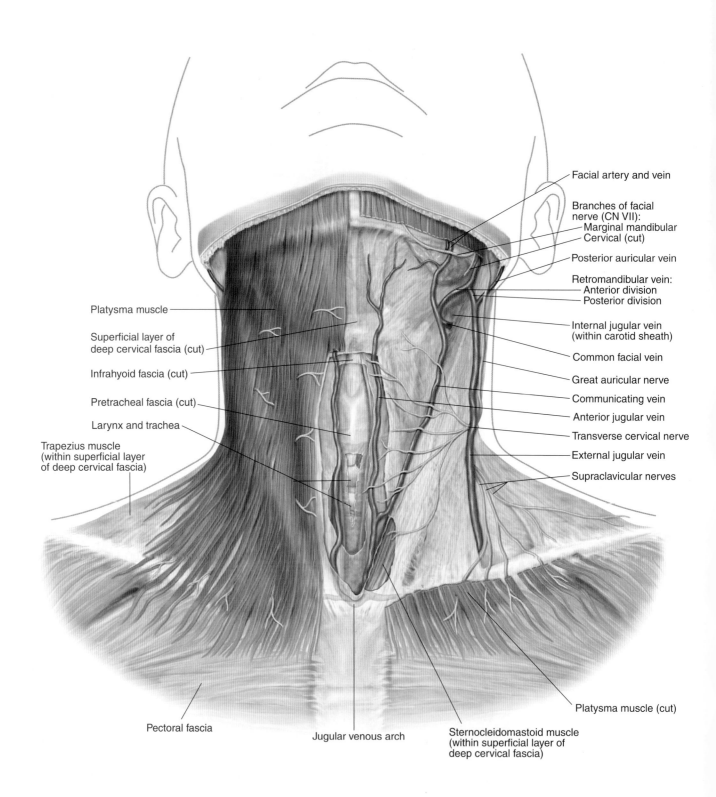

Facial artery and vein

Branches of facial nerve (CN VII):
Marginal mandibular
Cervical (cut)

Posterior auricular vein

Retromandibular vein:
Anterior division
Posterior division

Internal jugular vein (within carotid sheath)

Common facial vein

Great auricular nerve

Communicating vein

Anterior jugular vein

Transverse cervical nerve

External jugular vein

Supraclavicular nerves

Platysma muscle

Superficial layer of deep cervical fascia (cut)

Infrahyoid fascia (cut)

Pretracheal fascia (cut)

Larynx and trachea

Trapezius muscle (within superficial layer of deep cervical fascia)

Platysma muscle (cut)

Pectoral fascia

Jugular venous arch

Sternocleidomastoid muscle (within superficial layer of deep cervical fascia)

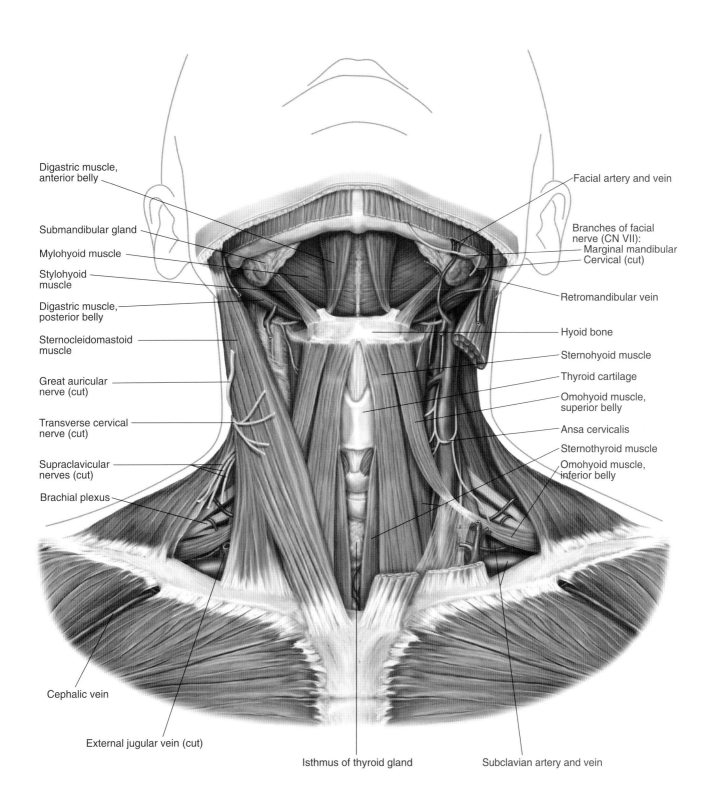

Digastric muscle, anterior belly

Submandibular gland

Mylohyoid muscle

Stylohyoid muscle

Digastric muscle, posterior belly

Sternocleidomastoid muscle

Great auricular nerve (cut)

Transverse cervical nerve (cut)

Supraclavicular nerves (cut)

Brachial plexus

Cephalic vein

External jugular vein (cut)

Isthmus of thyroid gland

Facial artery and vein

Branches of facial nerve (CN VII):
Marginal mandibular
Cervical (cut)

Retromandibular vein

Hyoid bone

Sternohyoid muscle

Thyroid cartilage

Omohyoid muscle, superior belly

Ansa cervicalis

Sternothyroid muscle

Omohyoid muscle, inferior belly

Subclavian artery and vein

PLATE 7-13 **Neck, Deep Dissection**

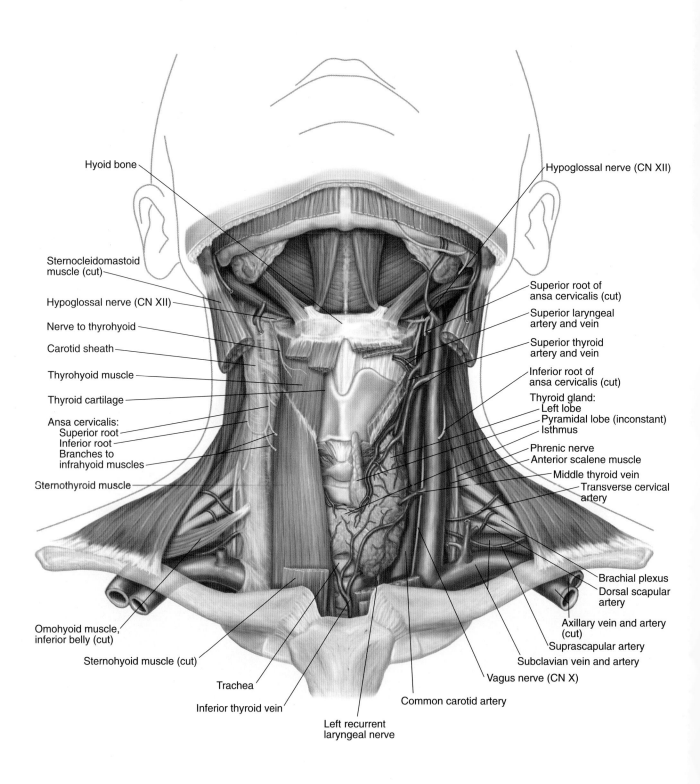

Hyoid bone

Hypoglossal nerve (CN XII)

Sternocleidomastoid muscle (cut)

Hypoglossal nerve (CN XII)

Nerve to thyrohyoid

Carotid sheath

Thyrohyoid muscle

Thyroid cartilage

Ansa cervicalis:
Superior root
Inferior root
Branches to
infrahyoid muscles

Sternothyroid muscle

Superior root of
ansa cervicalis (cut)

Superior laryngeal
artery and vein

Superior thyroid
artery and vein

Inferior root of
ansa cervicalis (cut)

Thyroid gland:
Left lobe
Pyramidal lobe (inconstant)
Isthmus

Phrenic nerve

Anterior scalene muscle

Middle thyroid vein

Transverse cervical
artery

Brachial plexus

Dorsal scapular
artery

Axillary vein and artery
(cut)

Suprascapular artery

Subclavian vein and artery

Vagus nerve (CN X)

Omohyoid muscle,
inferior belly (cut)

Sternohyoid muscle (cut)

Trachea

Inferior thyroid vein

Left recurrent
laryngeal nerve

Common carotid artery

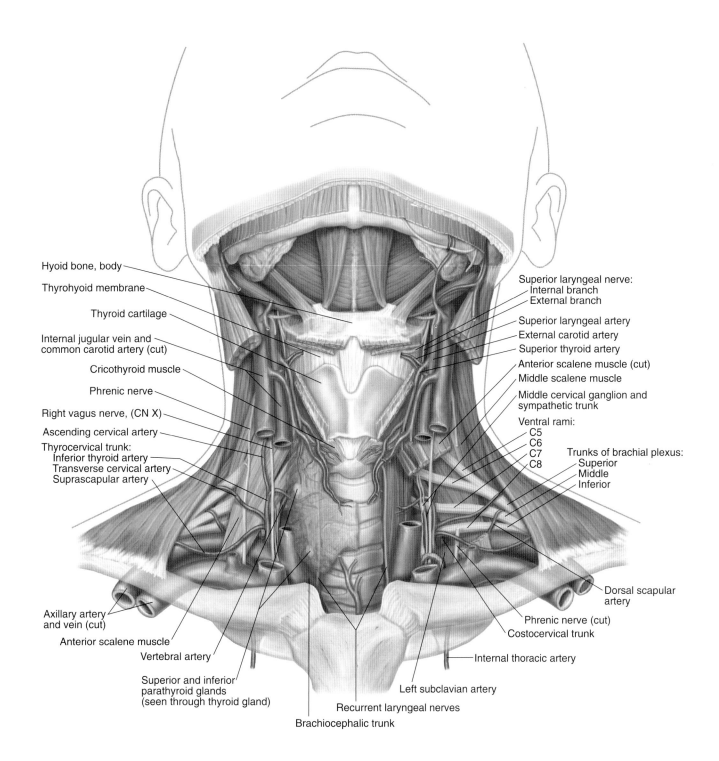

Hyoid bone, body

Thyrohyoid membrane

Thyroid cartilage

Internal jugular vein and
common carotid artery (cut)

Cricothyroid muscle

Phrenic nerve

Right vagus nerve, (CN X)

Ascending cervical artery

Thyrocervical trunk:
    Inferior thyroid artery
    Transverse cervical artery
    Suprascapular artery

Axillary artery
and vein (cut)

Anterior scalene muscle

Vertebral artery

Superior and inferior
parathyroid glands
(seen through thyroid gland)

Brachiocephalic trunk

Recurrent laryngeal nerves

Left subclavian artery

Internal thoracic artery

Costocervical trunk

Phrenic nerve (cut)

Dorsal scapular
artery

Trunks of brachial plexus:
    Superior
    Middle
    Inferior

Ventral rami:
    C5
    C6
    C7
    C8

Middle cervical ganglion and
sympathetic trunk

Middle scalene muscle

Anterior scalene muscle (cut)

Superior thyroid artery

External carotid artery

Superior laryngeal artery

Superior laryngeal nerve:
    Internal branch
    External branch

PLATE 7-15   Prevertebral Region

A. Dissection

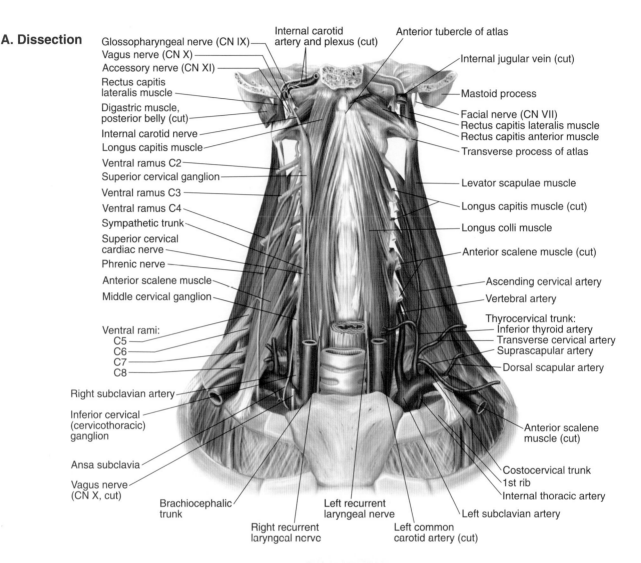

Glossopharyngeal nerve (CN IX)
Vagus nerve (CN X)
Accessory nerve (CN XI)
Rectus capitis lateralis muscle
Digastric muscle, posterior belly (cut)
Internal carotid nerve
Longus capitis muscle
Ventral ramus C2
Superior cervical ganglion
Ventral ramus C3
Ventral ramus C4
Sympathetic trunk
Superior cervical cardiac nerve
Phrenic nerve
Anterior scalene muscle
Middle cervical ganglion
Ventral rami:
C5
C6
C7
C8
Right subclavian artery
Inferior cervical (cervicothoracic) ganglion
Ansa subclavia
Vagus nerve (CN X, cut)
Brachiocephalic trunk
Right recurrent laryngeal nerve

Internal carotid artery and plexus (cut)
Anterior tubercle of atlas
Internal jugular vein (cut)
Mastoid process
Facial nerve (CN VII)
Rectus capitis lateralis muscle
Rectus capitis anterior muscle
Transverse process of atlas
Levator scapulae muscle
Longus capitis muscle (cut)
Longus colli muscle
Anterior scalene muscle (cut)
Ascending cervical artery
Vertebral artery
Thyrocervical trunk:
Inferior thyroid artery
Transverse cervical artery
Suprascapular artery
Dorsal scapular artery
Anterior scalene muscle (cut)
Costocervical trunk
1st rib
Internal thoracic artery
Left subclavian artery
Left recurrent laryngeal nerve
Left common carotid artery (cut)

B. Subclavian artery

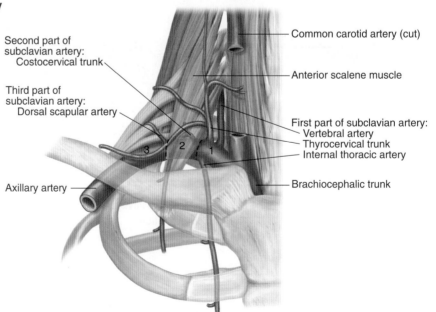

Second part of subclavian artery:
Costocervical trunk
Third part of subclavian artery:
Dorsal scapular artery
Axillary artery

Common carotid artery (cut)
Anterior scalene muscle
First part of subclavian artery:
Vertebral artery
Thyrocervical trunk
Internal thoracic artery
Brachiocephalic trunk

A. Superficial dissection

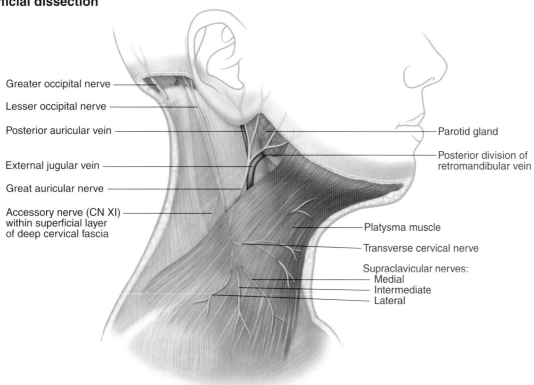

Greater occipital nerve

Lesser occipital nerve

Posterior auricular vein

External jugular vein

Great auricular nerve

Accessory nerve (CN XI)
within superficial layer
of deep cervical fascia

Parotid gland

Posterior division of
retromandibular vein

Platysma muscle

Transverse cervical nerve

Supraclavicular nerves:
Medial
Intermediate
Lateral

B. Intermediate dissection

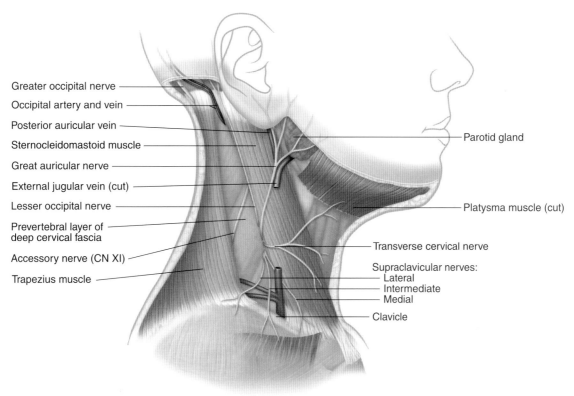

Greater occipital nerve

Occipital artery and vein

Posterior auricular vein

Sternocleidomastoid muscle

Great auricular nerve

External jugular vein (cut)

Lesser occipital nerve

Prevertebral layer of
deep cervical fascia

Accessory nerve (CN XI)

Trapezius muscle

Parotid gland

Platysma muscle (cut)

Transverse cervical nerve

Supraclavicular nerves:
Lateral
Intermediate
Medial

Clavicle

PLATE 7-17   Neck, Lateral View, Deeper Dissection

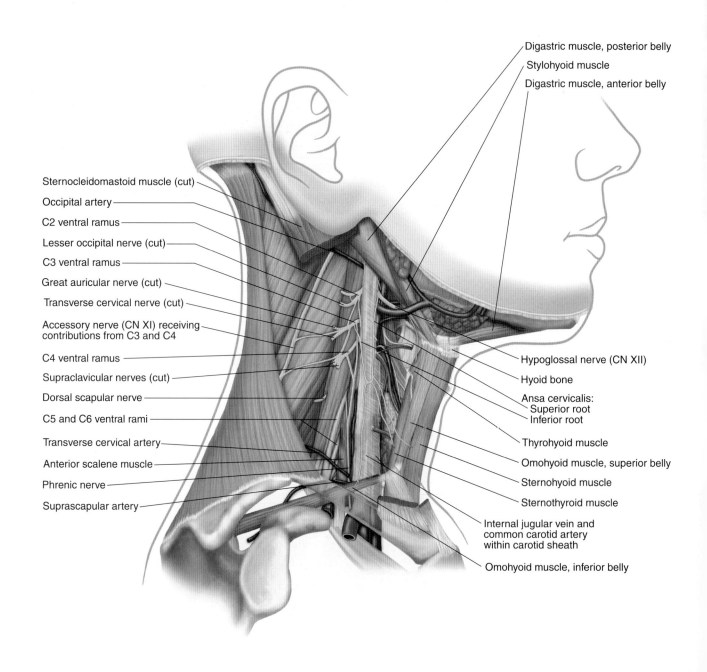

Digastric muscle, posterior belly

Stylohyoid muscle

Digastric muscle, anterior belly

Sternocleidomastoid muscle (cut)

Occipital artery

C2 ventral ramus

Lesser occipital nerve (cut)

C3 ventral ramus

Great auricular nerve (cut)

Transverse cervical nerve (cut)

Accessory nerve (CN XI) receiving contributions from C3 and C4

C4 ventral ramus

Supraclavicular nerves (cut)

Dorsal scapular nerve

C5 and C6 ventral rami

Transverse cervical artery

Anterior scalene muscle

Phrenic nerve

Suprascapular artery

Hypoglossal nerve (CN XII)

Hyoid bone

Ansa cervicalis:
  Superior root
  Inferior root

Thyrohyoid muscle

Omohyoid muscle, superior belly

Sternohyoid muscle

Sternothyroid muscle

Internal jugular vein and common carotid artery within carotid sheath

Omohyoid muscle, inferior belly

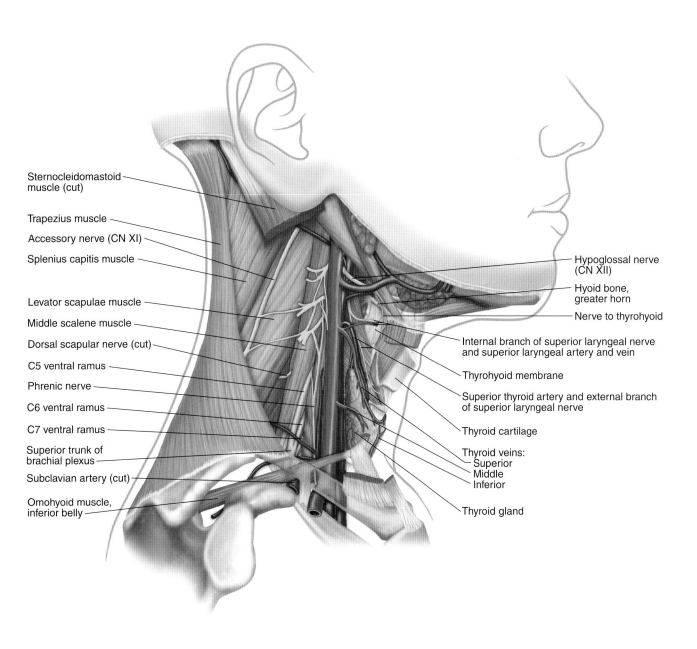

Sternocleidomastoid muscle (cut)

Trapezius muscle

Accessory nerve (CN XI)

Splenius capitis muscle

Levator scapulae muscle

Middle scalene muscle

Dorsal scapular nerve (cut)

C5 ventral ramus

Phrenic nerve

C6 ventral ramus

C7 ventral ramus

Superior trunk of brachial plexus

Subclavian artery (cut)

Omohyoid muscle, inferior belly

Hypoglossal nerve (CN XII)

Hyoid bone, greater horn

Nerve to thyrohyoid

Internal branch of superior laryngeal nerve and superior laryngeal artery and vein

Thyrohyoid membrane

Superior thyroid artery and external branch of superior laryngeal nerve

Thyroid cartilage

Thyroid veins:
Superior
Middle
Inferior

Thyroid gland

PLATE 7-19   **Neck, Lateral View, Larynx and Pharynx**

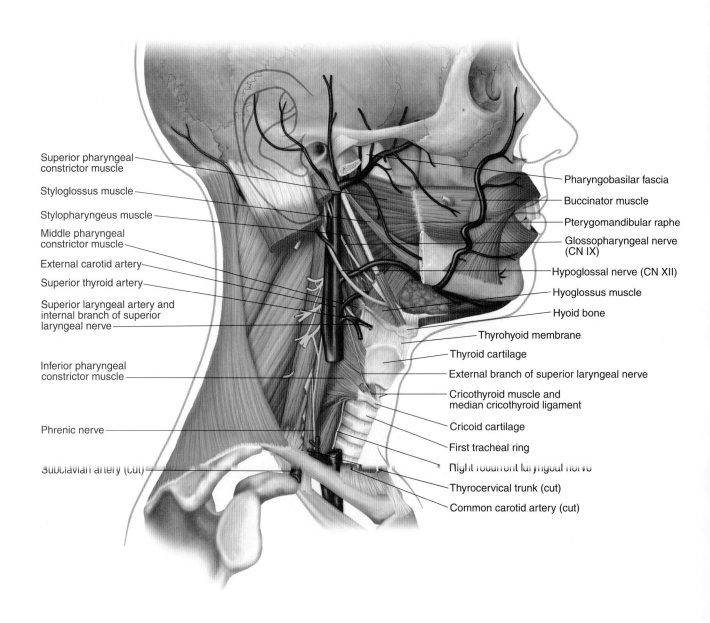

Superior pharyngeal
constrictor muscle

Styloglossus muscle

Stylopharyngeus muscle

Middle pharyngeal
constrictor muscle

External carotid artery

Superior thyroid artery

Superior laryngeal artery and
internal branch of superior
laryngeal nerve

Inferior pharyngeal
constrictor muscle

Phrenic nerve

Subclavian artery (cut)

Pharyngobasilar fascia

Buccinator muscle

Pterygomandibular raphe

Glossopharyngeal nerve
(CN IX)

Hypoglossal nerve (CN XII)

Hyoglossus muscle

Hyoid bone

Thyrohyoid membrane

Thyroid cartilage

External branch of superior laryngeal nerve

Cricothyroid muscle and
median cricothyroid ligament

Cricoid cartilage

First tracheal ring

Right recurrent laryngeal nerve

Thyrocervical trunk (cut)

Common carotid artery (cut)

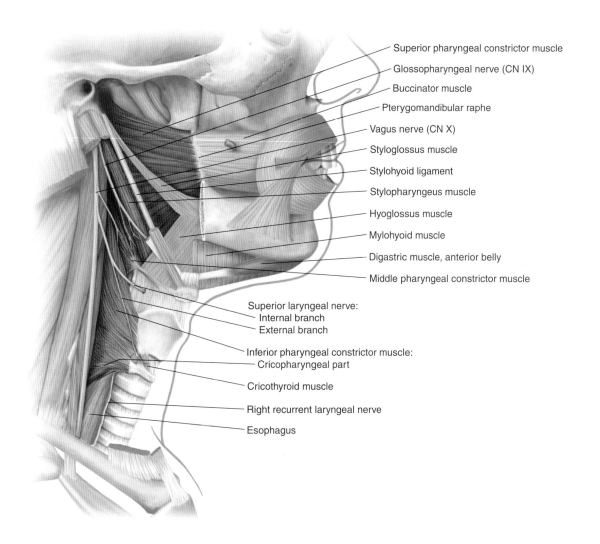

Superior pharyngeal constrictor muscle

Glossopharyngeal nerve (CN IX)

Buccinator muscle

Pterygomandibular raphe

Vagus nerve (CN X)

Styloglossus muscle

Stylohyoid ligament

Stylopharyngeus muscle

Hyoglossus muscle

Mylohyoid muscle

Digastric muscle, anterior belly

Middle pharyngeal constrictor muscle

Superior laryngeal nerve:
Internal branch
External branch

Inferior pharyngeal constrictor muscle:
Cricopharyngeal part

Cricothyroid muscle

Right recurrent laryngeal nerve

Esophagus

PLATE 7-21   **Pharynx, Posterior View**

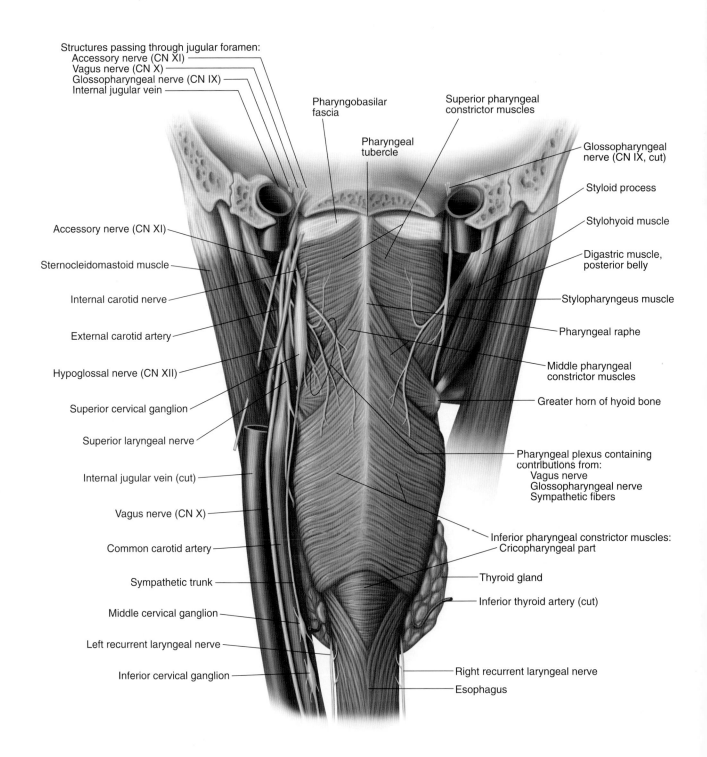

Structures passing through jugular foramen:
Accessory nerve (CN XI)
Vagus nerve (CN X)
Glossopharyngeal nerve (CN IX)
Internal jugular vein

Pharyngobasilar fascia

Pharyngeal tubercle

Superior pharyngeal constrictor muscles

Glossopharyngeal nerve (CN IX, cut)

Styloid process

Stylohyoid muscle

Digastric muscle, posterior belly

Accessory nerve (CN XI)

Sternocleidomastoid muscle

Internal carotid nerve

External carotid artery

Hypoglossal nerve (CN XII)

Superior cervical ganglion

Superior laryngeal nerve

Internal jugular vein (cut)

Vagus nerve (CN X)

Common carotid artery

Sympathetic trunk

Middle cervical ganglion

Left recurrent laryngeal nerve

Inferior cervical ganglion

Stylopharyngeus muscle

Pharyngeal raphe

Middle pharyngeal constrictor muscles

Greater horn of hyoid bone

Pharyngeal plexus containing contributions from:
Vagus nerve
Glossopharyngeal nerve
Sympathetic fibers

Inferior pharyngeal constrictor muscles:
Cricopharyngeal part

Thyroid gland

Inferior thyroid artery (cut)

Right recurrent laryngeal nerve

Esophagus

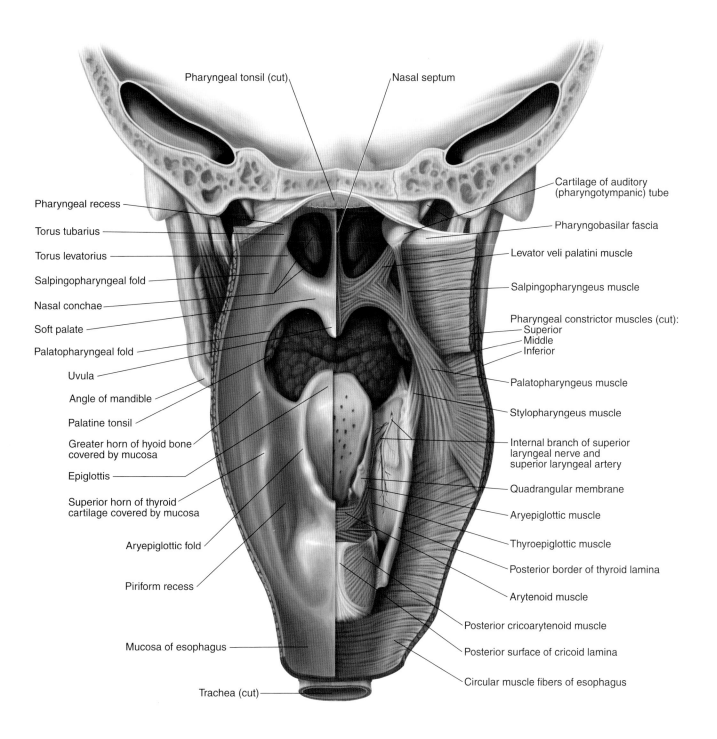

Pharyngeal tonsil (cut)

Nasal septum

Pharyngeal recess

Torus tubarius

Torus levatorius

Salpingopharyngeal fold

Nasal conchae

Soft palate

Palatopharyngeal fold

Uvula

Angle of mandible

Palatine tonsil

Greater horn of hyoid bone covered by mucosa

Epiglottis

Superior horn of thyroid cartilage covered by mucosa

Aryepiglottic fold

Piriform recess

Mucosa of esophagus

Trachea (cut)

Cartilage of auditory (pharyngotympanic) tube

Pharyngobasilar fascia

Levator veli palatini muscle

Salpingopharyngeus muscle

Pharyngeal constrictor muscles (cut):
Superior
Middle
Inferior

Palatopharyngeus muscle

Stylopharyngeus muscle

Internal branch of superior laryngeal nerve and superior laryngeal artery

Quadrangular membrane

Aryepiglottic muscle

Thyroepiglottic muscle

Posterior border of thyroid lamina

Arytenoid muscle

Posterior cricoarytenoid muscle

Posterior surface of cricoid lamina

Circular muscle fibers of esophagus

PLATE 7-23   **Interior of the Pharynx, Medial View**

A. Regions

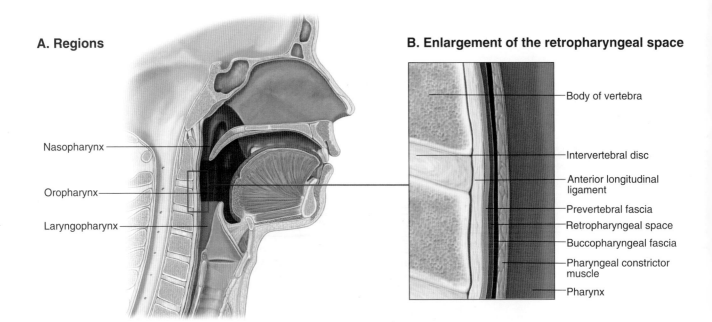

Nasopharynx

Oropharynx

Laryngopharynx

B. Enlargement of the retropharyngeal space

Body of vertebra

Intervertebral disc

Anterior longitudinal ligament

Prevertebral fascia

Retropharyngeal space

Buccopharyngeal fascia

Pharyngeal constrictor muscle

Pharynx

C. Mucosal features

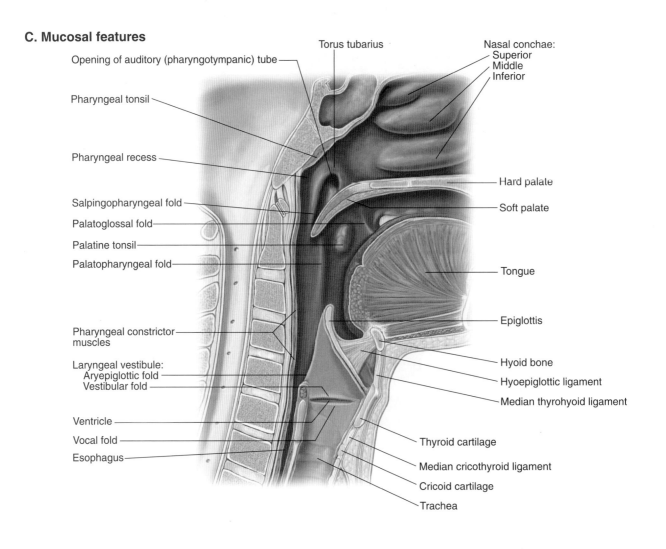

Torus tubarius

Nasal conchae:
Superior
Middle
Inferior

Opening of auditory (pharyngotympanic) tube

Pharyngeal tonsil

Pharyngeal recess

Hard palate

Salpingopharyngeal fold

Soft palate

Palatoglossal fold

Palatine tonsil

Palatopharyngeal fold

Tongue

Epiglottis

Pharyngeal constrictor muscles

Hyoid bone

Laryngeal vestibule:
Aryepiglottic fold
Vestibular fold

Hyoepiglottic ligament

Median thyrohyoid ligament

Ventricle

Vocal fold

Esophagus

Thyroid cartilage

Median cricothyroid ligament

Cricoid cartilage

Trachea

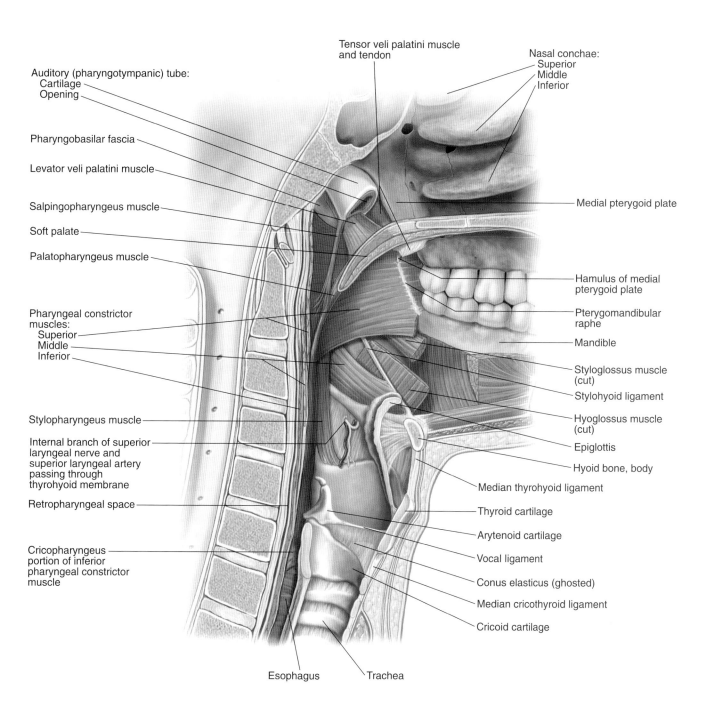

Tensor veli palatini muscle and tendon

Nasal conchae:
Superior
Middle
Inferior

Auditory (pharyngotympanic) tube:
Cartilage
Opening

Pharyngobasilar fascia

Levator veli palatini muscle

Salpingopharyngeus muscle

Soft palate

Palatopharyngeus muscle

Pharyngeal constrictor muscles:
Superior
Middle
Inferior

Stylopharyngeus muscle

Internal branch of superior laryngeal nerve and superior laryngeal artery passing through thyrohyoid membrane

Retropharyngeal space

Cricopharyngeus portion of inferior pharyngeal constrictor muscle

Esophagus

Trachea

Medial pterygoid plate

Hamulus of medial pterygoid plate

Pterygomandibular raphe

Mandible

Styloglossus muscle (cut)

Stylohyoid ligament

Hyoglossus muscle (cut)

Epiglottis

Hyoid bone, body

Median thyrohyoid ligament

Thyroid cartilage

Arytenoid cartilage

Vocal ligament

Conus elasticus (ghosted)

Median cricothyroid ligament

Cricoid cartilage

PLATE 7-25   Larynx, Anterior View

A. In situ

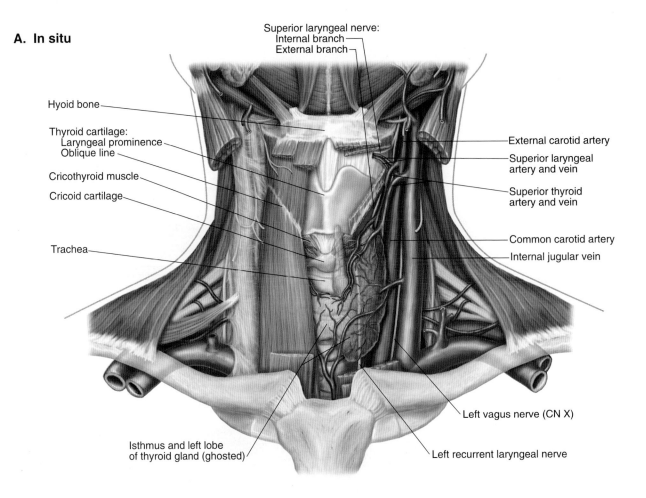

Superior laryngeal nerve:
Internal branch
External branch

Hyoid bone

Thyroid cartilage:
Laryngeal prominence
Oblique line

Cricothyroid muscle

Cricoid cartilage

Trachea

External carotid artery

Superior laryngeal
artery and vein

Superior thyroid
artery and vein

Common carotid artery

Internal jugular vein

Left vagus nerve (CN X)

Isthmus and left lobe
of thyroid gland (ghosted)

Left recurrent laryngeal nerve

B. Cartilages

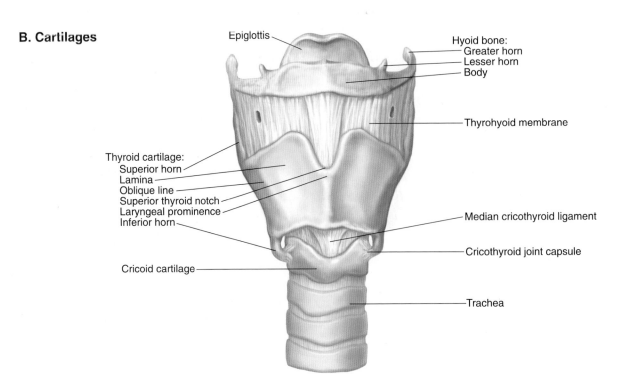

Epiglottis

Hyoid bone:
Greater horn
Lesser horn
Body

Thyrohyoid membrane

Thyroid cartilage:
Superior horn
Lamina
Oblique line
Superior thyroid notch
Laryngeal prominence
Inferior horn

Median cricothyroid ligament

Cricothyroid joint capsule

Cricoid cartilage

Trachea

A. Cartilages

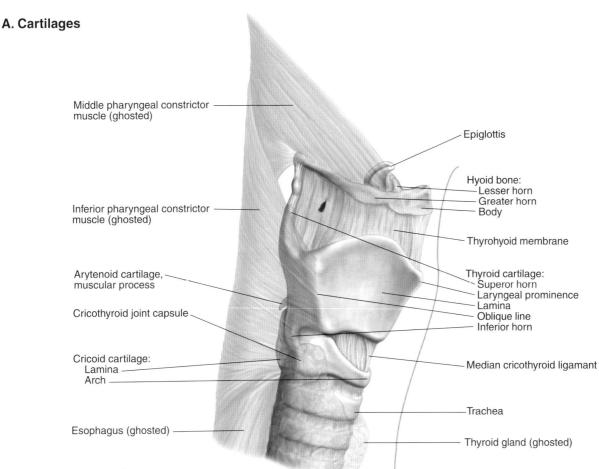

Middle pharyngeal constrictor muscle (ghosted)

Inferior pharyngeal constrictor muscle (ghosted)

Arytenoid cartilage, muscular process

Cricothyroid joint capsule

Cricoid cartilage:
Lamina
Arch

Esophagus (ghosted)

Epiglottis

Hyoid bone:
Lesser horn
Greater horn
Body

Thyrohyoid membrane

Thyroid cartilage:
Superor horn
Laryngeal prominence
Lamina
Oblique line
Inferior horn

Median cricothyroid ligamant

Trachea

Thyroid gland (ghosted)

B. Muscles, external view

C. Muscles, thyroid lamina removed

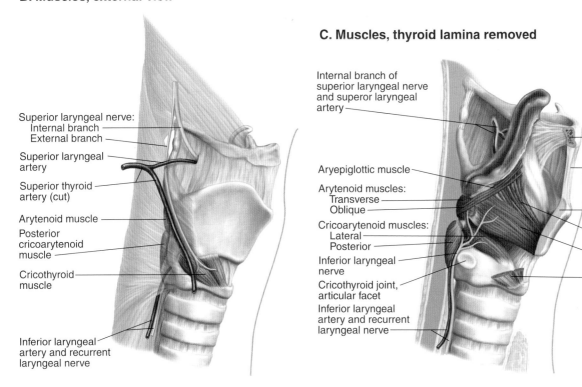

Superior laryngeal nerve:
Internal branch
External branch
Superior laryngeal artery
Superior thyroid artery (cut)
Arytenoid muscle
Posterior cricoarytenoid muscle
Cricothyroid muscle
Inferior laryngeal artery and recurrent laryngeal nerve

Internal branch of superior laryngeal nerve and superor laryngeal artery

Aryepiglottic muscle

Arytenoid muscles:
Transverse
Oblique

Cricoarytenoid muscles:
Lateral
Posterior

Inferior laryngeal nerve

Cricothyroid joint, articular facet

Inferior laryngeal artery and recurrent laryngeal nerve

Hyoid bone (cut)
Thyrohyoid membrane (cut)
Thyroid cartilage (cut)
Thyroepiglottic muscle
Thyroarytenoid muscle
Cricothyroid muscle (cut)

PLATE 7-27   Larynx, Sagittal Section

A. Cartilages

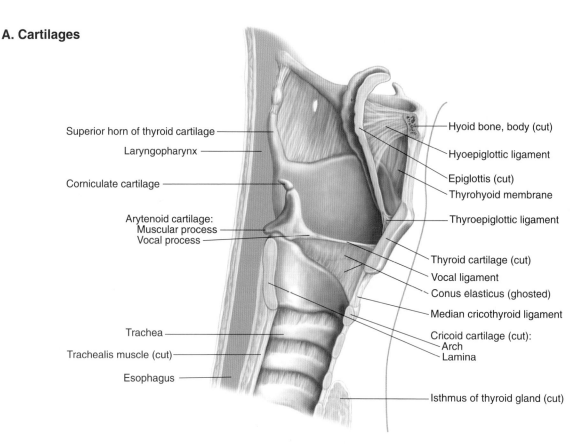

Superior horn of thyroid cartilage

Laryngopharynx

Corniculate cartilage

Arytenoid cartilage:
   Muscular process
   Vocal process

Trachea

Trachealis muscle (cut)

Esophagus

Hyoid bone, body (cut)

Hyoepiglottic ligament

Epiglottis (cut)
Thyrohyoid membrane

Thyroepiglottic ligament

Thyroid cartilage (cut)
Vocal ligament
Conus elasticus (ghosted)
Median cricothyroid ligament
Cricoid cartilage (cut):
   Arch
   Lamina

Isthmus of thyroid gland (cut)

B. Muscles, left side of larynx

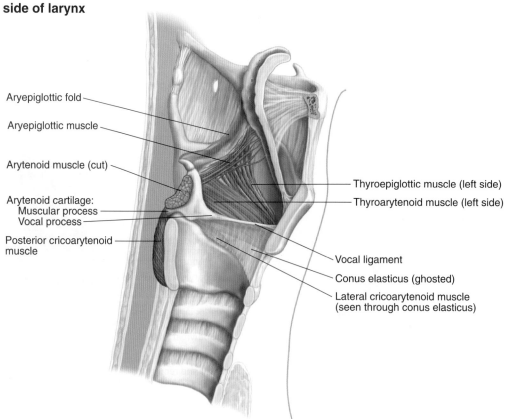

Aryepiglottic fold

Aryepiglottic muscle

Arytenoid muscle (cut)

Arytenoid cartilage:
   Muscular process
   Vocal process

Posterior cricoarytenoid
muscle

Thyroepiglottic muscle (left side)

Thyroarytenoid muscle (left side)

Vocal ligament

Conus elasticus (ghosted)

Lateral cricoarytenoid muscle
(seen through conus elasticus)

A. Cartilages

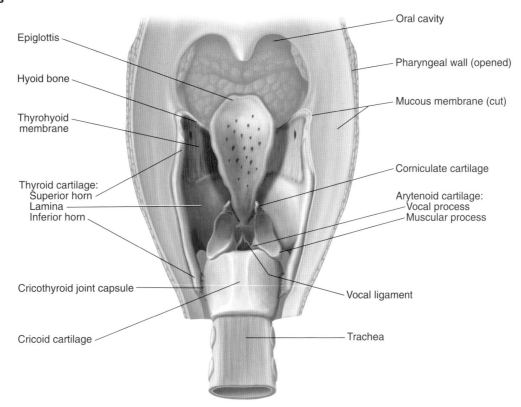

Epiglottis

Hyoid bone

Thyrohyoid membrane

Thyroid cartilage:
  Superior horn
  Lamina
  Inferior horn

Cricothyroid joint capsule

Cricoid cartilage

Oral cavity

Pharyngeal wall (opened)

Mucous membrane (cut)

Corniculate cartilage

Arytenoid cartilage:
  Vocal process
  Muscular process

Vocal ligament

Trachea

B. Muscles

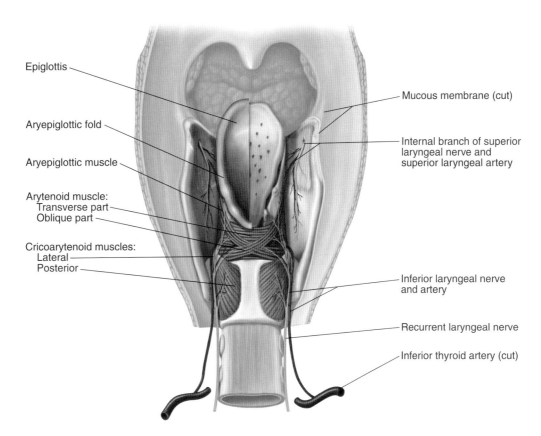

Epiglottis

Aryepiglottic fold

Aryepiglottic muscle

Arytenoid muscle:
  Transverse part
  Oblique part

Cricoarytenoid muscles:
  Lateral
  Posterior

Mucous membrane (cut)

Internal branch of superior laryngeal nerve and superior laryngeal artery

Inferior laryngeal nerve and artery

Recurrent laryngeal nerve

Inferior thyroid artery (cut)

PLATE 7-29   **Face, Anterior View**

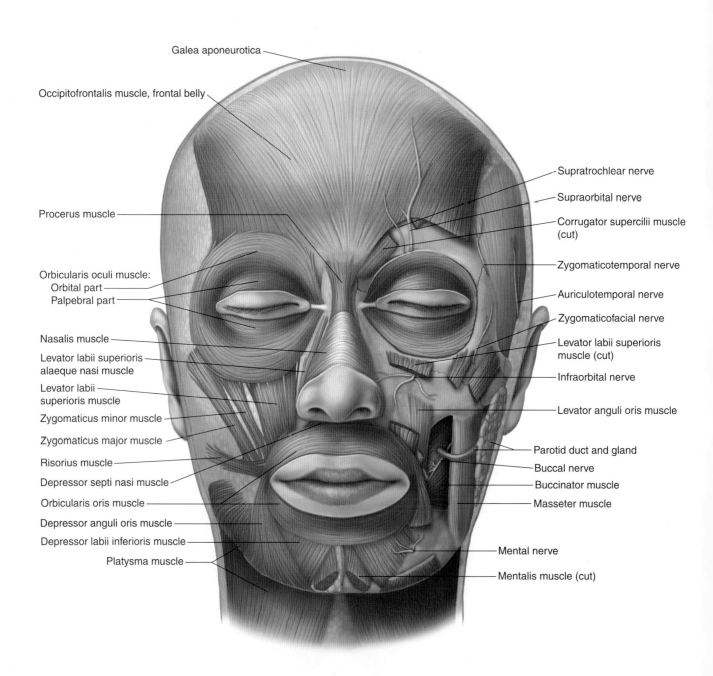

Galea aponeurotica

Occipitofrontalis muscle, frontal belly

Procerus muscle

Orbicularis oculi muscle:
  Orbital part
  Palpebral part

Nasalis muscle

Levator labii superioris
alaeque nasi muscle

Levator labii
superioris muscle

Zygomaticus minor muscle

Zygomaticus major muscle

Risorius muscle

Depressor septi nasi muscle

Orbicularis oris muscle

Depressor anguli oris muscle

Depressor labii inferioris muscle

Platysma muscle

Supratrochlear nerve

Supraorbital nerve

Corrugator supercilii muscle
(cut)

Zygomaticotemporal nerve

Auriculotemporal nerve

Zygomaticofacial nerve

Levator labii superioris
muscle (cut)

Infraorbital nerve

Levator anguli oris muscle

Parotid duct and gland

Buccal nerve

Buccinator muscle

Masseter muscle

Mental nerve

Mentalis muscle (cut)

A. Superficial dissection

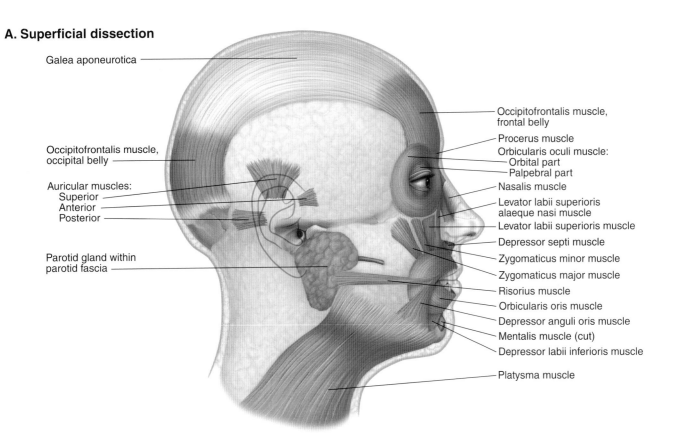

Galea aponeurotica

Occipitofrontalis muscle, occipital belly

Auricular muscles:
Superior
Anterior
Posterior

Parotid gland within parotid fascia

Occipitofrontalis muscle, frontal belly
Procerus muscle
Orbicularis oculi muscle:
Orbital part
Palpebral part
Nasalis muscle
Levator labii superioris alaeque nasi muscle
Levator labii superioris muscle
Depressor septi muscle
Zygomaticus minor muscle
Zygomaticus major muscle
Risorius muscle
Orbicularis oris muscle
Depressor anguli oris muscle
Mentalis muscle (cut)
Depressor labii inferioris muscle
Platysma muscle

B. Deep dissection

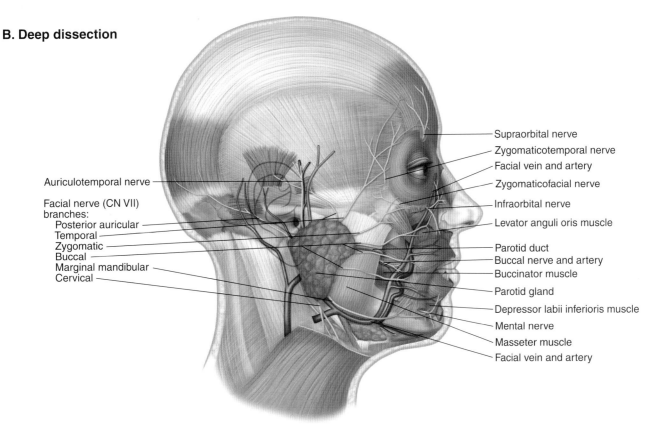

Auriculotemporal nerve

Facial nerve (CN VII) branches:
Posterior auricular
Temporal
Zygomatic
Buccal
Marginal mandibular
Cervical

Supraorbital nerve
Zygomaticotemporal nerve
Facial vein and artery
Zygomaticofacial nerve
Infraorbital nerve
Levator anguli oris muscle
Parotid duct
Buccal nerve and artery
Buccinator muscle
Parotid gland
Depressor labii inferioris muscle
Mental nerve
Masseter muscle
Facial vein and artery

PLATE 7-31 | Face, Lateral View II

A. Parotid gland and facial nerve

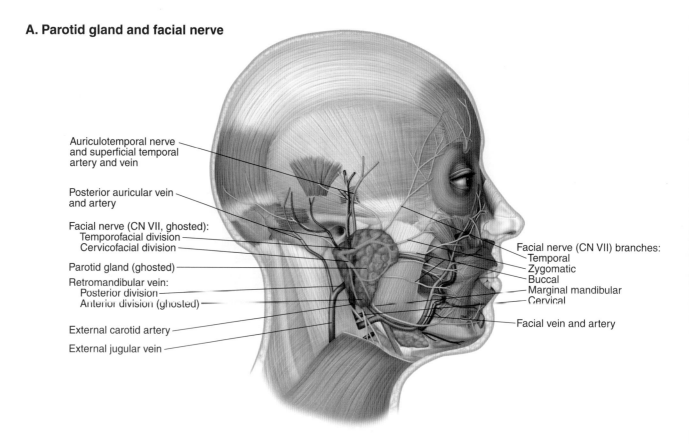

Auriculotemporal nerve
and superficial temporal
artery and vein

Posterior auricular vein
and artery

Facial nerve (CN VII, ghosted):
  Temporofacial division
  Cervicofacial division

Parotid gland (ghosted)

Retromandibular vein:
  Posterior division
  Anterior division (ghosted)

External carotid artery

External jugular vein

Facial nerve (CN VII) branches:
  Temporal
  Zygomatic
  Buccal
  Marginal mandibular
  Cervical

Facial vein and artery

B. Muscles innervated by trigeminal nerve (CN V), superficial dissection

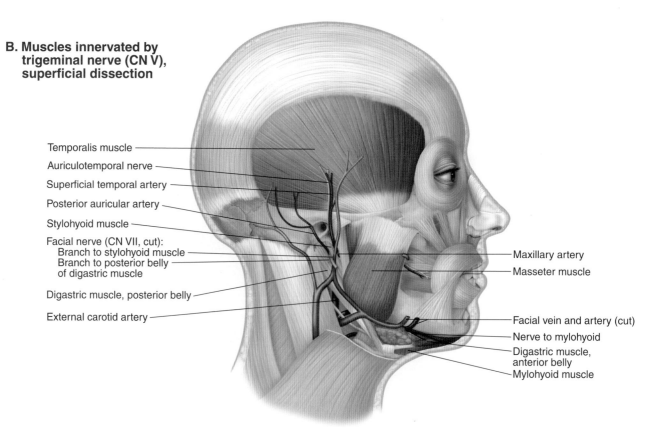

Temporalis muscle

Auriculotemporal nerve

Superficial temporal artery

Posterior auricular artery

Stylohyoid muscle

Facial nerve (CN VII, cut):
  Branch to stylohyoid muscle
  Branch to posterior belly
  of digastric muscle

Digastric muscle, posterior belly

External carotid artery

Maxillary artery

Masseter muscle

Facial vein and artery (cut)

Nerve to mylohyoid

Digastric muscle,
anterior belly

Mylohyoid muscle

A. Temporal and infratemporal fossae

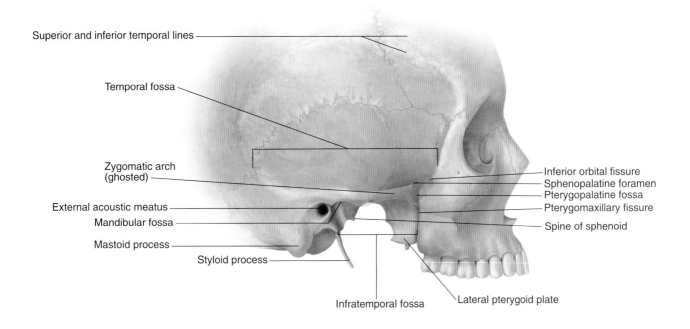

Superior and inferior temporal lines

Temporal fossa

Zygomatic arch (ghosted)

External acoustic meatus

Mandibular fossa

Mastoid process

Styloid process

Infratemporal fossa

Inferior orbital fissure
Sphenopalatine foramen
Pterygopalatine fossa
Pterygomaxillary fissure
Spine of sphenoid

Lateral pterygoid plate

C. Mandible, medial view

Coronoid process

Condyle

Mandibular notch

Lingula
Mandibular foramen

I_1 I_2

C P_1 P_2 M_1 M_2 M_3

Alveolar process

Groove for nerve to mylohyoid
Angle

Mylohyoid line

Digastric fossa

Mental spine

B. Mandible, lateral view

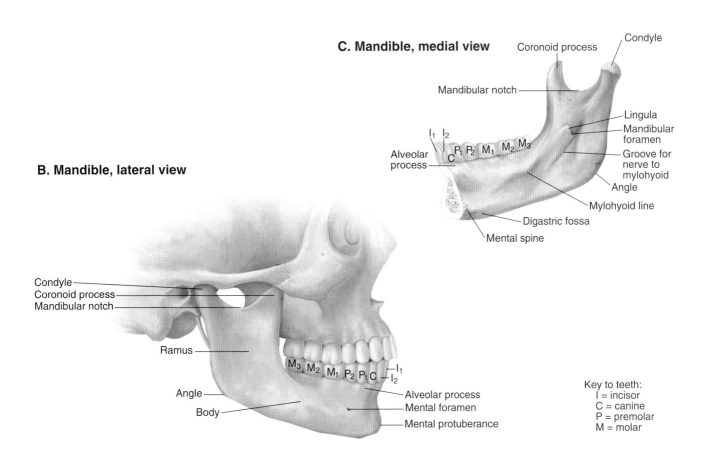

Condyle
Coronoid process
Mandibular notch

Ramus

Angle

Body

M_3 M_2 M_1 P_2 P_1 C I_1 I_2

Alveolar process
Mental foramen

Mental protuberance

Key to teeth:
I = incisor
C = canine
P = premolar
M = molar

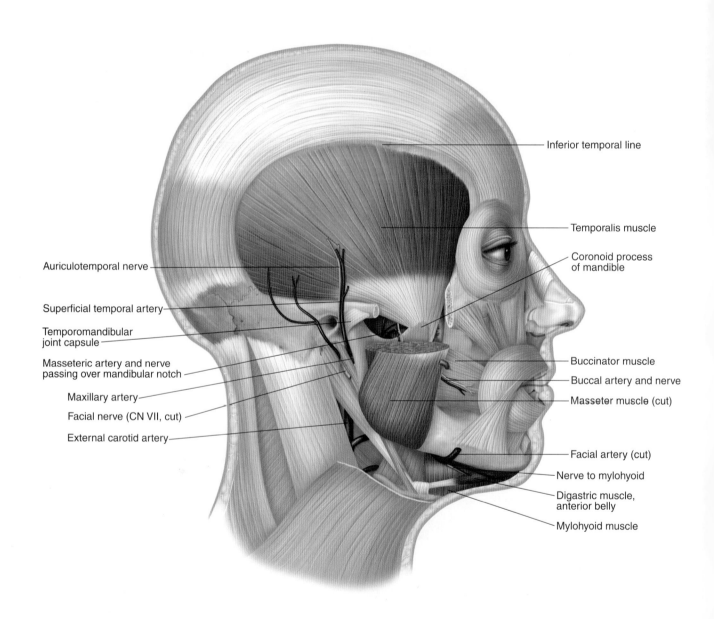

Inferior temporal line

Temporalis muscle

Coronoid process
of mandible

Auriculotemporal nerve

Superficial temporal artery

Temporomandibular
joint capsule

Masseteric artery and nerve
passing over mandibular notch

Maxillary artery

Facial nerve (CN VII, cut)

External carotid artery

Buccinator muscle

Buccal artery and nerve

Masseter muscle (cut)

Facial artery (cut)

Nerve to mylohyoid

Digastric muscle,
anterior belly

Mylohyoid muscle

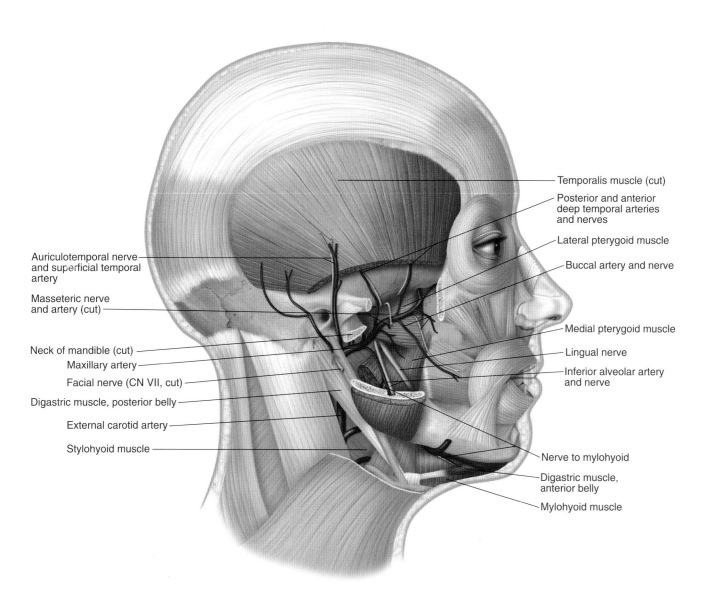

Temporalis muscle (cut)

Posterior and anterior
deep temporal arteries
and nerves

Lateral pterygoid muscle

Buccal artery and nerve

Auriculotemporal nerve
and superficial temporal
artery

Masseteric nerve
and artery (cut)

Neck of mandible (cut)

Maxillary artery

Facial nerve (CN VII, cut)

Digastric muscle, posterior belly

External carotid artery

Stylohyoid muscle

Medial pterygoid muscle

Lingual nerve

Inferior alveolar artery
and nerve

Nerve to mylohyoid

Digastric muscle,
anterior belly

Mylohyoid muscle

PLATE 7-35   **Arteries of the Infratemporal Region**

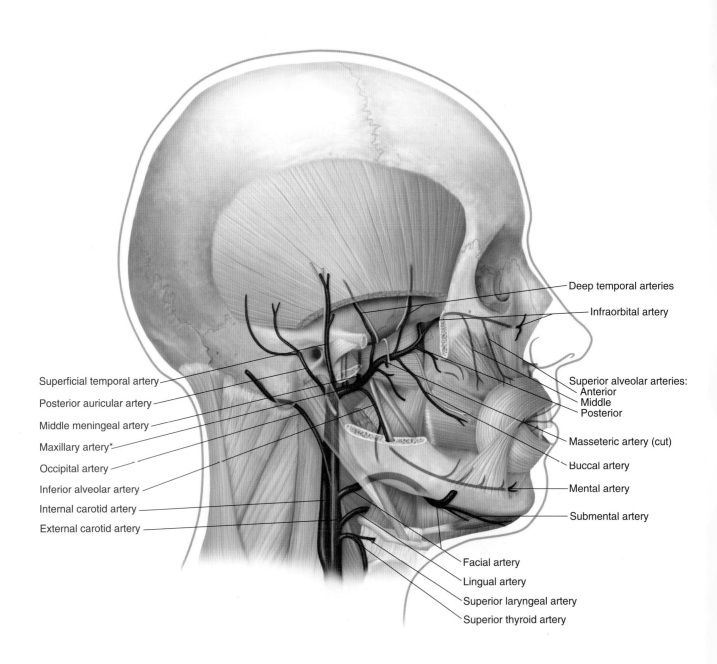

Deep temporal arteries

Infraorbital artery

Superficial temporal artery

Posterior auricular artery

Middle meningeal artery

Maxillary artery*

Occipital artery

Inferior alveolar artery

Internal carotid artery

External carotid artery

Superior alveolar arteries:
Anterior
Middle
Posterior

Masseteric artery (cut)

Buccal artery

Mental artery

Submental artery

Facial artery

Lingual artery

Superior laryngeal artery

Superior thyroid artery

* The maxillary artery may pass medial (42%) or
lateral to lateral pterygoid muscle

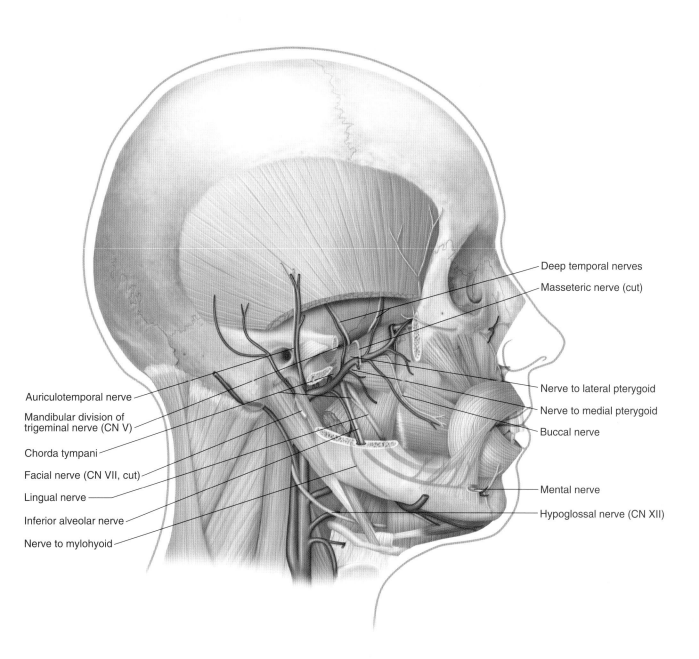

Deep temporal nerves

Masseteric nerve (cut)

Auriculotemporal nerve

Mandibular division of
trigeminal nerve (CN V)

Chorda tympani

Facial nerve (CN VII, cut)

Lingual nerve

Inferior alveolar nerve

Nerve to mylohyoid

Nerve to lateral pterygoid

Nerve to medial pterygoid

Buccal nerve

Mental nerve

Hypoglossal nerve (CN XII)

PLATE 7-37 **Submandibular and Sublingual Regions**

A. Lateral view

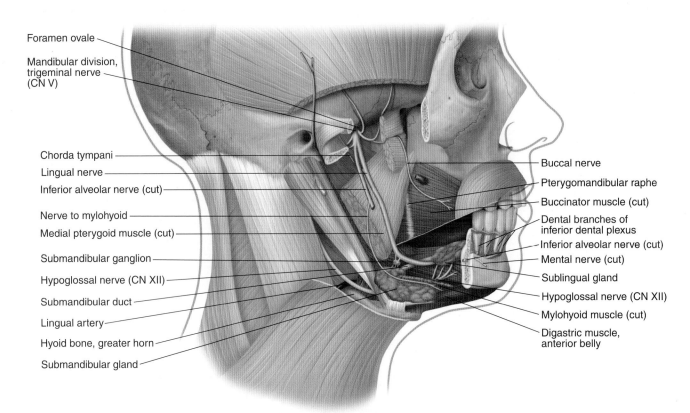

Foramen ovale

Mandibular division, trigeminal nerve (CN V)

Chorda tympani

Lingual nerve

Inferior alveolar nerve (cut)

Nerve to mylohyoid

Medial pterygoid muscle (cut)

Submandibular ganglion

Hypoglossal nerve (CN XII)

Submandibular duct

Lingual artery

Hyoid bone, greater horn

Submandibular gland

Buccal nerve

Pterygomandibular raphe

Buccinator muscle (cut)

Dental branches of inferior dental plexus

Inferior alveolar nerve (cut)

Mental nerve (cut)

Sublingual gland

Hypoglossal nerve (CN XII)

Mylohyoid muscle (cut)

Digastric muscle, anterior belly

B. Medial view

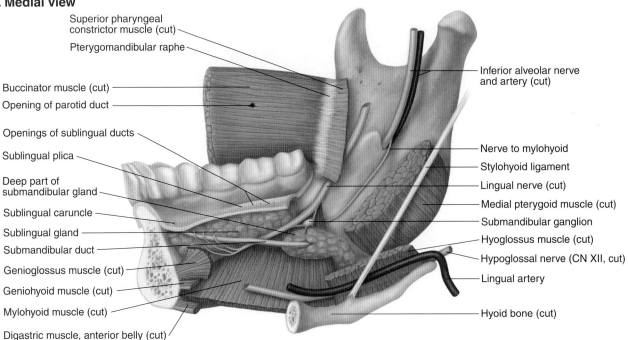

Superior pharyngeal constrictor muscle (cut)

Pterygomandibular raphe

Buccinator muscle (cut)

Opening of parotid duct

Openings of sublingual ducts

Sublingual plica

Deep part of submandibular gland

Sublingual caruncle

Sublingual gland

Submandibular duct

Genioglossus muscle (cut)

Geniohyoid muscle (cut)

Mylohyoid muscle (cut)

Digastric muscle, anterior belly (cut)

Inferior alveolar nerve and artery (cut)

Nerve to mylohyoid

Stylohyoid ligament

Lingual nerve (cut)

Medial pterygoid muscle (cut)

Submandibular ganglion

Hyoglossus muscle (cut)

Hypoglossal nerve (CN XII, cut)

Lingual artery

Hyoid bone (cut)

A. Mucosal features

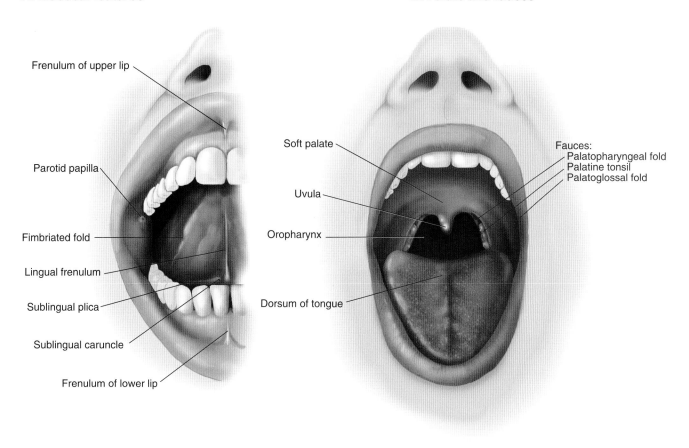

Frenulum of upper lip

Parotid papilla

Fimbriated fold

Lingual frenulum

Sublingual plica

Sublingual caruncle

Frenulum of lower lip

B. Palate and fauces

Soft palate

Uvula

Oropharynx

Dorsum of tongue

Fauces:
Palatopharyngeal fold
Palatine tonsil
Palatoglossal fold

C. Coronal section

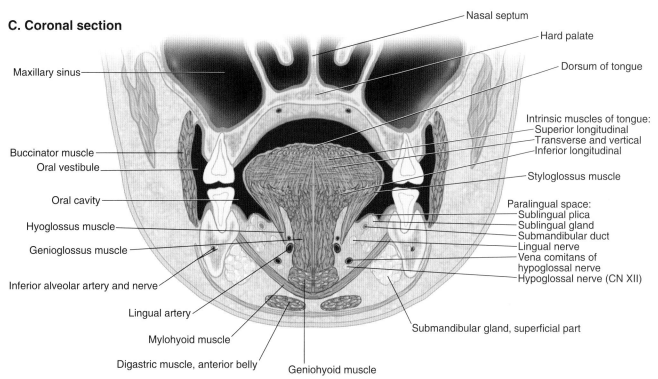

Nasal septum

Hard palate

Dorsum of tongue

Maxillary sinus

Buccinator muscle

Oral vestibule

Oral cavity

Hyoglossus muscle

Genioglossus muscle

Inferior alveolar artery and nerve

Lingual artery

Mylohyoid muscle

Digastric muscle, anterior belly

Geniohyoid muscle

Intrinsic muscles of tongue:
Superior longitudinal
Transverse and vertical
Inferior longitudinal

Styloglossus muscle

Paralingual space:
Sublingual plica
Sublingual gland
Submandibular duct
Lingual nerve
Vena comitans of
hypoglossal nerve
Hypoglossal nerve (CN XII)

Submandibular gland, superficial part

PLATE 7-39   **Dorsum of Tongue**

A. Surface features

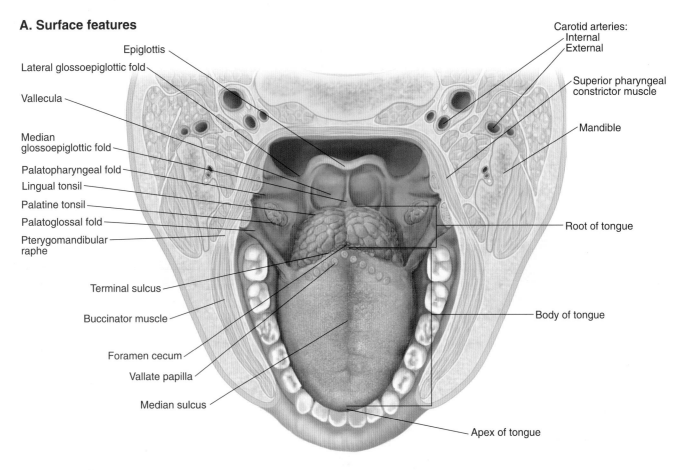

Epiglottis

Lateral glossoepiglottic fold

Vallecula

Median glossoepiglottic fold

Palatopharyngeal fold

Lingual tonsil

Palatine tonsil

Palatoglossal fold

Pterygomandibular raphe

Terminal sulcus

Buccinator muscle

Foramen cecum

Vallate papilla

Median sulcus

Carotid arteries:
Internal
External

Superior pharyngeal constrictor muscle

Mandible

Root of tongue

Body of tongue

Apex of tongue

B. Innervation

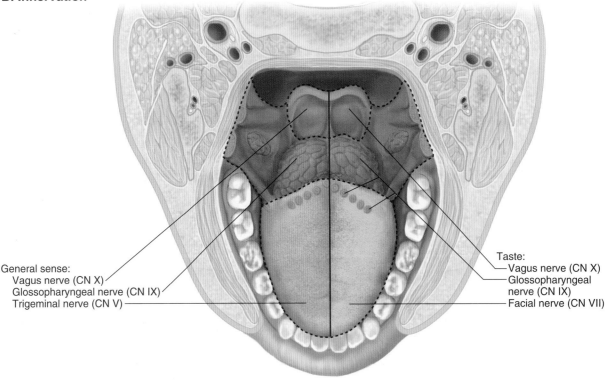

General sense:
Vagus nerve (CN X)
Glossopharyngeal nerve (CN IX)
Trigeminal nerve (CN V)

Taste:
Vagus nerve (CN X)
Glossopharyngeal nerve (CN IX)
Facial nerve (CN VII)

A. Extrinsic muscles

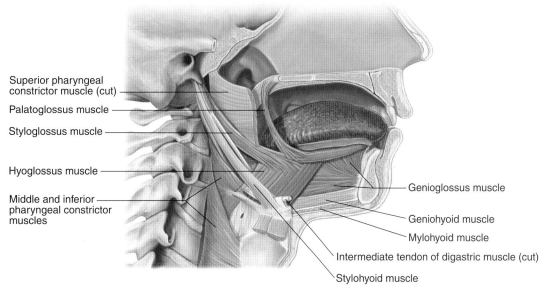

Superior pharyngeal constrictor muscle (cut)

Palatoglossus muscle

Styloglossus muscle

Hyoglossus muscle

Middle and inferior pharyngeal constrictor muscles

Genioglossus muscle

Geniohyoid muscle

Mylohyoid muscle

Intermediate tendon of digastric muscle (cut)

Stylohyoid muscle

B. Blood supply

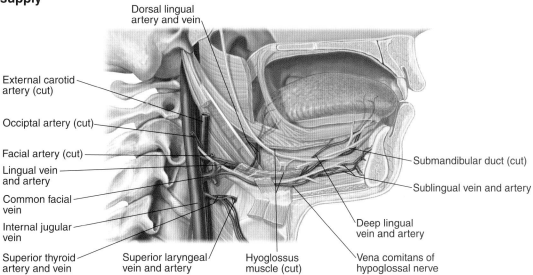

Dorsal lingual artery and vein

External carotid artery (cut)

Occiptal artery (cut)

Facial artery (cut)

Lingual vein and artery

Common facial vein

Internal jugular vein

Superior thyroid artery and vein

Superior laryngeal vein and artery

Hyoglossus muscle (cut)

Submandibular duct (cut)

Sublingual vein and artery

Deep lingual vein and artery

Vena comitans of hypoglossal nerve

C. Nerve supply

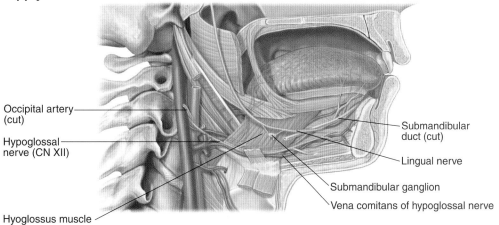

Occipital artery (cut)

Hypoglossal nerve (CN XII)

Hyoglossus muscle

Submandibular duct (cut)

Lingual nerve

Submandibular ganglion

Vena comitans of hypoglossal nerve

PLATE 7-41 | Nasal Septum and Palate

A. Bones and cartilages

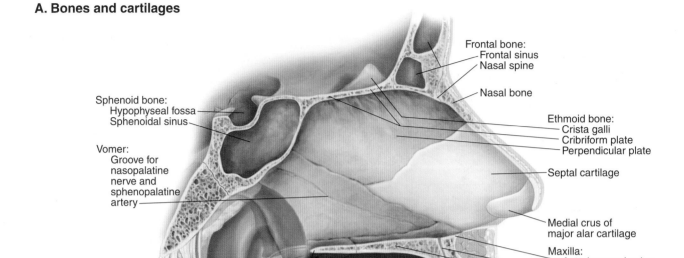

Frontal bone:
Frontal sinus
Nasal spine

Nasal bone

Sphenoid bone:
Hypophyseal fossa
Sphenoidal sinus

Ethmoid bone:
Crista galli
Cribriform plate
Perpendicular plate

Vomer:
Groove for
nasopalatine
nerve and
sphenopalatine
artery

Septal cartilage

Medial crus of
major alar cartilage

Maxilla:
Anterior nasal spine
Incisive canal
Palatine process
Alveolar process

Palatine bone:
Horizontal plate
Lesser palatine foramen

Greater palatine foramen

B. Mucosal features

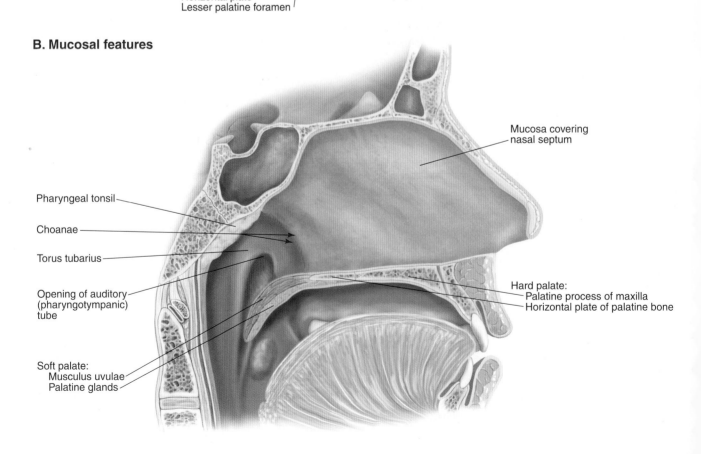

Mucosa covering
nasal septum

Pharyngeal tonsil

Choanae

Torus tubarius

Opening of auditory
(pharyngotympanic)
tube

Hard palate:
Palatine process of maxilla
Horizontal plate of palatine bone

Soft palate:
Musculus uvulae
Palatine glands

A. Bones

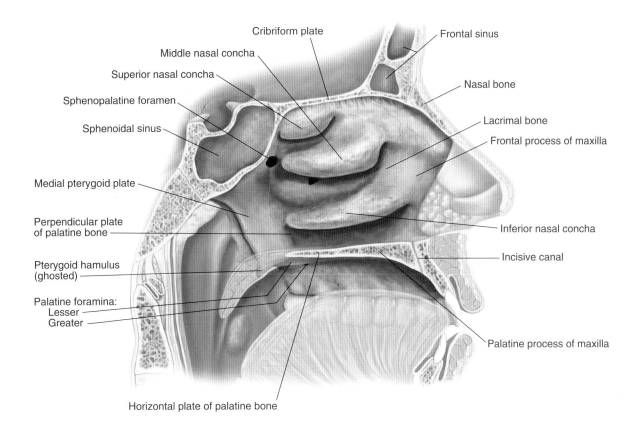

Cribriform plate
Middle nasal concha
Superior nasal concha
Sphenopalatine foramen
Sphenoidal sinus
Medial pterygoid plate
Perpendicular plate of palatine bone
Pterygoid hamulus (ghosted)
Palatine foramina:
  Lesser
  Greater
Horizontal plate of palatine bone
Frontal sinus
Nasal bone
Lacrimal bone
Frontal process of maxilla
Inferior nasal concha
Incisive canal
Palatine process of maxilla

B. Bones of the middle meatus

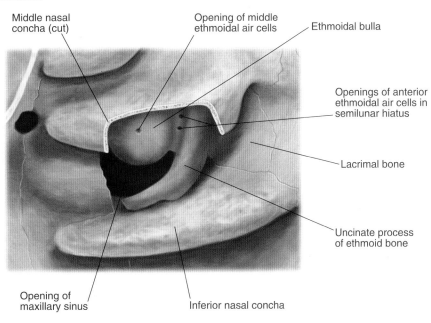

Middle nasal concha (cut)
Opening of middle ethmoidal air cells
Ethmoidal bulla
Openings of anterior ethmoidal air cells in semilunar hiatus
Lacrimal bone
Uncinate process of ethmoid bone
Opening of maxillary sinus
Inferior nasal concha

PLATE 7-43 | Lateral Wall of Nasal Cavity II

A. Nasal conchae and meatuses

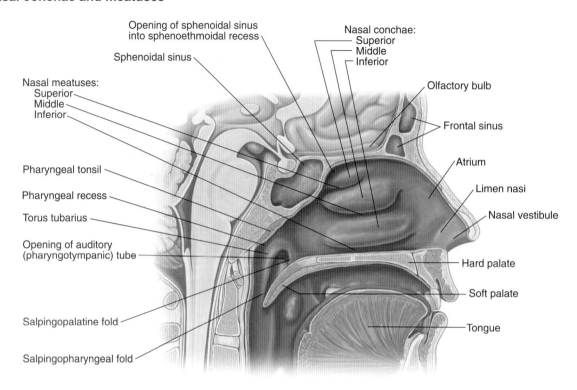

Opening of sphenoidal sinus into sphenoethmoidal recess

Sphenoidal sinus

Nasal conchae:
Superior
Middle
Inferior

Olfactory bulb

Frontal sinus

Nasal meatuses:
Superior
Middle
Inferior

Atrium

Limen nasi

Pharyngeal tonsil

Nasal vestibule

Pharyngeal recess

Torus tubarius

Opening of auditory (pharyngotympanic) tube

Hard palate

Soft palate

Salpingopalatine fold

Tongue

Salpingopharyngeal fold

B. Openings in the lateral wall of the nasal cavity

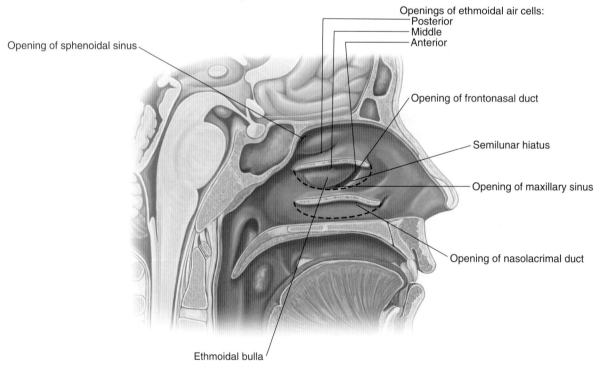

Openings of ethmoidal air cells:
Posterior
Middle
Anterior

Opening of sphenoidal sinus

Opening of frontonasal duct

Semilunar hiatus

Opening of maxillary sinus

Opening of nasolacrimal duct

Ethmoidal bulla

A. Medial view

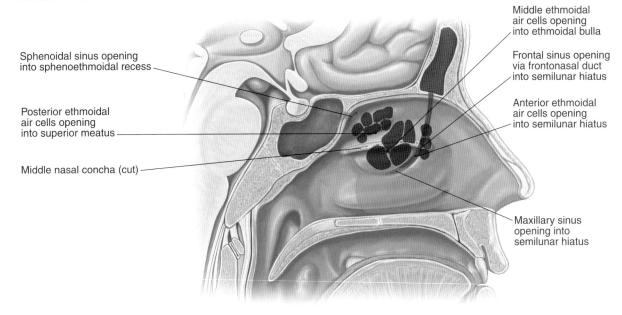

Middle ethmoidal
air cells opening
into ethmoidal bulla

Frontal sinus opening
via frontonasal duct
into semilunar hiatus

Anterior ethmoidal
air cells opening
into semilunar hiatus

Sphenoidal sinus opening
into sphenoethmoidal recess

Posterior ethmoidal
air cells opening
into superior meatus

Middle nasal concha (cut)

Maxillary sinus
opening into
semilunar hiatus

B. Anterior view

C. Lateral view

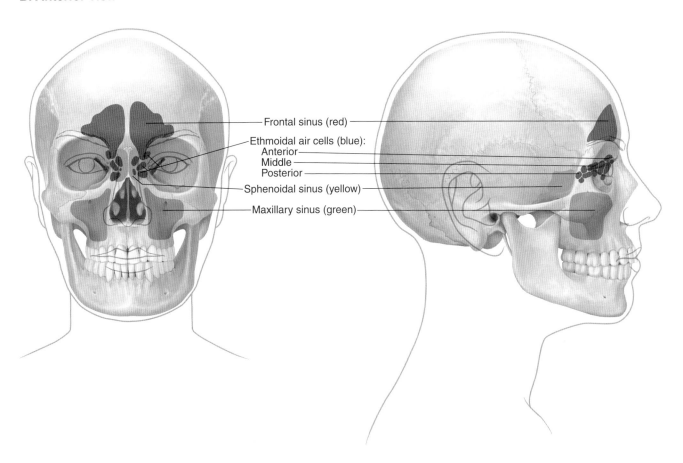

Frontal sinus (red)

Ethmoidal air cells (blue):
Anterior
Middle
Posterior

Sphenoidal sinus (yellow)

Maxillary sinus (green)

PLATE 7-45   **Blood Supply and Innervation of the Nasal Cavity**

A. Blood supply of lateral wall

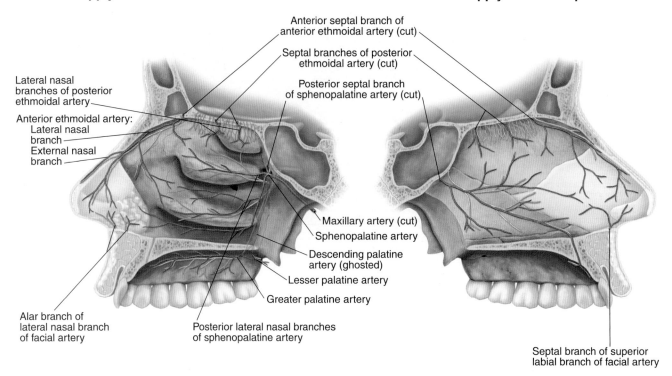

Anterior septal branch of anterior ethmoidal artery (cut)

Septal branches of posterior ethmoidal artery (cut)

Posterior septal branch of sphenopalatine artery (cut)

Lateral nasal branches of posterior ethmoidal artery

Anterior ethmoidal artery:
Lateral nasal branch
External nasal branch

Maxillary artery (cut)

Sphenopalatine artery

Descending palatine artery (ghosted)

Lesser palatine artery

Greater palatine artery

Alar branch of lateral nasal branch of facial artery

Posterior lateral nasal branches of sphenopalatine artery

B. Blood supply of nasal septum

Septal branch of superior labial branch of facial artery

C. Nerves of lateral wall

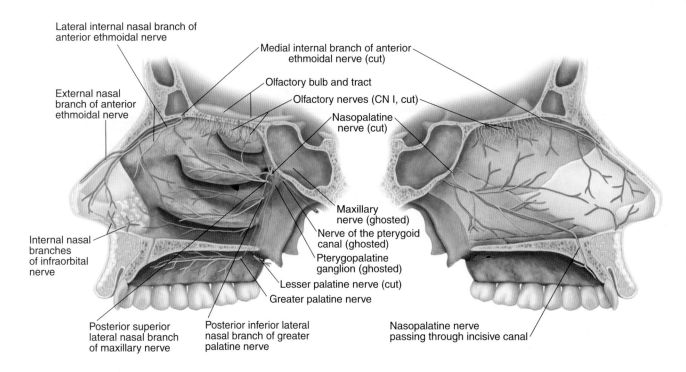

Lateral internal nasal branch of anterior ethmoidal nerve

Medial internal branch of anterior ethmoidal nerve (cut)

Olfactory bulb and tract

External nasal branch of anterior ethmoidal nerve

Olfactory nerves (CN I, cut)

Nasopalatine nerve (cut)

Maxillary nerve (ghosted)

Nerve of the pterygoid canal (ghosted)

Internal nasal branches of infraorbital nerve

Pterygopalatine ganglion (ghosted)

Lesser palatine nerve (cut)

Greater palatine nerve

Posterior superior lateral nasal branch of maxillary nerve

Posterior inferior lateral nasal branch of greater palatine nerve

D. Nerves of nasal septum

Nasopalatine nerve passing through incisive canal

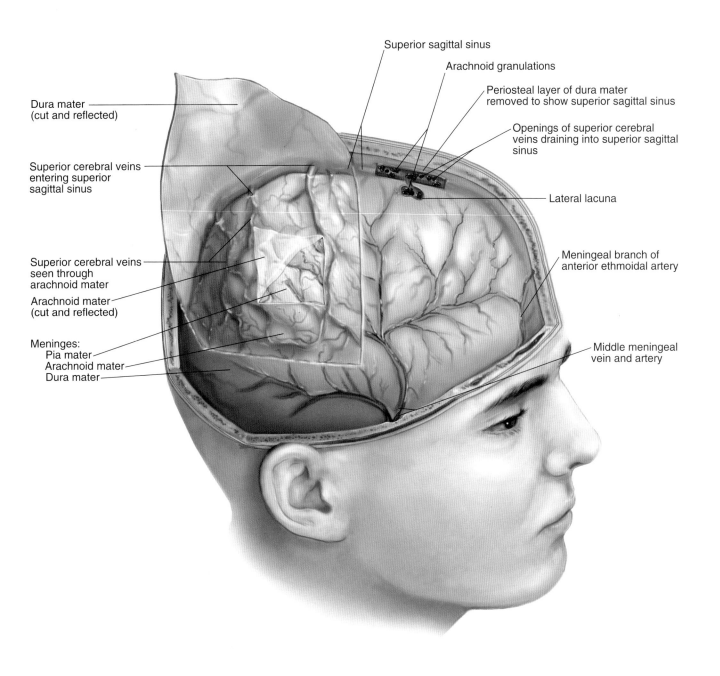

Superior sagittal sinus

Arachnoid granulations

Periosteal layer of dura mater
removed to show superior sagittal sinus

Openings of superior cerebral
veins draining into superior sagittal
sinus

Dura mater
(cut and reflected)

Superior cerebral veins
entering superior
sagittal sinus

Lateral lacuna

Superior cerebral veins
seen through
arachnoid mater

Arachnoid mater
(cut and reflected)

Meninges:
 Pia mater
 Arachnoid mater
 Dura mater

Meningeal branch of
anterior ethmoidal artery

Middle meningeal
vein and artery

PLATE 7-47 **Dural Venous Sinuses, Superior View**

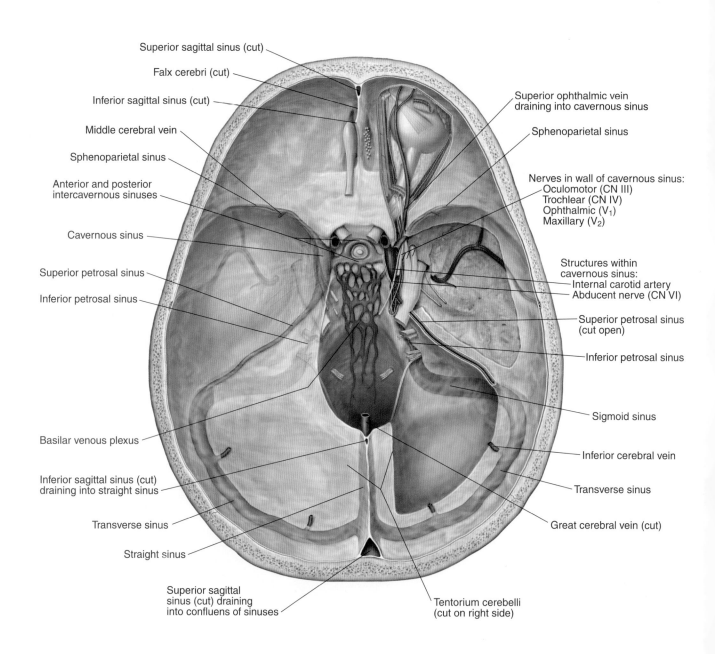

Superior sagittal sinus (cut)

Falx cerebri (cut)

Inferior sagittal sinus (cut)

Middle cerebral vein

Sphenoparietal sinus

Anterior and posterior
intercavernous sinuses

Cavernous sinus

Superior petrosal sinus

Inferior petrosal sinus

Basilar venous plexus

Inferior sagittal sinus (cut)
draining into straight sinus

Transverse sinus

Straight sinus

Superior sagittal
sinus (cut) draining
into confluens of sinuses

Superior ophthalmic vein
draining into cavernous sinus

Sphenoparietal sinus

Nerves in wall of cavernous sinus:
Oculomotor (CN III)
Trochlear (CN IV)
Ophthalmic (V₁)
Maxillary (V₂)

Structures within
cavernous sinus:
Internal carotid artery
Abducent nerve (CN VI)

Superior petrosal sinus
(cut open)

Inferior petrosal sinus

Sigmoid sinus

Inferior cerebral vein

Transverse sinus

Great cerebral vein (cut)

Tentorium cerebelli
(cut on right side)

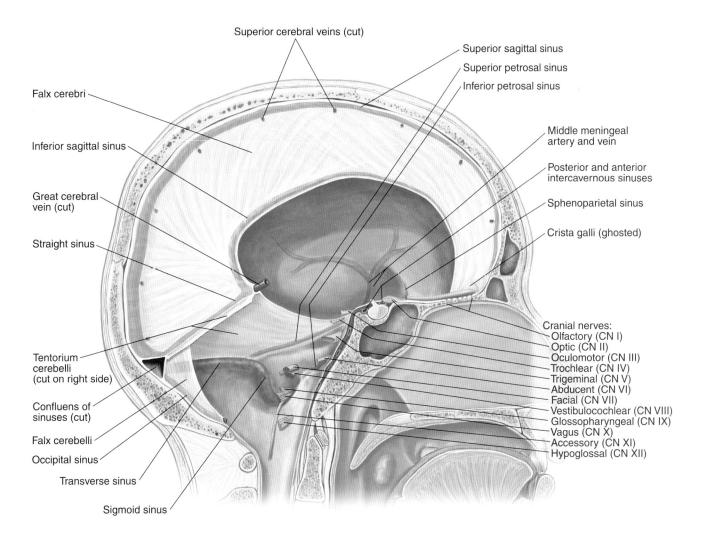

Superior cerebral veins (cut)

Falx cerebri

Inferior sagittal sinus

Great cerebral vein (cut)

Straight sinus

Tentorium cerebelli (cut on right side)

Confluens of sinuses (cut)

Falx cerebelli

Occipital sinus

Transverse sinus

Sigmoid sinus

Superior sagittal sinus

Superior petrosal sinus

Inferior petrosal sinus

Middle meningeal artery and vein

Posterior and anterior intercavernous sinuses

Sphenoparietal sinus

Crista galli (ghosted)

Cranial nerves:
Olfactory (CN I)
Optic (CN II)
Oculomotor (CN III)
Trochlear (CN IV)
Trigeminal (CN V)
Abducent (CN VI)
Facial (CN VII)
Vestibulocochlear (CN VIII)
Glossopharyngeal (CN IX)
Vagus (CN X)
Accessory (CN XI)
Hypoglossal (CN XII)

PLATE 7-49   **Dural Venous Sinuses, Sectioned**

A. Sagittal section

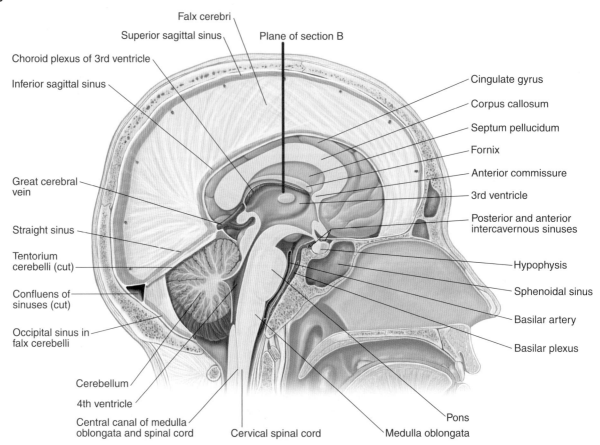

Falx cerebri

Superior sagittal sinus

Plane of section B

Choroid plexus of 3rd ventricle

Inferior sagittal sinus

Cingulate gyrus

Corpus callosum

Septum pellucidum

Fornix

Anterior commissure

Great cerebral vein

3rd ventricle

Posterior and anterior intercavernous sinuses

Straight sinus

Tentorium cerebelli (cut)

Hypophysis

Sphenoidal sinus

Confluens of sinuses (cut)

Basilar artery

Occipital sinus in falx cerebelli

Basilar plexus

Cerebellum

4th ventricle

Central canal of medulla oblongata and spinal cord

Cervical spinal cord

Pons

Medulla oblongata

B. Coronal section

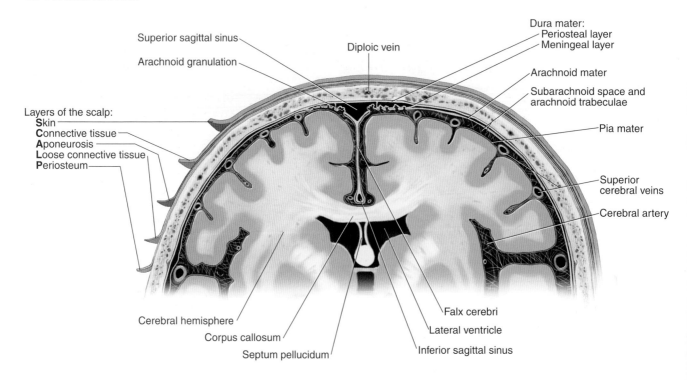

Superior sagittal sinus

Arachnoid granulation

Diploic vein

Dura mater:
  Periosteal layer
  Meningeal layer

Arachnoid mater

Subarachnoid space and arachnoid trabeculae

Layers of the scalp:
Skin
Connective tissue
Aponeurosis
Loose connective tissue
Periosteum

Pia mater

Superior cerebral veins

Cerebral artery

Cerebral hemisphere

Corpus callosum

Septum pellucidum

Falx cerebri

Lateral ventricle

Inferior sagittal sinus

A. Location of ventricles

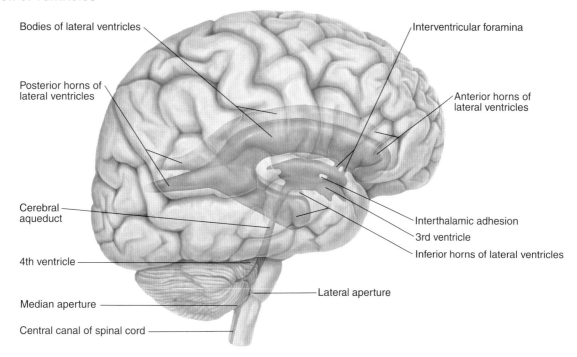

Bodies of lateral ventricles

Interventricular foramina

Posterior horns of lateral ventricles

Anterior horns of lateral ventricles

Cerebral aqueduct

Interthalamic adhesion

3rd ventricle

Inferior horns of lateral ventricles

4th ventricle

Lateral aperture

Median aperture

Central canal of spinal cord

B. Circulation of cerebrospinal fluid

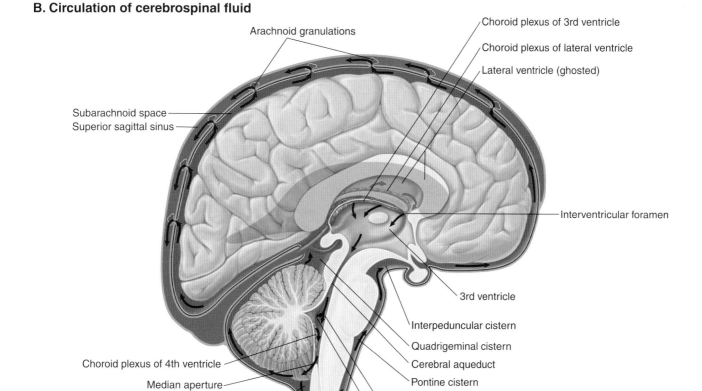

Arachnoid granulations

Choroid plexus of 3rd ventricle

Choroid plexus of lateral ventricle

Lateral ventricle (ghosted)

Subarachnoid space

Superior sagittal sinus

Interventricular foramen

3rd ventricle

Interpeduncular cistern

Quadrigeminal cistern

Cerebral aqueduct

Pontine cistern

Choroid plexus of 4th ventricle

Median aperture

Cerebellomedullary cistern

4th ventricle

Central canal of spinal cord

Lateral aperture

PLATE 7-51   **Cranial Nerves in the Cranial Cavity**

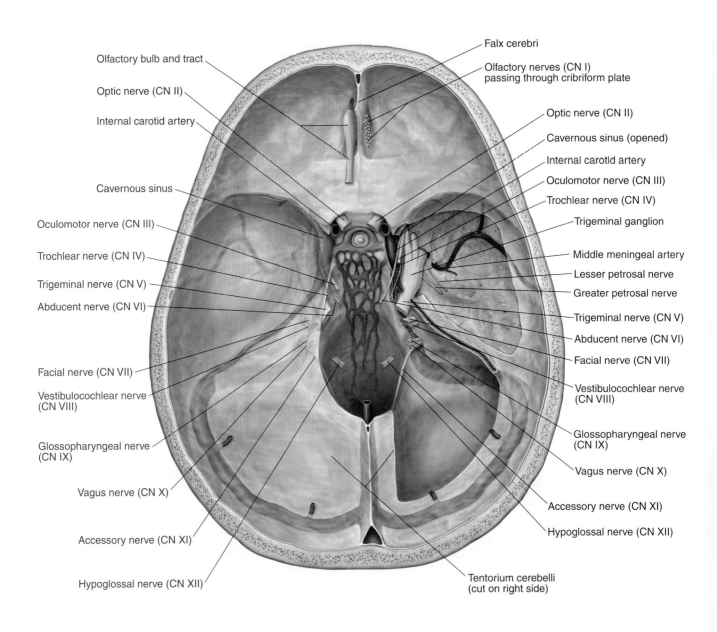

Olfactory bulb and tract

Optic nerve (CN II)

Internal carotid artery

Cavernous sinus

Oculomotor nerve (CN III)

Trochlear nerve (CN IV)

Trigeminal nerve (CN V)

Abducent nerve (CN VI)

Facial nerve (CN VII)

Vestibulocochlear nerve
(CN VIII)

Glossopharyngeal nerve
(CN IX)

Vagus nerve (CN X)

Accessory nerve (CN XI)

Hypoglossal nerve (CN XII)

Falx cerebri

Olfactory nerves (CN I)
passing through cribriform plate

Optic nerve (CN II)

Cavernous sinus (opened)

Internal carotid artery

Oculomotor nerve (CN III)

Trochlear nerve (CN IV)

Trigeminal ganglion

Middle meningeal artery

Lesser petrosal nerve

Greater petrosal nerve

Trigeminal nerve (CN V)

Abducent nerve (CN VI)

Facial nerve (CN VII)

Vestibulocochlear nerve
(CN VIII)

Glossopharyngeal nerve
(CN IX)

Vagus nerve (CN X)

Accessory nerve (CN XI)

Hypoglossal nerve (CN XII)

Tentorium cerebelli
(cut on right side)

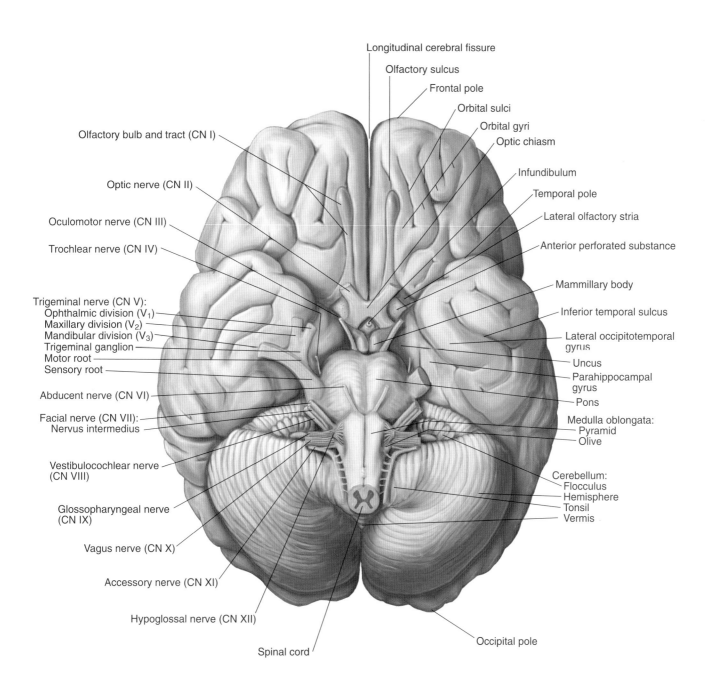

Longitudinal cerebral fissure

Olfactory sulcus

Frontal pole

Orbital sulci

Orbital gyri

Optic chiasm

Infundibulum

Temporal pole

Lateral olfactory stria

Anterior perforated substance

Mammillary body

Inferior temporal sulcus

Lateral occipitotemporal gyrus

Uncus

Parahippocampal gyrus

Pons

Medulla oblongata:
Pyramid
Olive

Cerebellum:
Flocculus
Hemisphere
Tonsil
Vermis

Occipital pole

Olfactory bulb and tract (CN I)

Optic nerve (CN II)

Oculomotor nerve (CN III)

Trochlear nerve (CN IV)

Trigeminal nerve (CN V):
Ophthalmic division (V$_1$)
Maxillary division (V$_2$)
Mandibular division (V$_3$)
Trigeminal ganglion
Motor root
Sensory root

Abducent nerve (CN VI)

Facial nerve (CN VII):
Nervus intermedius

Vestibulocochlear nerve (CN VIII)

Glossopharyngeal nerve (CN IX)

Vagus nerve (CN X)

Accessory nerve (CN XI)

Hypoglossal nerve (CN XII)

Spinal cord

PLATE 7-53   Brain, Brainstem, and Cerebellum

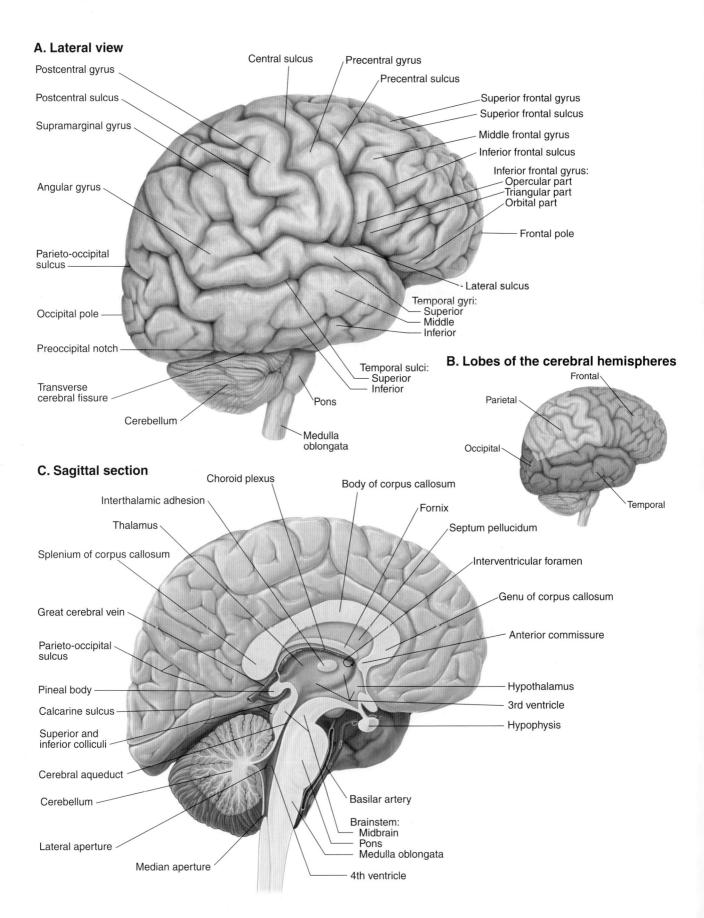

A. Lateral view

Postcentral gyrus

Central sulcus

Precentral gyrus

Precentral sulcus

Postcentral sulcus

Superior frontal gyrus

Supramarginal gyrus

Superior frontal sulcus

Middle frontal gyrus

Inferior frontal sulcus

Inferior frontal gyrus:
Opercular part
Triangular part
Orbital part

Angular gyrus

Frontal pole

Parieto-occipital
sulcus

Lateral sulcus

Temporal gyri:
Superior
Middle
Inferior

Occipital pole

Preoccipital notch

Temporal sulci:
Superior
Inferior

B. Lobes of the cerebral hemispheres

Frontal

Parietal

Occipital

Temporal

Transverse
cerebral fissure

Cerebellum

Pons

Medulla
oblongata

C. Sagittal section

Choroid plexus

Body of corpus callosum

Interthalamic adhesion

Fornix

Thalamus

Septum pellucidum

Splenium of corpus callosum

Interventricular foramen

Genu of corpus callosum

Great cerebral vein

Anterior commissure

Parieto-occipital
sulcus

Hypothalamus

Pineal body

3rd ventricle

Calcarine sulcus

Hypophysis

Superior and
inferior colliculi

Cerebral aqueduct

Basilar artery

Cerebellum

Brainstem:
Midbrain
Pons
Medulla oblongata

Lateral aperture

Median aperture

4th ventricle

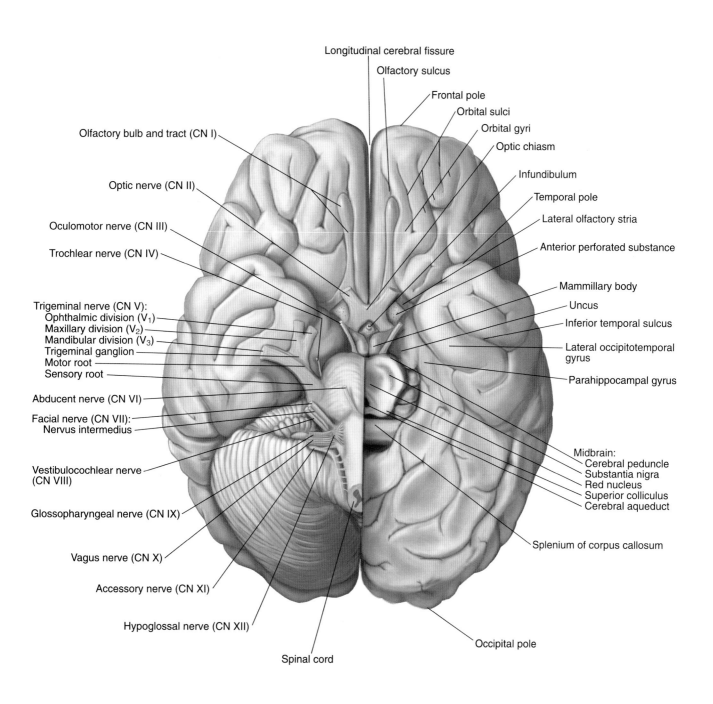

Longitudinal cerebral fissure

Olfactory sulcus

Frontal pole

Orbital sulci

Orbital gyri

Optic chiasm

Infundibulum

Temporal pole

Lateral olfactory stria

Anterior perforated substance

Mammillary body

Uncus

Inferior temporal sulcus

Lateral occipitotemporal gyrus

Parahippocampal gyrus

Midbrain:
Cerebral peduncle
Substantia nigra
Red nucleus
Superior colliculus
Cerebral aqueduct

Splenium of corpus callosum

Occipital pole

Olfactory bulb and tract (CN I)

Optic nerve (CN II)

Oculomotor nerve (CN III)

Trochlear nerve (CN IV)

Trigeminal nerve (CN V):
Ophthalmic division (V$_1$)
Maxillary division (V$_2$)
Mandibular division (V$_3$)
Trigeminal ganglion
Motor root
Sensory root

Abducent nerve (CN VI)

Facial nerve (CN VII):
Nervus intermedius

Vestibulocochlear nerve (CN VIII)

Glossopharyngeal nerve (CN IX)

Vagus nerve (CN X)

Accessory nerve (CN XI)

Hypoglossal nerve (CN XII)

Spinal cord

PLATE 7-55   Cranial Nerves and Brainstem

A. Anterior view

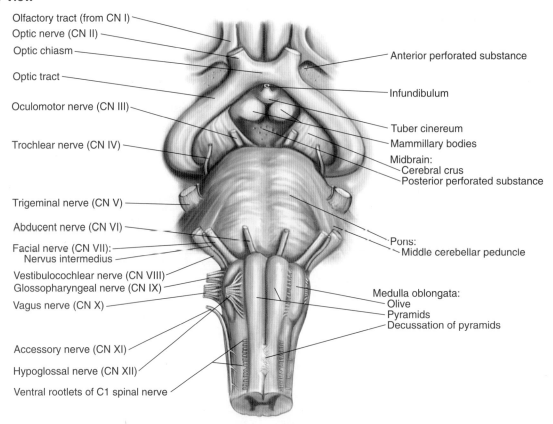

Olfactory tract (from CN I)
Optic nerve (CN II)
Optic chiasm
Optic tract
Oculomotor nerve (CN III)
Trochlear nerve (CN IV)
Trigeminal nerve (CN V)
Abducent nerve (CN VI)
Facial nerve (CN VII):
  Nervus intermedius
Vestibulocochlear nerve (CN VIII)
Glossopharyngeal nerve (CN IX)
Vagus nerve (CN X)
Accessory nerve (CN XI)
Hypoglossal nerve (CN XII)
Ventral rootlets of C1 spinal nerve

Anterior perforated substance
Infundibulum
Tuber cinereum
Mammillary bodies
Midbrain:
  Cerebral crus
  Posterior perforated substance
Pons:
  Middle cerebellar peduncle
Medulla oblongata:
  Olive
  Pyramids
  Decussation of pyramids

B. Posterior view

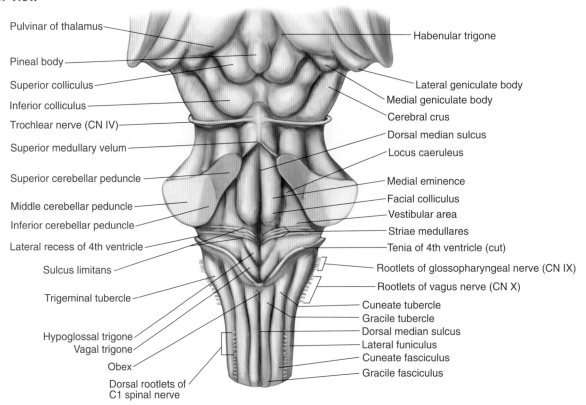

Pulvinar of thalamus
Pineal body
Superior colliculus
Inferior colliculus
Trochlear nerve (CN IV)
Superior medullary velum
Superior cerebellar peduncle
Middle cerebellar peduncle
Inferior cerebellar peduncle
Lateral recess of 4th ventricle
Sulcus limitans
Trigeminal tubercle
Hypoglossal trigone
Vagal trigone
Obex
Dorsal rootlets of
C1 spinal nerve

Habenular trigone
Lateral geniculate body
Medial geniculate body
Cerebral crus
Dorsal median sulcus
Locus caeruleus
Medial eminence
Facial colliculus
Vestibular area
Striae medullares
Tenia of 4th ventricle (cut)
Rootlets of glossopharyngeal nerve (CN IX)
Rootlets of vagus nerve (CN X)
Cuneate tubercle
Gracile tubercle
Dorsal median sulcus
Lateral funiculus
Cuneate fasciculus
Gracile fasciculus

A. Inferior view

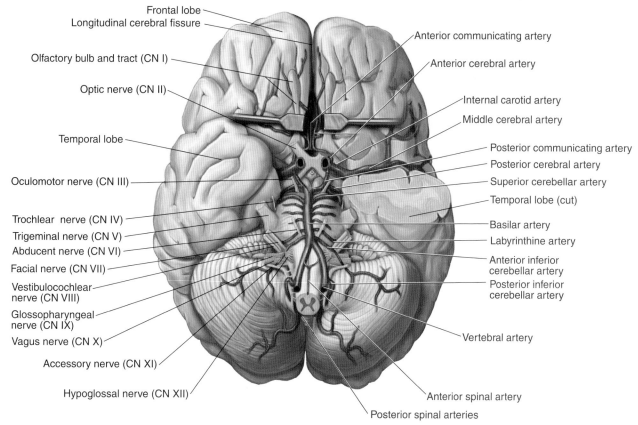

Frontal lobe
Longitudinal cerebral fissure
Olfactory bulb and tract (CN I)
Optic nerve (CN II)
Temporal lobe
Oculomotor nerve (CN III)
Trochlear nerve (CN IV)
Trigeminal nerve (CN V)
Abducent nerve (CN VI)
Facial nerve (CN VII)
Vestibulocochlear nerve (CN VIII)
Glossopharyngeal nerve (CN IX)
Vagus nerve (CN X)
Accessory nerve (CN XI)
Hypoglossal nerve (CN XII)

Anterior communicating artery
Anterior cerebral artery
Internal carotid artery
Middle cerebral artery
Posterior communicating artery
Posterior cerebral artery
Superior cerebellar artery
Temporal lobe (cut)
Basilar artery
Labyrinthine artery
Anterior inferior cerebellar artery
Posterior inferior cerebellar artery
Vertebral artery
Anterior spinal artery
Posterior spinal arteries

B. Schematic, inferior view

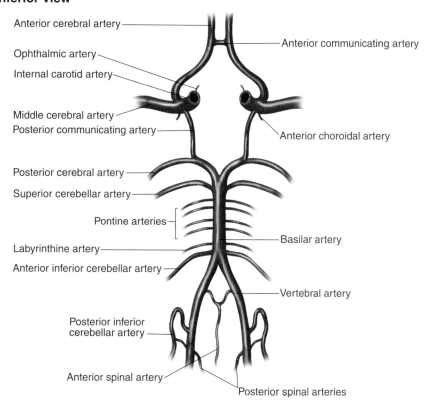

Anterior cerebral artery
Ophthalmic artery
Internal carotid artery
Middle cerebral artery
Posterior communicating artery
Posterior cerebral artery
Superior cerebellar artery
Pontine arteries
Labyrinthine artery
Anterior inferior cerebellar artery
Posterior inferior cerebellar artery
Anterior spinal artery

Anterior communicating artery
Anterior choroidal artery
Basilar artery
Vertebral artery
Posterior spinal arteries

PLATE 7-57   Orbit, Anterior View I

A. Surface projection

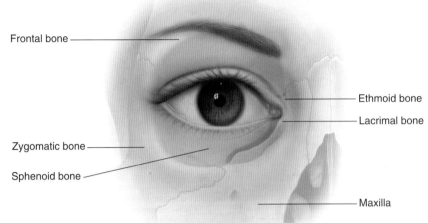

Frontal bone

Ethmoid bone

Lacrimal bone

Zygomatic bone

Sphenoid bone

Maxilla

B. Bones

Frontal bone:
Lacrimal fossa
Supraorbital notch
Orbital plate

Posterior and anterior
ethmoidal foramina

Ethmoid bone (orbital plate)

Sphenoid bone:
Lesser wing
Superior orbital fissure
Optic canal
Greater wing

Lacrimal bone

Lacrimal groove

Zygomatic bone:
Frontal process
Zygomaticofacial foramen

Inferior orbital fissure

Maxilla:
Frontal process
Infraorbital foramen

C. Muscles and orbital septum

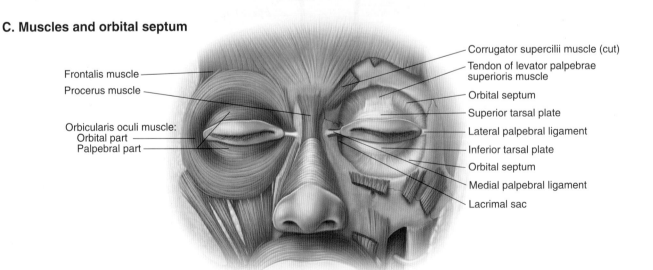

Frontalis muscle

Procerus muscle

Orbicularis oculi muscle:
Orbital part
Palpebral part

Corrugator supercilii muscle (cut)

Tendon of levator palpebrae
superioris muscle

Orbital septum

Superior tarsal plate

Lateral palpebral ligament

Inferior tarsal plate

Orbital septum

Medial palpebral ligament

Lacrimal sac

A. Surface anatomy of the eye

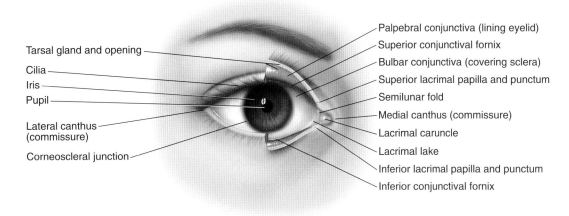

Tarsal gland and opening
Cilia
Iris
Pupil
Lateral canthus (commissure)
Corneoscleral junction

Palpebral conjunctiva (lining eyelid)
Superior conjunctival fornix
Bulbar conjunctiva (covering sclera)
Superior lacrimal papilla and punctum
Semilunar fold
Medial canthus (commissure)
Lacrimal caruncle
Lacrimal lake
Inferior lacrimal papilla and punctum
Inferior conjunctival fornix

B. Lacrimal apparatus

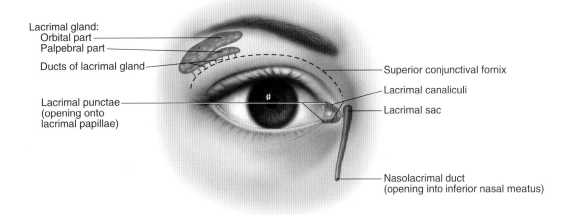

Lacrimal gland:
Orbital part
Palpebral part
Ducts of lacrimal gland
Lacrimal punctae (opening onto lacrimal papillae)

Superior conjunctival fornix
Lacrimal canaliculi
Lacrimal sac
Nasolacrimal duct (opening into inferior nasal meatus)

C. Sagittal section of eye

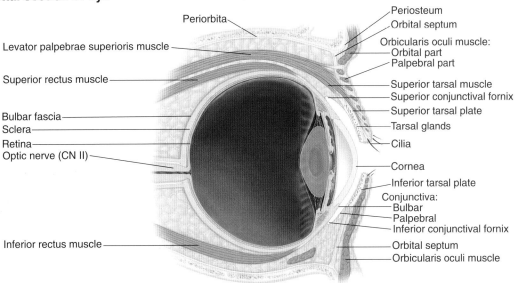

Periorbita
Levator palpebrae superioris muscle
Superior rectus muscle
Bulbar fascia
Sclera
Retina
Optic nerve (CN II)
Inferior rectus muscle

Periosteum
Orbital septum
Orbicularis oculi muscle:
Orbital part
Palpebral part
Superior tarsal muscle
Superior conjunctival fornix
Superior tarsal plate
Tarsal glands
Cilia
Cornea
Inferior tarsal plate
Conjunctiva:
Bulbar
Palpebral
Inferior conjunctival fornix
Orbital septum
Orbicularis oculi muscle

PLATE 7-59   **Orbit, Anterior View II**

A. Extraocular muscles

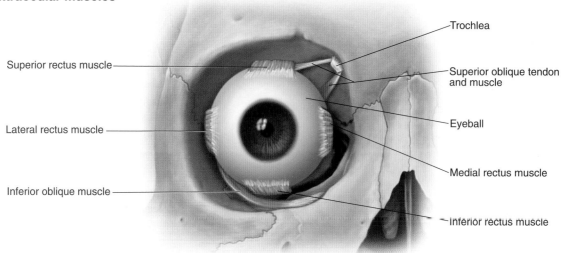

Superior rectus muscle

Lateral rectus muscle

Inferior oblique muscle

Trochlea

Superior oblique tendon and muscle

Eyeball

Medial rectus muscle

Inferior rectus muscle

B. Coronal section

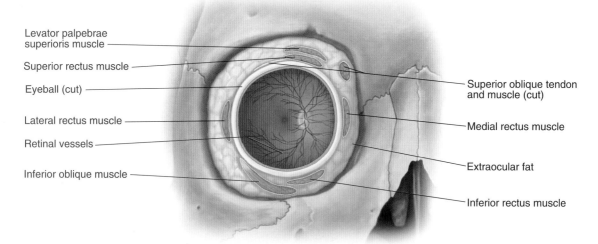

Levator palpebrae superioris muscle

Superior rectus muscle

Eyeball (cut)

Lateral rectus muscle

Retinal vessels

Inferior oblique muscle

Superior oblique tendon and muscle (cut)

Medial rectus muscle

Extraocular fat

Inferior rectus muscle

C. Apex

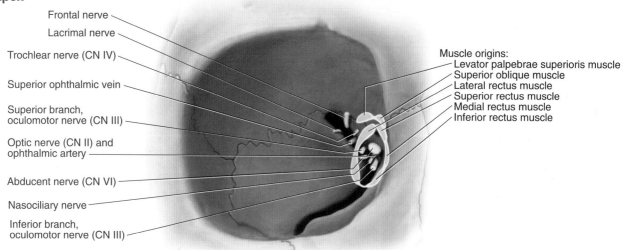

Frontal nerve

Lacrimal nerve

Trochlear nerve (CN IV)

Superior ophthalmic vein

Superior branch, oculomotor nerve (CN III)

Optic nerve (CN II) and ophthalmic artery

Abducent nerve (CN VI)

Nasociliary nerve

Inferior branch, oculomotor nerve (CN III)

Muscle origins:
Levator palpebrae superioris muscle
Superior oblique muscle
Lateral rectus muscle
Superior rectus muscle
Medial rectus muscle
Inferior rectus muscle

A. Superior view

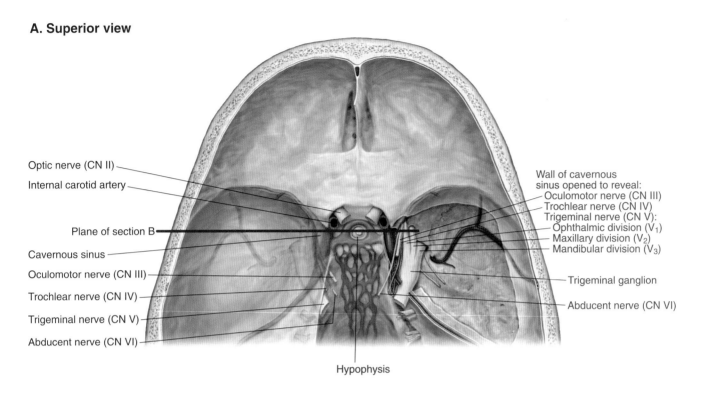

Optic nerve (CN II)

Internal carotid artery

Plane of section B

Cavernous sinus

Oculomotor nerve (CN III)

Trochlear nerve (CN IV)

Trigeminal nerve (CN V)

Abducent nerve (CN VI)

Wall of cavernous
sinus opened to reveal:
Oculomotor nerve (CN III)
Trochlear nerve (CN IV)
Trigeminal nerve (CN V):
Ophthalmic division (V_1)
Maxillary division (V_2)
Mandibular division (V_3)

Trigeminal ganglion

Abducent nerve (CN VI)

Hypophysis

B. Coronal section

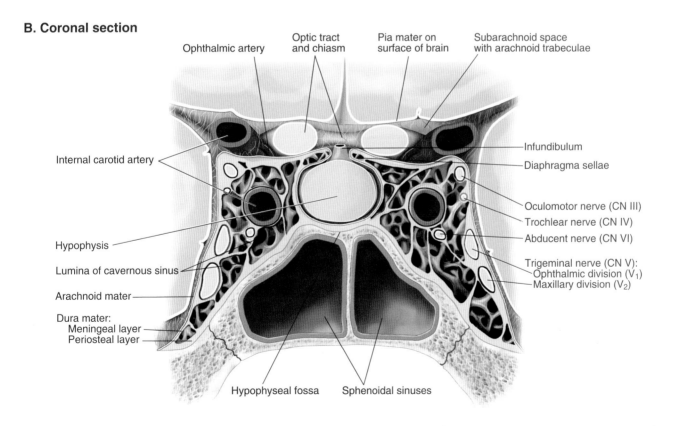

Ophthalmic artery

Optic tract
and chiasm

Pia mater on
surface of brain

Subarachnoid space
with arachnoid trabeculae

Internal carotid artery

Infundibulum

Diaphragma sellae

Oculomotor nerve (CN III)

Trochlear nerve (CN IV)

Abducent nerve (CN VI)

Hypophysis

Trigeminal nerve (CN V):
Ophthalmic division (V_1)
Maxillary division (V_2)

Lumina of cavernous sinus

Arachnoid mater

Dura mater:
  Meningeal layer
  Periosteal layer

Hypophyseal fossa

Sphenoidal sinuses

PLATE 7-61   **Orbit, Superior View I**

A. Layer I

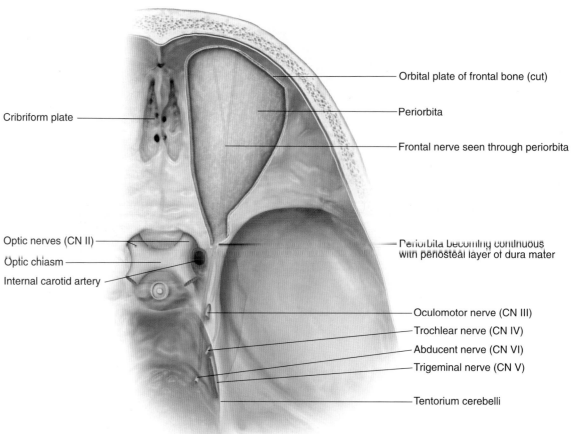

Cribriform plate

Optic nerves (CN II)
Optic chiasm
Internal carotid artery

Orbital plate of frontal bone (cut)

Periorbita

Frontal nerve seen through periorbita

Periorbita becoming continuous
with periosteal layer of dura mater

Oculomotor nerve (CN III)
Trochlear nerve (CN IV)
Abducent nerve (CN VI)
Trigeminal nerve (CN V)

Tentorium cerebelli

B. Layer II

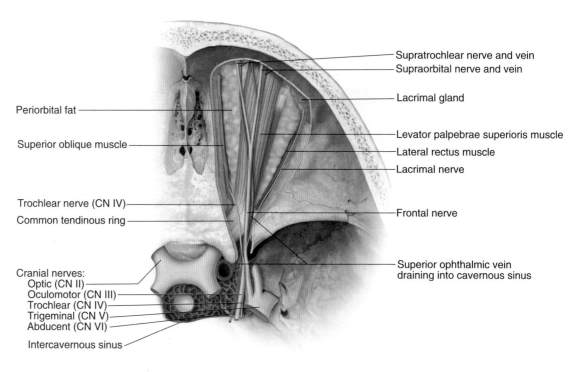

Periorbital fat

Superior oblique muscle

Trochlear nerve (CN IV)
Common tendinous ring

Cranial nerves:
Optic (CN II)
Oculomotor (CN III)
Trochlear (CN IV)
Trigeminal (CN V)
Abducent (CN VI)

Intercavernous sinus

Supratrochlear nerve and vein
Supraorbital nerve and vein

Lacrimal gland

Levator palpebrae superioris muscle
Lateral rectus muscle
Lacrimal nerve

Frontal nerve

Superior ophthalmic vein
draining into cavernous sinus

A. Layer III

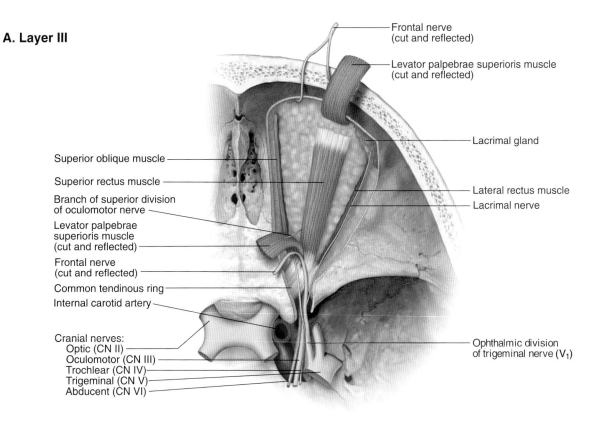

Frontal nerve
(cut and reflected)

Levator palpebrae superioris muscle
(cut and reflected)

Lacrimal gland

Superior oblique muscle

Superior rectus muscle

Branch of superior division
of oculomotor nerve

Levator palpebrae
superioris muscle
(cut and reflected)

Frontal nerve
(cut and reflected)

Common tendinous ring

Internal carotid artery

Lateral rectus muscle
Lacrimal nerve

Cranial nerves:
Optic (CN II)
Oculomotor (CN III)
Trochlear (CN IV)
Trigeminal (CN V)
Abducent (CN VI)

Ophthalmic division
of trigeminal nerve (V$_1$)

B. Layer IV

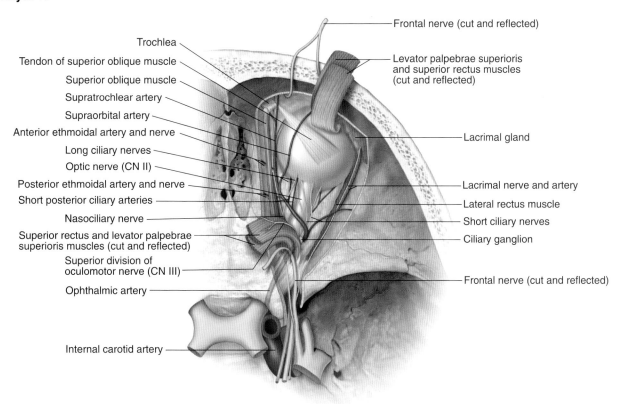

Frontal nerve (cut and reflected)

Trochlea

Tendon of superior oblique muscle

Superior oblique muscle

Supratrochlear artery

Supraorbital artery

Anterior ethmoidal artery and nerve

Long ciliary nerves

Optic nerve (CN II)

Posterior ethmoidal artery and nerve

Short posterior ciliary arteries

Nasociliary nerve

Superior rectus and levator palpebrae
superioris muscles (cut and reflected)

Superior division of
oculomotor nerve (CN III)

Ophthalmic artery

Internal carotid artery

Levator palpebrae superioris
and superior rectus muscles
(cut and reflected)

Lacrimal gland

Lacrimal nerve and artery

Lateral rectus muscle

Short ciliary nerves

Ciliary ganglion

Frontal nerve (cut and reflected)

PLATE 7-63   Orbit, Superior View III

A. Layer V

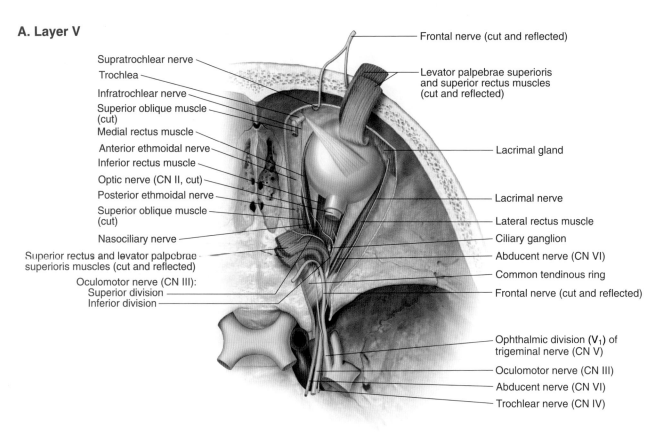

Supratrochlear nerve

Trochlea

Infratrochlear nerve

Superior oblique muscle (cut)

Medial rectus muscle

Anterior ethmoidal nerve

Inferior rectus muscle

Optic nerve (CN II, cut)

Posterior ethmoidal nerve

Superior oblique muscle (cut)

Nasociliary nerve

Superior rectus and levator palpebrae superioris muscles (cut and reflected)

Oculomotor nerve (CN III):
Superior division
Inferior division

Frontal nerve (cut and reflected)

Levator palpebrae superioris and superior rectus muscles (cut and reflected)

Lacrimal gland

Lacrimal nerve

Lateral rectus muscle

Ciliary ganglion

Abducent nerve (CN VI)

Common tendinous ring

Frontal nerve (cut and reflected)

Ophthalmic division (V₁) of trigeminal nerve (CN V)

Oculomotor nerve (CN III)

Abducent nerve (CN VI)

Trochlear nerve (CN IV)

B. Layer VI

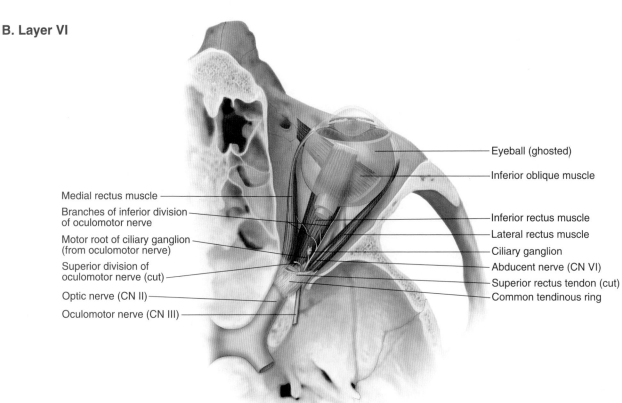

Medial rectus muscle

Branches of inferior division of oculomotor nerve

Motor root of ciliary ganglion (from oculomotor nerve)

Superior division of oculomotor nerve (cut)

Optic nerve (CN II)

Oculomotor nerve (CN III)

Eyeball (ghosted)

Inferior oblique muscle

Inferior rectus muscle

Lateral rectus muscle

Ciliary ganglion

Abducent nerve (CN VI)

Superior rectus tendon (cut)

Common tendinous ring

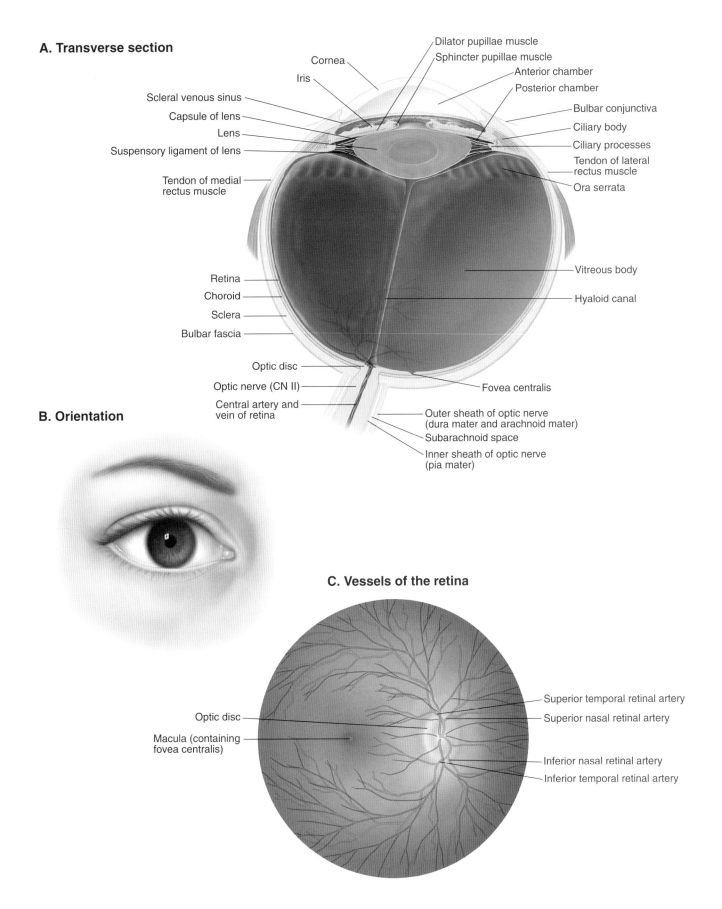

A. Transverse section

Dilator pupillae muscle
Sphincter pupillae muscle
Cornea
Anterior chamber
Iris
Posterior chamber
Scleral venous sinus
Capsule of lens
Bulbar conjunctiva
Lens
Ciliary body
Suspensory ligament of lens
Ciliary processes
Tendon of lateral rectus muscle
Tendon of medial rectus muscle
Ora serrata
Retina
Vitreous body
Choroid
Hyaloid canal
Sclera
Bulbar fascia
Optic disc
Optic nerve (CN II)
Fovea centralis
Central artery and vein of retina
Outer sheath of optic nerve (dura mater and arachnoid mater)
Subarachnoid space
Inner sheath of optic nerve (pia mater)

B. Orientation

C. Vessels of the retina

Optic disc
Superior temporal retinal artery
Superior nasal retinal artery
Macula (containing fovea centralis)
Inferior nasal retinal artery
Inferior temporal retinal artery

PLATE 7-65 | **Ear I**

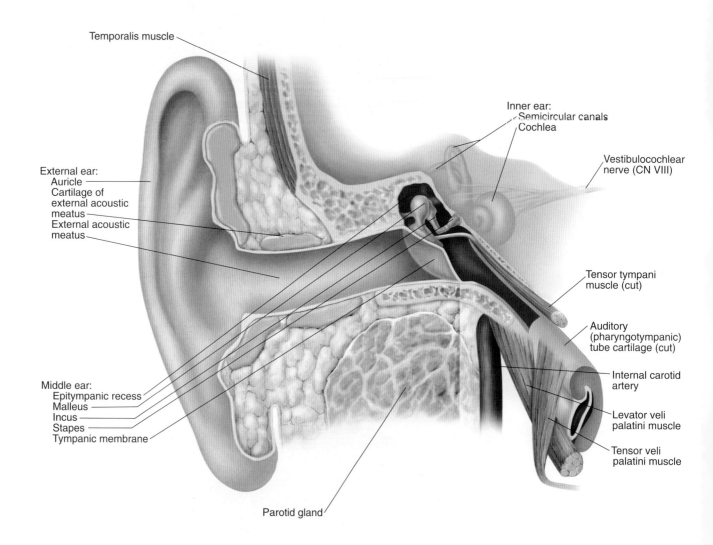

Temporalis muscle

Inner ear:
Semicircular canals
Cochlea

Vestibulocochlear
nerve (CN VIII)

External ear:
Auricle
Cartilage of
external acoustic
meatus
External acoustic
meatus

Tensor tympani
muscle (cut)

Auditory
(pharyngotympanic)
tube cartilage (cut)

Internal carotid
artery

Middle ear:
Epitympanic recess
Malleus
Incus
Stapes
Tympanic membrane

Levator veli
palatini muscle

Tensor veli
palatini muscle

Parotid gland

A. Auricle

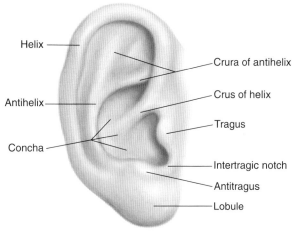

Helix

Crura of antihelix

Crus of helix

Antihelix

Tragus

Concha

Intertragic notch

Antitragus

Lobule

B. Tympanic membrane, lateral view

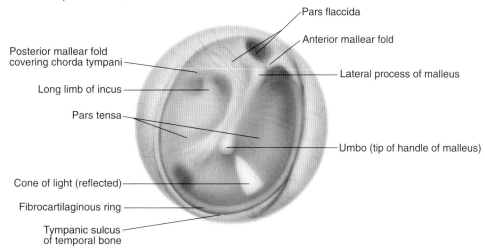

Pars flaccida

Anterior mallear fold

Posterior mallear fold covering chorda tympani

Lateral process of malleus

Long limb of incus

Pars tensa

Umbo (tip of handle of malleus)

Cone of light (reflected)

Fibrocartilaginous ring

Tympanic sulcus of temporal bone

C. Ossicles of ear seen through tympanic membrane

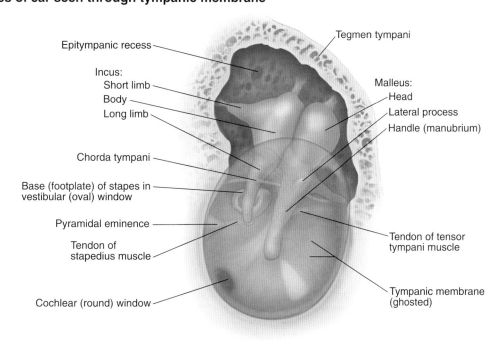

Epitympanic recess

Tegmen tympani

Incus:
Short limb
Body
Long limb

Malleus:
Head
Lateral process
Handle (manubrium)

Chorda tympani

Base (footplate) of stapes in vestibular (oval) window

Pyramidal eminence

Tendon of stapedius muscle

Tendon of tensor tympani muscle

Tympanic membrane (ghosted)

Cochlear (round) window

PLATE 7-67   Ear III

A. Orientation

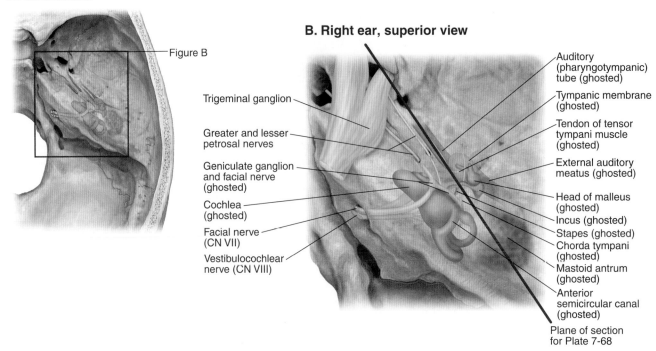

Figure B

B. Right ear, superior view

Trigeminal ganglion

Greater and lesser petrosal nerves

Geniculate ganglion and facial nerve (ghosted)

Cochlea (ghosted)

Facial nerve (CN VII)

Vestibulocochlear nerve (CN VIII)

Auditory (pharyngotympanic) tube (ghosted)

Tympanic membrane (ghosted)

Tendon of tensor tympani muscle (ghosted)

External auditory meatus (ghosted)

Head of malleus (ghosted)

Incus (ghosted)

Stapes (ghosted)

Chorda tympani (ghosted)

Mastoid antrum (ghosted)

Anterior semicircular canal (ghosted)

Plane of section for Plate 7-68

C. Right ear, inferior view

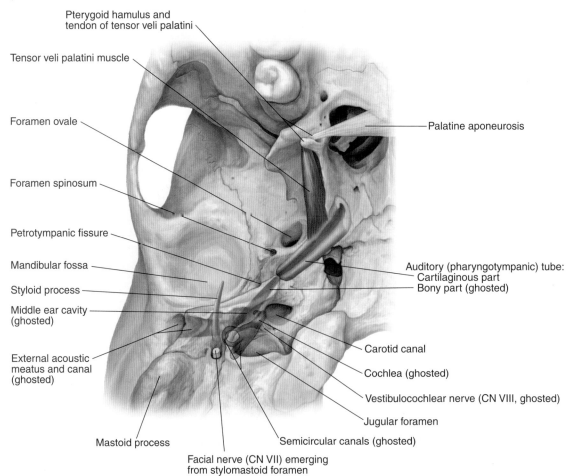

Pterygoid hamulus and tendon of tensor veli palatini

Tensor veli palatini muscle

Foramen ovale

Foramen spinosum

Petrotympanic fissure

Mandibular fossa

Styloid process

Middle ear cavity (ghosted)

External acoustic meatus and canal (ghosted)

Mastoid process

Facial nerve (CN VII) emerging from stylomastoid foramen

Semicircular canals (ghosted)

Jugular foramen

Vestibulocochlear nerve (CN VIII, ghosted)

Cochlea (ghosted)

Carotid canal

Auditory (pharyngotympanic) tube:
Cartilaginous part
Bony part (ghosted)

Palatine aponeurosis

A. Lateral wall of middle ear, right

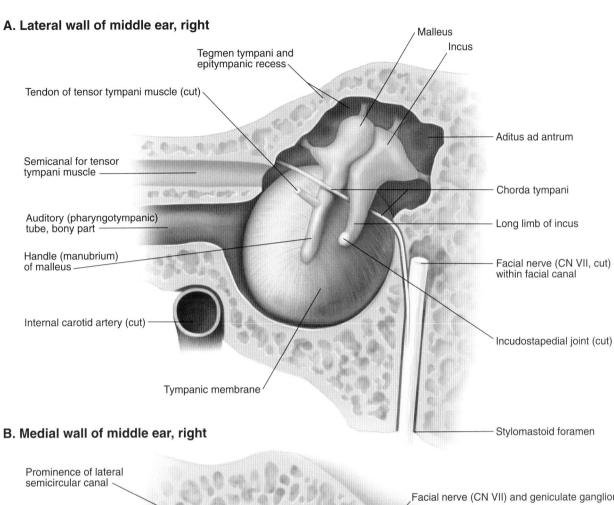

Tegmen tympani and epitympanic recess

Malleus

Incus

Tendon of tensor tympani muscle (cut)

Aditus ad antrum

Semicanal for tensor tympani muscle

Chorda tympani

Long limb of incus

Auditory (pharyngotympanic) tube, bony part

Facial nerve (CN VII, cut) within facial canal

Handle (manubrium) of malleus

Internal carotid artery (cut)

Incudostapedial joint (cut)

Tympanic membrane

Stylomastoid foramen

B. Medial wall of middle ear, right

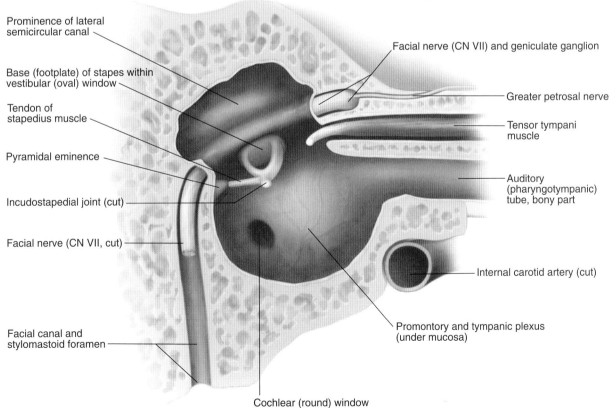

Prominence of lateral semicircular canal

Facial nerve (CN VII) and geniculate ganglion

Base (footplate) of stapes within vestibular (oval) window

Greater petrosal nerve

Tendon of stapedius muscle

Tensor tympani muscle

Pyramidal eminence

Auditory (pharyngotympanic) tube, bony part

Incudostapedial joint (cut)

Facial nerve (CN VII, cut)

Internal carotid artery (cut)

Facial canal and stylomastoid foramen

Promontory and tympanic plexus (under mucosa)

Cochlear (round) window

PLATE 7-69   **Ear V**

A. Ossicles in situ, right ear, lateral view

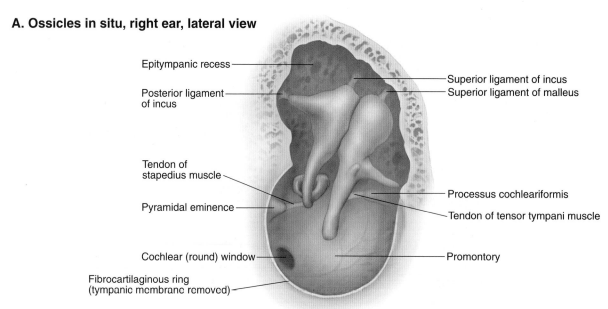

Epitympanic recess

Posterior ligament of incus

Tendon of stapedius muscle

Pyramidal eminence

Cochlear (round) window

Fibrocartilaginous ring (tympanic membrane removed)

Superior ligament of incus

Superior ligament of malleus

Processus cochleariformis

Tendon of tensor tympani muscle

Promontory

B. Malleus

Head

Neck

Lateral process

Anterior process

Handle (manubrium)

C. Incus

Short limb

Body

Long limb

D. Stapes

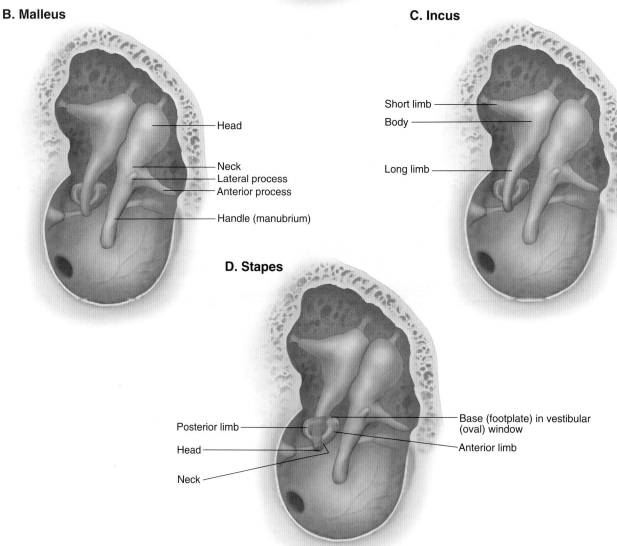

Posterior limb

Head

Neck

Base (footplate) in vestibular (oval) window

Anterior limb

A. Orientation, right ear, lateral view

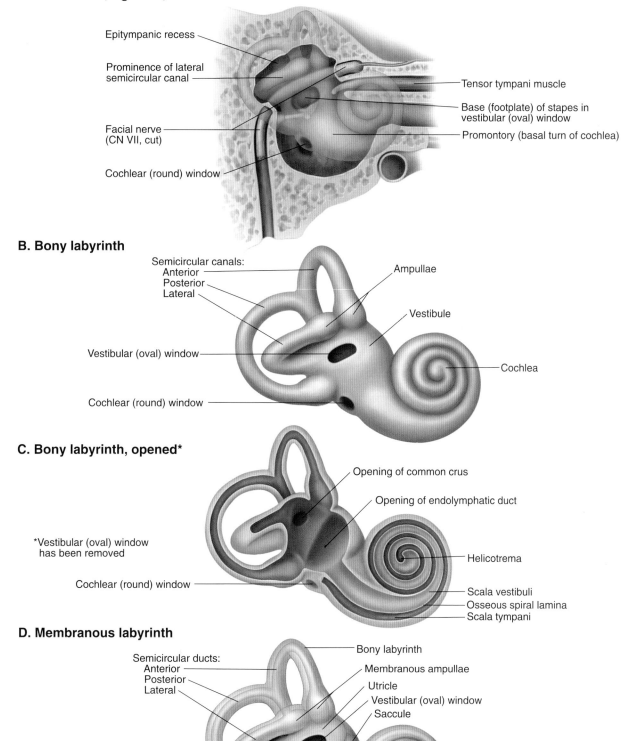

Epitympanic recess

Prominence of lateral
semicircular canal

Facial nerve
(CN VII, cut)

Cochlear (round) window

Tensor tympani muscle

Base (footplate) of stapes in
vestibular (oval) window

Promontory (basal turn of cochlea)

B. Bony labyrinth

Semicircular canals:
  Anterior
  Posterior
  Lateral

Vestibular (oval) window

Cochlear (round) window

Ampullae

Vestibule

Cochlea

C. Bony labyrinth, opened*

*Vestibular (oval) window
has been removed

Cochlear (round) window

Opening of common crus

Opening of endolymphatic duct

Helicotrema

Scala vestibuli
Osseous spiral lamina
Scala tympani

D. Membranous labyrinth

Semicircular ducts:
  Anterior
  Posterior
  Lateral

Endolymphatic sac

Endolymphatic duct

Ductus reuniens

Bony labyrinth

Membranous ampullae

Utricle

Vestibular (oval) window

Saccule

Cochlear duct

Cochlear (round) window

PLATE 7-71 **External Carotid Artery, Overview**

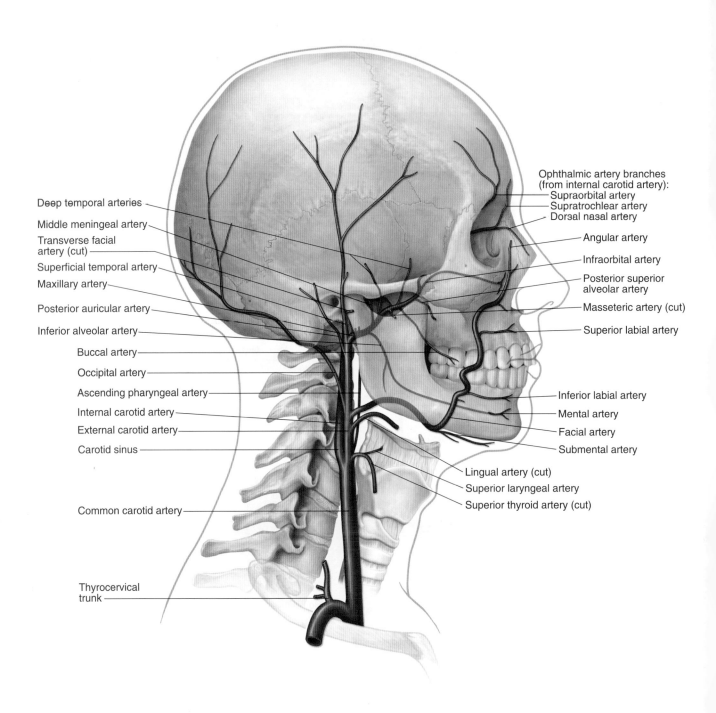

Deep temporal arteries

Middle meningeal artery

Transverse facial artery (cut)

Superficial temporal artery

Maxillary artery

Posterior auricular artery

Inferior alveolar artery

Buccal artery

Occipital artery

Ascending pharyngeal artery

Internal carotid artery

External carotid artery

Carotid sinus

Common carotid artery

Thyrocervical trunk

Ophthalmic artery branches (from internal carotid artery):
Supraorbital artery
Supratrochlear artery
Dorsal nasal artery

Angular artery

Infraorbital artery

Posterior superior alveolar artery

Masseteric artery (cut)

Superior labial artery

Inferior labial artery

Mental artery

Facial artery

Submental artery

Lingual artery (cut)

Superior laryngeal artery

Superior thyroid artery (cut)

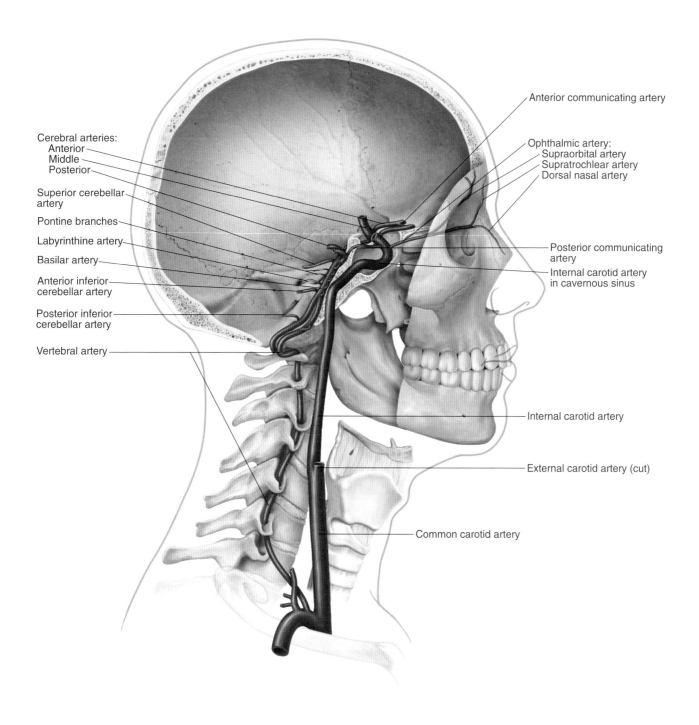

Cerebral arteries:
  Anterior
  Middle
  Posterior

Superior cerebellar artery

Pontine branches

Labyrinthine artery

Basilar artery

Anterior inferior cerebellar artery

Posterior inferior cerebellar artery

Vertebral artery

Anterior communicating artery

Ophthalmic artery:
  Supraorbital artery
  Supratrochlear artery
  Dorsal nasal artery

Posterior communicating artery

Internal carotid artery in cavernous sinus

Internal carotid artery

External carotid artery (cut)

Common carotid artery

PLATE 7-73 **Veins of the Head and Neck**

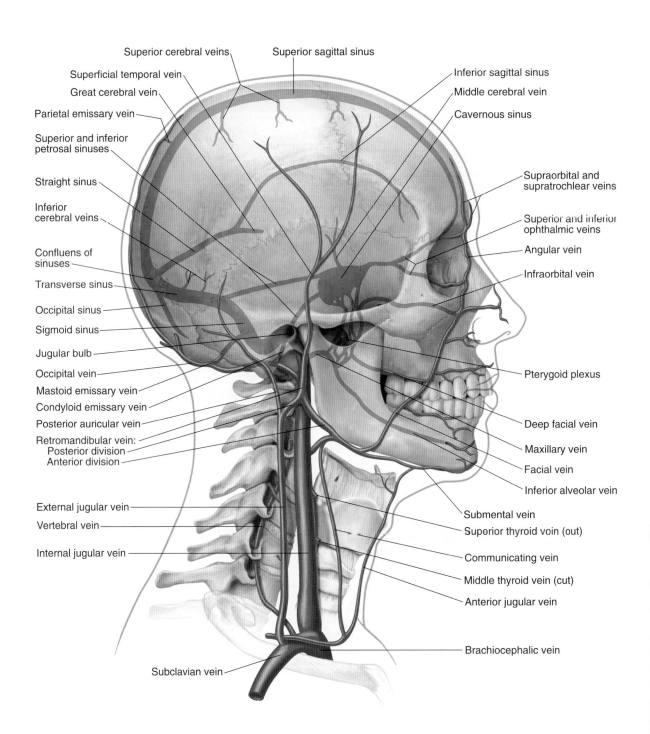

Superior cerebral veins

Superficial temporal vein

Great cerebral vein

Parietal emissary vein

Superior and inferior petrosal sinuses

Straight sinus

Inferior cerebral veins

Confluens of sinuses

Transverse sinus

Occipital sinus

Sigmoid sinus

Jugular bulb

Occipital vein

Mastoid emissary vein

Condyloid emissary vein

Posterior auricular vein

Retromandibular vein:
    Posterior division
    Anterior division

External jugular vein

Vertebral vein

Internal jugular vein

Subclavian vein

Superior sagittal sinus

Inferior sagittal sinus

Middle cerebral vein

Cavernous sinus

Supraorbital and supratrochlear veins

Superior and inferior ophthalmic veins

Angular vein

Infraorbital vein

Pterygoid plexus

Deep facial vein

Maxillary vein

Facial vein

Inferior alveolar vein

Submental vein

Superior thyroid vein (cut)

Communicating vein

Middle thyroid vein (cut)

Anterior jugular vein

Brachiocephalic vein

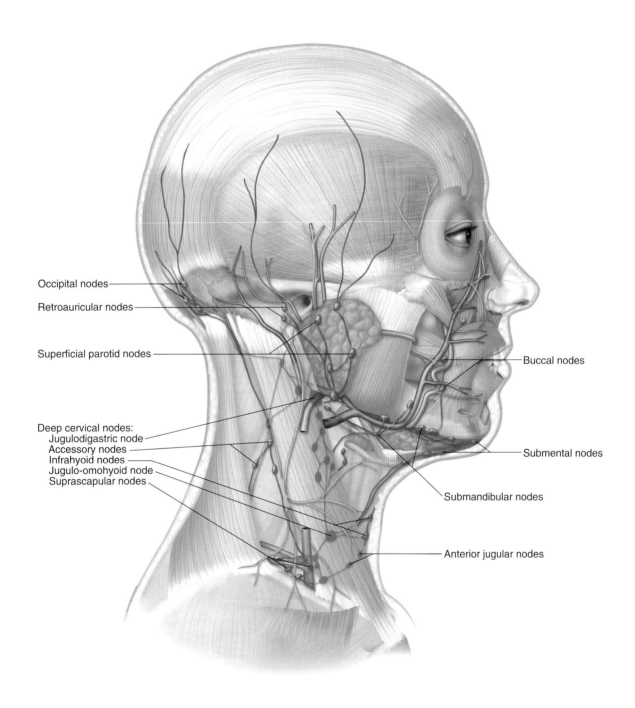

Occipital nodes

Retroauricular nodes

Superficial parotid nodes

Deep cervical nodes:
  Jugulodigastric node
  Accessory nodes
  Infrahyoid nodes
  Jugulo-omohyoid node
  Suprascapular nodes

Buccal nodes

Submental nodes

Submandibular nodes

Anterior jugular nodes

PLATE 7-75 | **Cranial Nerve Summary I**

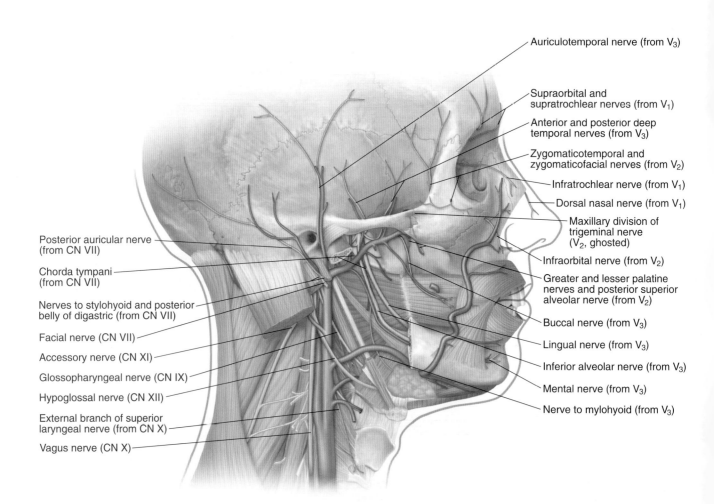

Auriculotemporal nerve (from V₃)

Supraorbital and supratrochlear nerves (from V₁)

Anterior and posterior deep temporal nerves (from V₃)

Zygomaticotemporal and zygomaticofacial nerves (from V₂)

Infratrochlear nerve (from V₁)

Dorsal nasal nerve (from V₁)

Maxillary division of trigeminal nerve (V₂, ghosted)

Infraorbital nerve (from V₂)

Greater and lesser palatine nerves and posterior superior alveolar nerve (from V₂)

Buccal nerve (from V₃)

Lingual nerve (from V₃)

Inferior alveolar nerve (from V₃)

Mental nerve (from V₃)

Nerve to mylohyoid (from V₃)

Posterior auricular nerve (from CN VII)

Chorda tympani (from CN VII)

Nerves to stylohyoid and posterior belly of digastric (from CN VII)

Facial nerve (CN VII)

Accessory nerve (CN XI)

Glossopharyngeal nerve (CN IX)

Hypoglossal nerve (CN XII)

External branch of superior laryngeal nerve (from CN X)

Vagus nerve (CN X)

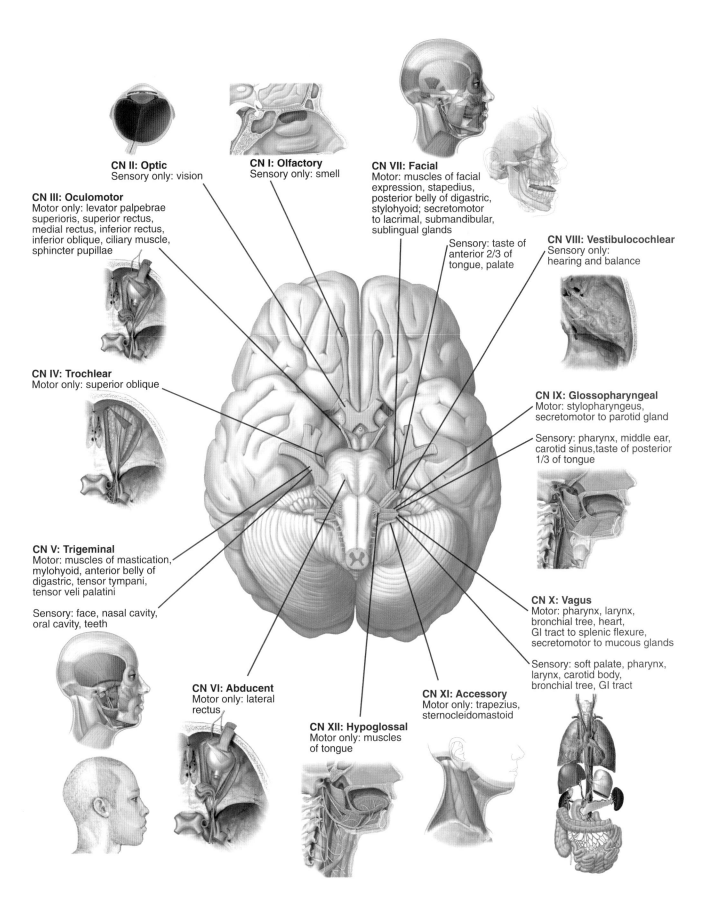

CN II: Optic
Sensory only: vision

CN I: Olfactory
Sensory only: smell

CN VII: Facial
Motor: muscles of facial
expression, stapedius,
posterior belly of digastric,
stylohyoid; secretomotor
to lacrimal, submandibular,
sublingual glands

Sensory: taste of
anterior 2/3 of
tongue, palate

CN VIII: Vestibulocochlear
Sensory only:
hearing and balance

CN III: Oculomotor
Motor only: levator palpebrae
superioris, superior rectus,
medial rectus, inferior rectus,
inferior oblique, ciliary muscle,
sphincter pupillae

CN IV: Trochlear
Motor only: superior oblique

CN IX: Glossopharyngeal
Motor: stylopharyngeus,
secretomotor to parotid gland

Sensory: pharynx, middle ear,
carotid sinus,taste of posterior
1/3 of tongue

CN V: Trigeminal
Motor: muscles of mastication,
mylohyoid, anterior belly of
digastric, tensor tympani,
tensor veli palatini

Sensory: face, nasal cavity,
oral cavity, teeth

CN X: Vagus
Motor: pharynx, larynx,
bronchial tree, heart,
GI tract to splenic flexure,
secretomotor to mucous glands

Sensory: soft palate, pharynx,
larynx, carotid body,
bronchial tree, GI tract

CN VI: Abducent
Motor only: lateral
rectus

CN XI: Accessory
Motor only: trapezius,
sternocleidomastoid

CN XII: Hypoglossal
Motor only: muscles
of tongue

PLATE 7-77   **Olfactory Nerve, Cranial Nerve I**

A. Origin from brain

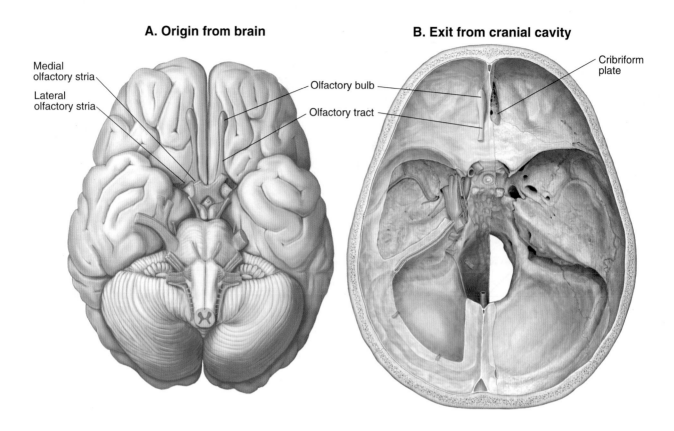

Medial
olfactory stria

Lateral
olfactory stria

Olfactory bulb

Olfactory tract

B. Exit from cranial cavity

Cribriform
plate

C. Sensory innervation, sagittal section

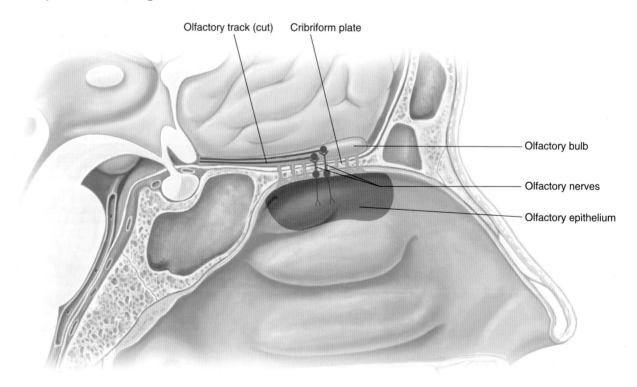

Olfactory track (cut)

Cribriform plate

Olfactory bulb

Olfactory nerves

Olfactory epithelium

A. Origin from brain

B. Exit from cranial cavity

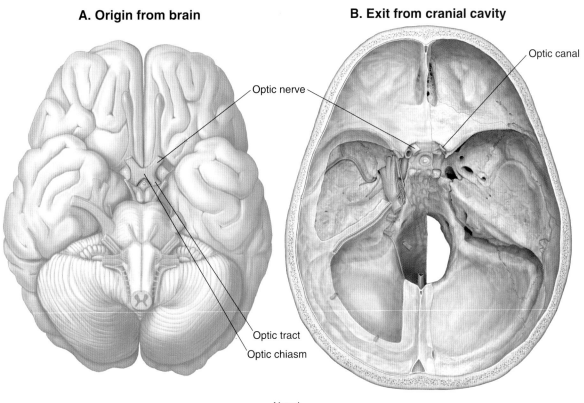

Optic canal

Optic nerve

Optic tract

Optic chiasm

C. Sensory innervation, transverse section, inferior view

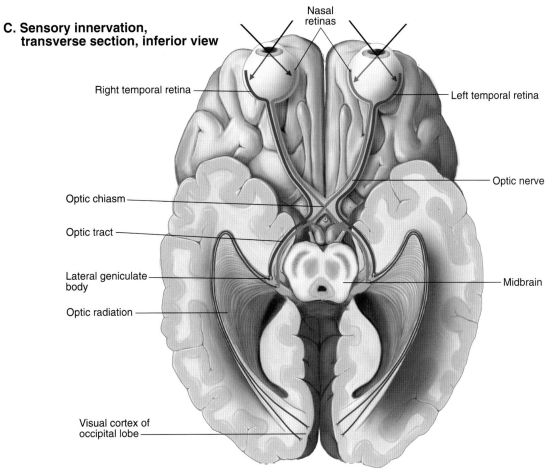

Nasal retinas

Right temporal retina

Left temporal retina

Optic nerve

Optic chiasm

Optic tract

Lateral geniculate body

Midbrain

Optic radiation

Visual cortex of occipital lobe

PLATE 7-79   Oculomotor Nerve, Cranial Nerve III

A. Origin from brain

B. Exit from cranial cavity

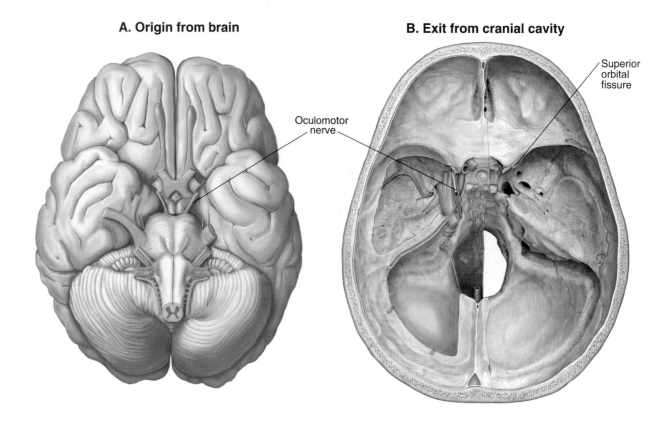

Oculomotor nerve

Superior orbital fissure

C. Skeletal muscle innervation

D. Parasympathetic innervation

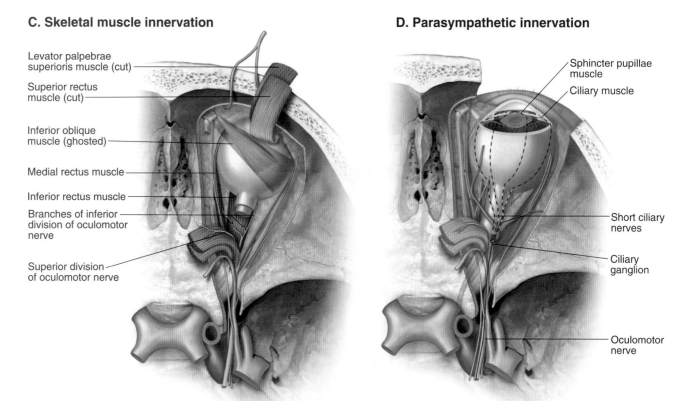

Levator palpebrae superioris muscle (cut)

Superior rectus muscle (cut)

Inferior oblique muscle (ghosted)

Medial rectus muscle

Inferior rectus muscle

Branches of inferior division of oculomotor nerve

Superior division of oculomotor nerve

Sphincter pupillae muscle

Ciliary muscle

Short ciliary nerves

Ciliary ganglion

Oculomotor nerve

A. Origin from brain

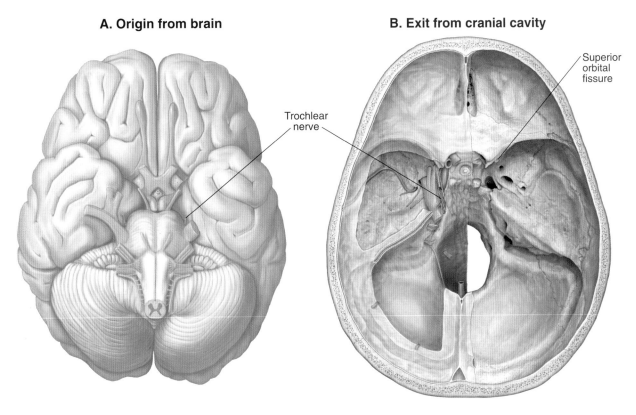

Trochlear nerve

B. Exit from cranial cavity

Superior orbital fissure

Trochlear nerve

C. Skeletal muscle innervation

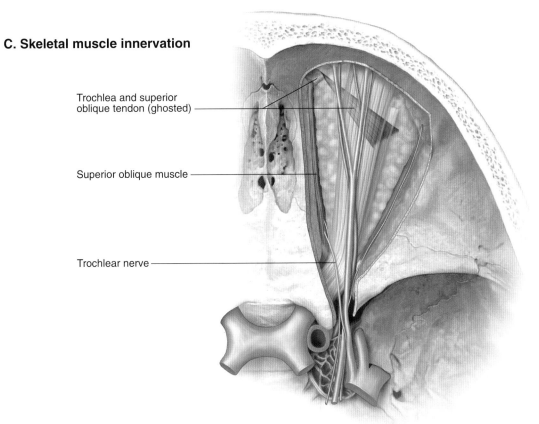

Trochlea and superior oblique tendon (ghosted)

Superior oblique muscle

Trochlear nerve

PLATE 7-81   Trigeminal Nerve, Cranial Nerve V

A. Origin from brain

B. Exit from cranial cavity

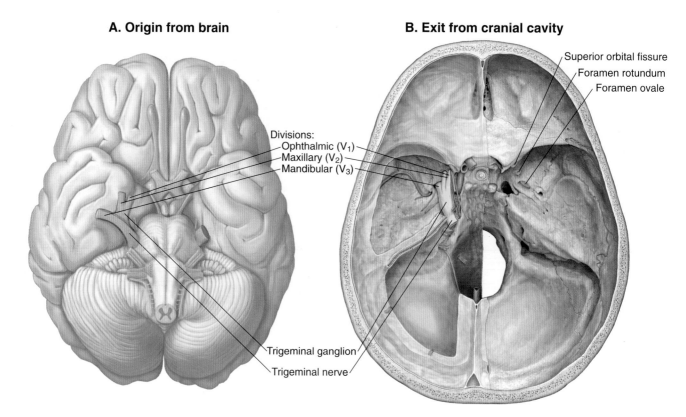

Divisions:
- Ophthalmic (V₁)
- Maxillary (V₂)
- Mandibular (V₃)

Superior orbital fissure
Foramen rotundum
Foramen ovale

Trigeminal ganglion
Trigeminal nerve

C. Overview of divisions

D. Cutaneous distribution

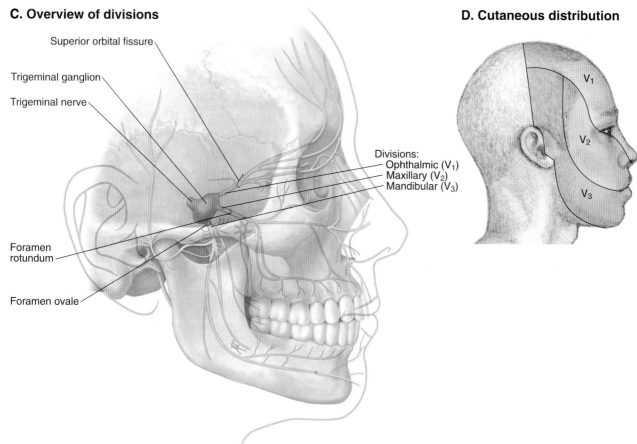

Superior orbital fissure

Trigeminal ganglion

Trigeminal nerve

Divisions:
- Ophthalmic (V₁)
- Maxillary (V₂)
- Mandibular (V₃)

Foramen
rotundum

Foramen ovale

V₁
V₂
V₃

A. Sensory innervation

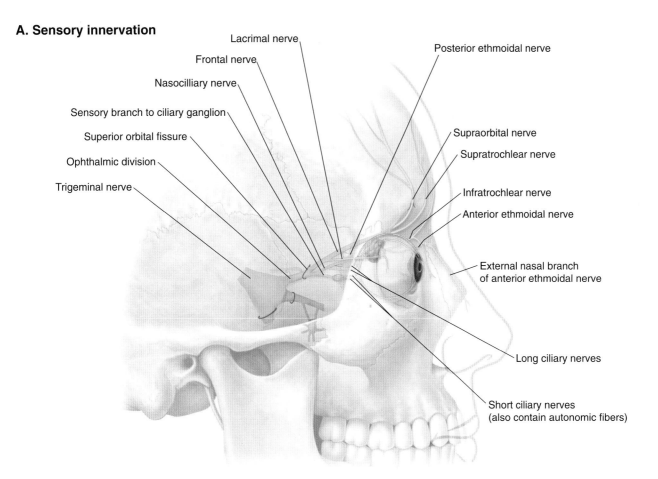

Lacrimal nerve

Frontal nerve

Nasocilliary nerve

Sensory branch to ciliary ganglion

Superior orbital fissure

Ophthalmic division

Trigeminal nerve

Posterior ethmoidal nerve

Supraorbital nerve

Supratrochlear nerve

Infratrochlear nerve

Anterior ethmoidal nerve

External nasal branch
of anterior ethmoidal nerve

Long ciliary nerves

Short ciliary nerves
(also contain autonomic fibers)

B. Cutaneous distribution

C. Branches that carry parasympathetic innervation

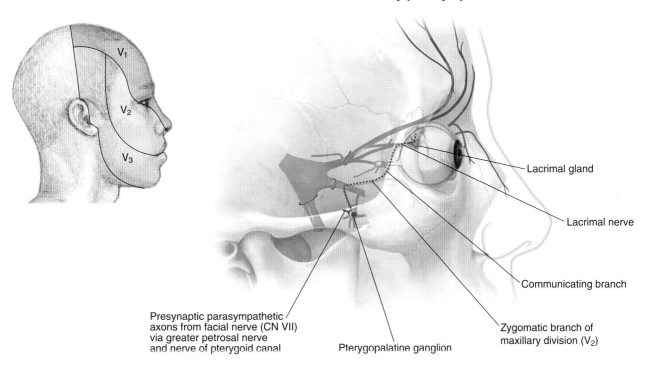

V₁

V₂

V₃

Lacrimal gland

Lacrimal nerve

Communicating branch

Presynaptic parasympathetic
axons from facial nerve (CN VII)
via greater petrosal nerve
and nerve of pterygoid canal

Pterygopalatine ganglion

Zygomatic branch of
maxillary division (V₂)

PLATE 7-83   **Maxillary Division of Trigeminal Nerve (V₂)**

A. Sensory innervation

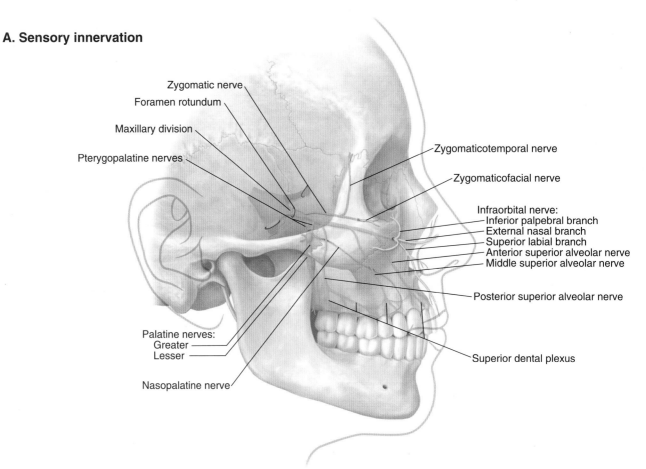

Zygomatic nerve
Foramen rotundum
Maxillary division
Pterygopalatine nerves

Zygomaticotemporal nerve
Zygomaticofacial nerve

Infraorbital nerve:
Inferior palpebral branch
External nasal branch
Superior labial branch
Anterior superior alveolar nerve
Middle superior alveolar nerve

Posterior superior alveolar nerve

Superior dental plexus

Palatine nerves:
Greater
Lesser

Nasopalatine nerve

B. Cutaneous distribution

C. Branches that carry parasympathetic innervation

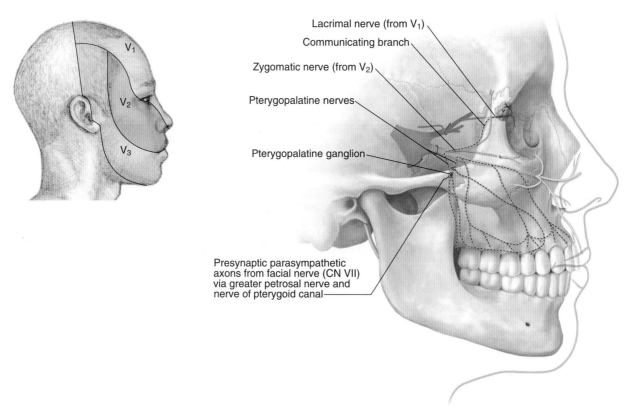

V₁
V₂
V₃

Lacrimal nerve (from V₁)
Communicating branch
Zygomatic nerve (from V₂)
Pterygopalatine nerves
Pterygopalatine ganglion

Presynaptic parasympathetic
axons from facial nerve (CN VII)
via greater petrosal nerve and
nerve of pterygoid canal

A. Sensory innervation

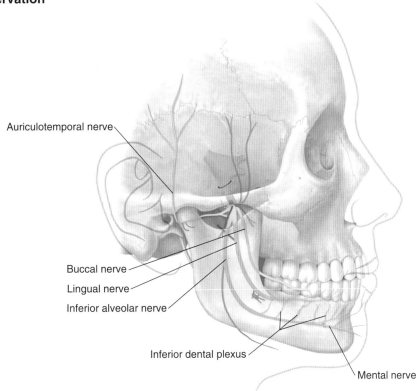

Auriculotemporal nerve

Buccal nerve

Lingual nerve

Inferior alveolar nerve

Inferior dental plexus

Mental nerve

B. Cutaneous distribution

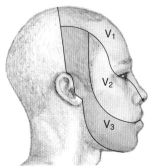

V₁

V₂

V₃

C. Branches that carry parasympathetic innervation

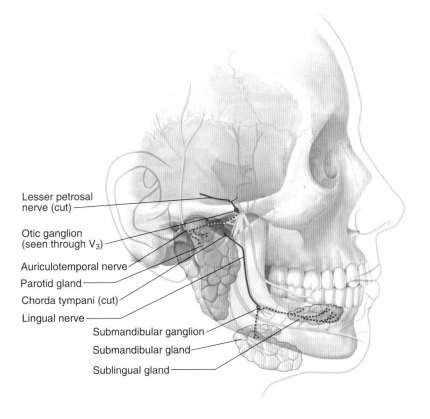

Lesser petrosal nerve (cut)

Otic ganglion (seen through V₃)

Auriculotemporal nerve

Parotid gland

Chorda tympani (cut)

Lingual nerve

Submandibular ganglion

Submandibular gland

Sublingual gland

PLATE 7-85   Mandibular Division of Trigeminal Nerve (V₃) II

A. Skeletal muscle innervation I

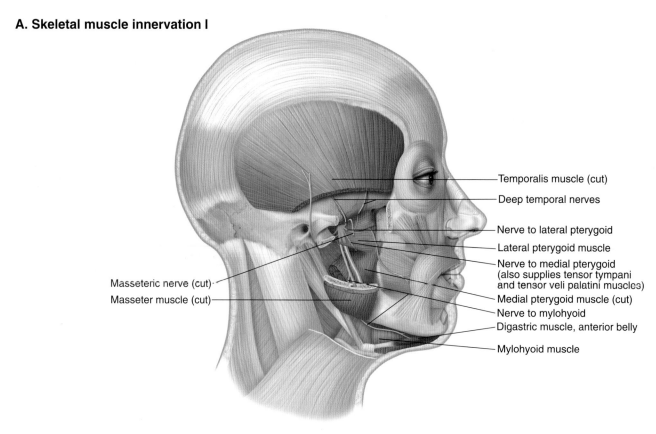

Temporalis muscle (cut)

Deep temporal nerves

Nerve to lateral pterygoid

Lateral pterygoid muscle

Nerve to medial pterygoid
(also supplies tensor tympani
and tensor veli palatini muscles)

Medial pterygoid muscle (cut)

Nerve to mylohyoid

Digastric muscle, anterior belly

Mylohyoid muscle

Masseteric nerve (cut)

Masseter muscle (cut)

B. Skeletal muscle innervation II

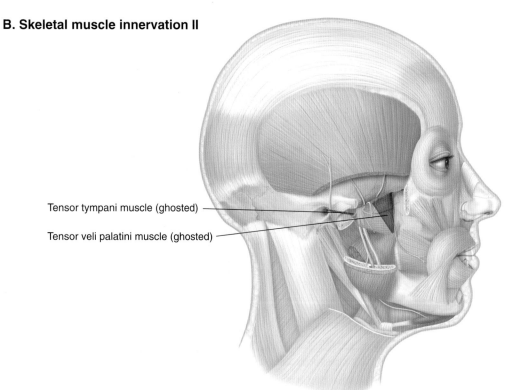

Tensor tympani muscle (ghosted)

Tensor veli palatini muscle (ghosted)

A. Origin from brain

B. Exit from cranial cavity

C. Skeletal muscle innervation

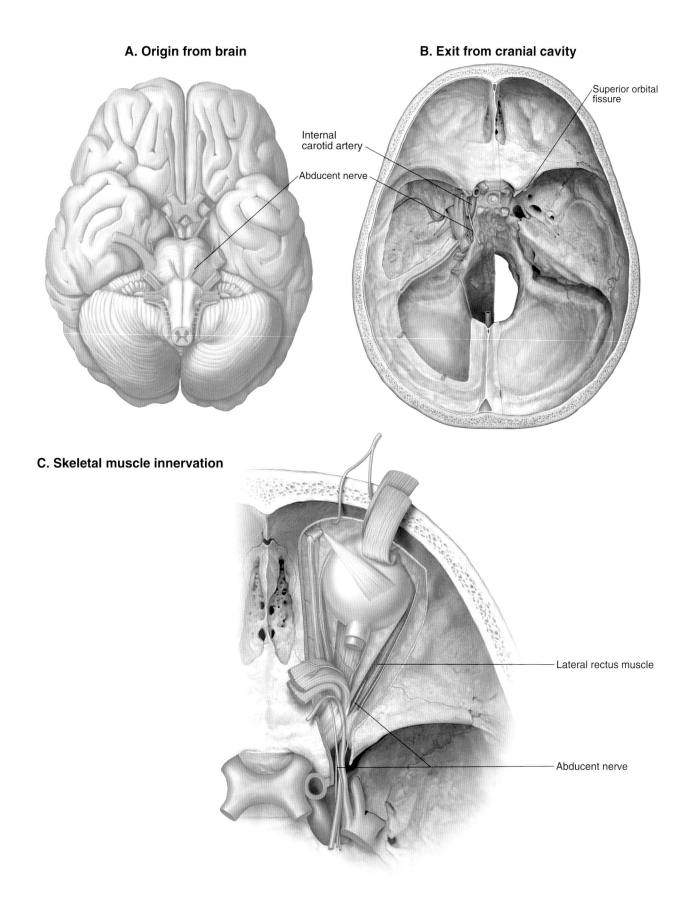

Superior orbital fissure

Internal carotid artery

Abducent nerve

Lateral rectus muscle

Abducent nerve

PLATE 7-87 Facial Nerve, Cranial Nerve VII, I

A. Origin from brain

B. Exit from cranial cavity

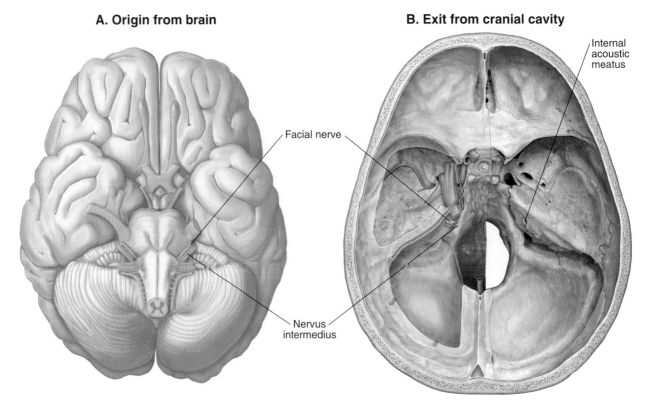

Internal
acoustic
meatus

Facial nerve

Nervus
intermedius

C. Skeletal muscle innervation

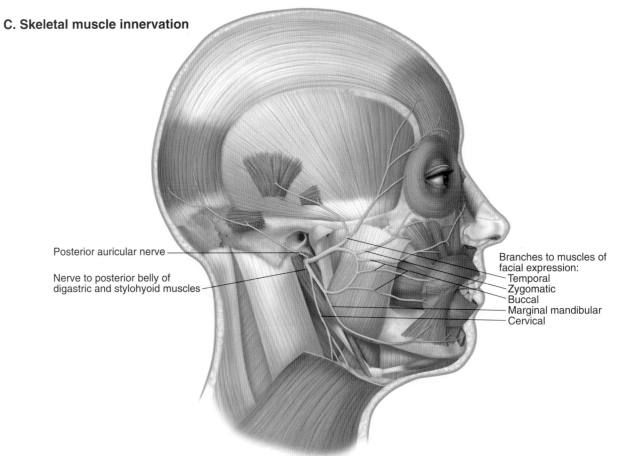

Posterior auricular nerve

Nerve to posterior belly of
digastric and stylohyoid muscles

Branches to muscles of
facial expression:
Temporal
Zygomatic
Buccal
Marginal mandibular
Cervical

A. Sensory innervation

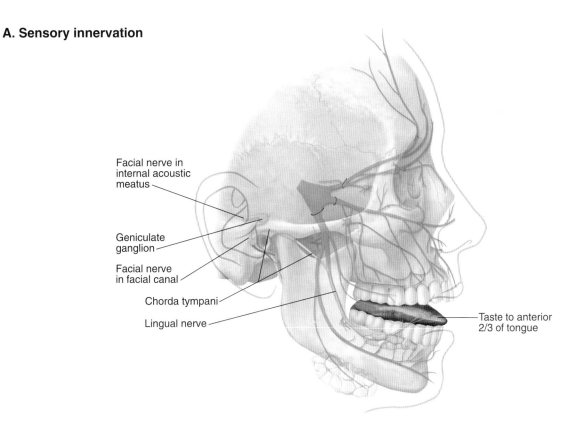

Facial nerve in
internal acoustic
meatus

Geniculate
ganglion

Facial nerve
in facial canal

Chorda tympani

Lingual nerve

Taste to anterior
2/3 of tongue

B. Parasympathetic innervation

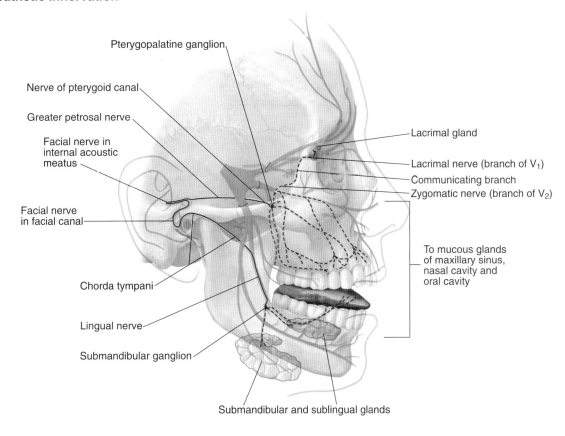

Pterygopalatine ganglion

Nerve of pterygoid canal

Greater petrosal nerve

Facial nerve in
internal acoustic
meatus

Facial nerve
in facial canal

Chorda tympani

Lingual nerve

Submandibular ganglion

Lacrimal gland

Lacrimal nerve (branch of V_1)

Communicating branch

Zygomatic nerve (branch of V_2)

To mucous glands
of maxillary sinus,
nasal cavity and
oral cavity

Submandibular and sublingual glands

PLATE 7-89   **Vestibulocochlear Nerve, Cranial Nerve VIII**

A. Origin from brain

B. Exit from cranial cavity

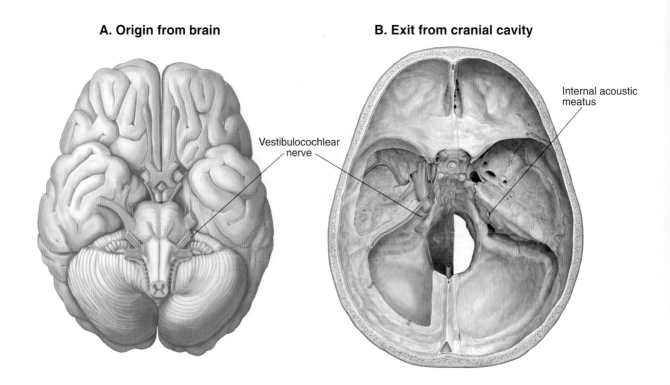

Vestibulocochlear nerve

Internal acoustic meatus

C. Sensory innervation

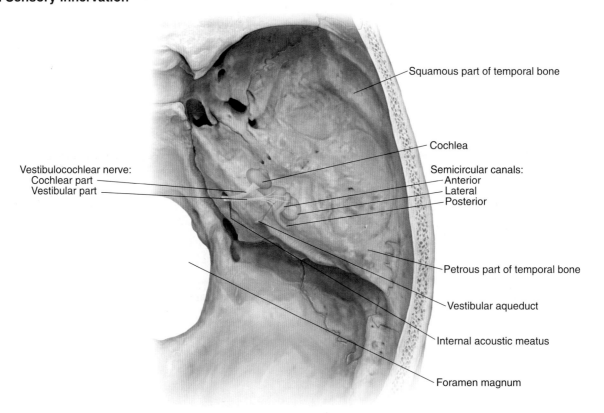

Squamous part of temporal bone

Cochlea

Semicircular canals:
- Anterior
- Lateral
- Posterior

Vestibulocochlear nerve:
- Cochlear part
- Vestibular part

Petrous part of temporal bone

Vestibular aqueduct

Internal acoustic meatus

Foramen magnum

A. Origin from brain

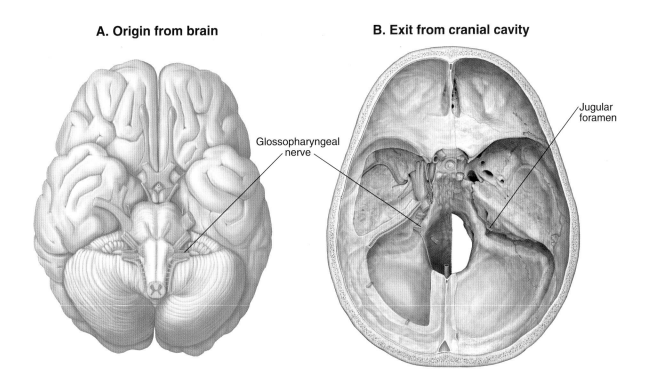

Glossopharyngeal nerve

B. Exit from cranial cavity

Jugular foramen

C. Sensory and skeletal muscle innervation

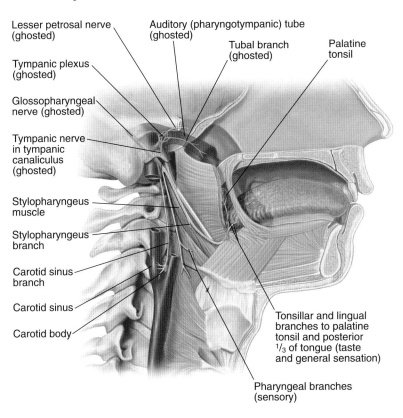

Lesser petrosal nerve (ghosted)

Tympanic plexus (ghosted)

Glossopharyngeal nerve (ghosted)

Tympanic nerve in tympanic canaliculus (ghosted)

Stylopharyngeus muscle

Stylopharyngeus branch

Carotid sinus branch

Carotid sinus

Carotid body

Auditory (pharyngotympanic) tube (ghosted)

Tubal branch (ghosted)

Palatine tonsil

Tonsillar and lingual branches to palatine tonsil and posterior $1/3$ of tongue (taste and general sensation)

Pharyngeal branches (sensory)

D. Parasympathetic innervation

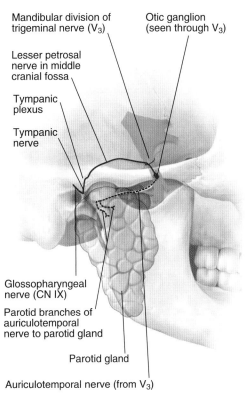

Mandibular division of trigeminal nerve (V_3)

Otic ganglion (seen through V_3)

Lesser petrosal nerve in middle cranial fossa

Tympanic plexus

Tympanic nerve

Glossopharyngeal nerve (CN IX)

Parotid branches of auriculotemporal nerve to parotid gland

Parotid gland

Auriculotemporal nerve (from V_3)

PLATE 7-91   Vagus Nerve, Cranial Nerve X

A. Origin from brain

B. Exit from cranial cavity

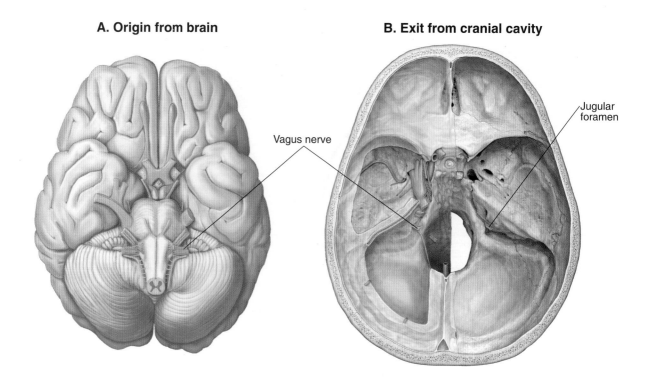

Vagus nerve

Jugular foramen

C. Skeletal muscle innervation

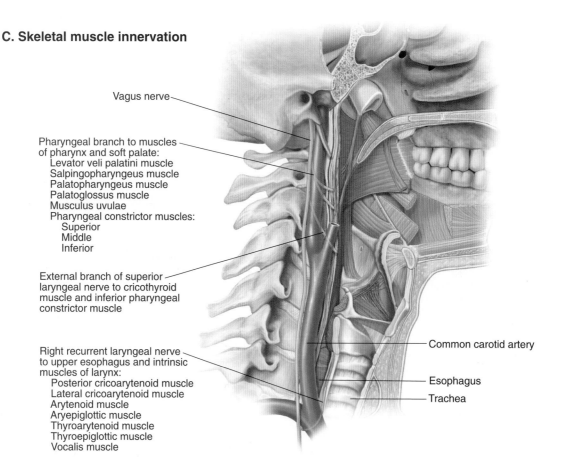

Vagus nerve

Pharyngeal branch to muscles of pharynx and soft palate:
    Levator veli palatini muscle
    Salpingopharyngeus muscle
    Palatopharyngeus muscle
    Palatoglossus muscle
    Musculus uvulae
    Pharyngeal constrictor muscles:
        Superior
        Middle
        Inferior

External branch of superior laryngeal nerve to cricothyroid muscle and inferior pharyngeal constrictor muscle

Right recurrent laryngeal nerve to upper esophagus and intrinsic muscles of larynx:
    Posterior cricoarytenoid muscle
    Lateral cricoarytenoid muscle
    Arytenoid muscle
    Aryepiglottic muscle
    Thyroarytenoid muscle
    Thyroepiglottic muscle
    Vocalis muscle

Common carotid artery

Esophagus

Trachea

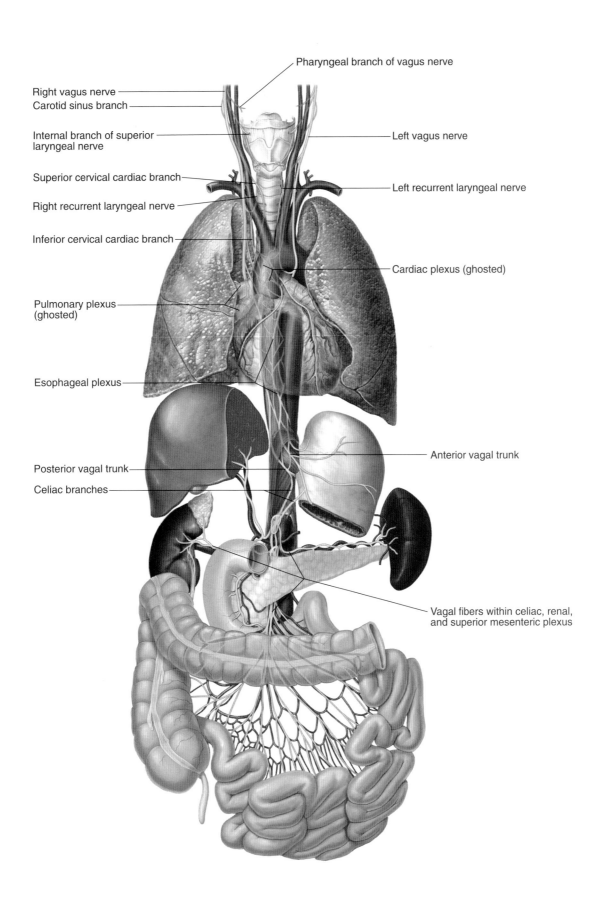

Pharyngeal branch of vagus nerve

Right vagus nerve

Carotid sinus branch

Internal branch of superior laryngeal nerve

Left vagus nerve

Superior cervical cardiac branch

Left recurrent laryngeal nerve

Right recurrent laryngeal nerve

Inferior cervical cardiac branch

Cardiac plexus (ghosted)

Pulmonary plexus (ghosted)

Esophageal plexus

Anterior vagal trunk

Posterior vagal trunk

Celiac branches

Vagal fibers within celiac, renal, and superior mesenteric plexus

PLATE 7-93   **Accessory Nerve, Cranial Nerve XI**

A. Origin from spinal cord

B. Exit from cranial cavity

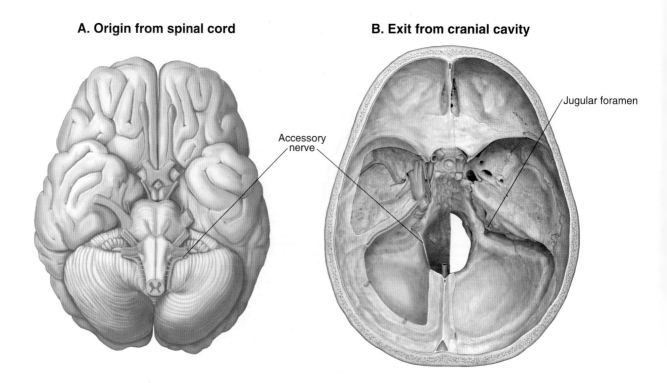

Jugular foramen

Accessory nerve

C. Skeletal muscle innervation

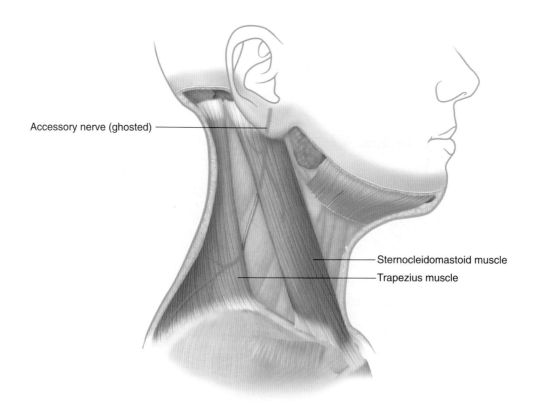

Accessory nerve (ghosted)

Sternocleidomastoid muscle

Trapezius muscle

A. Origin from brain

B. Exit from cranial cavity

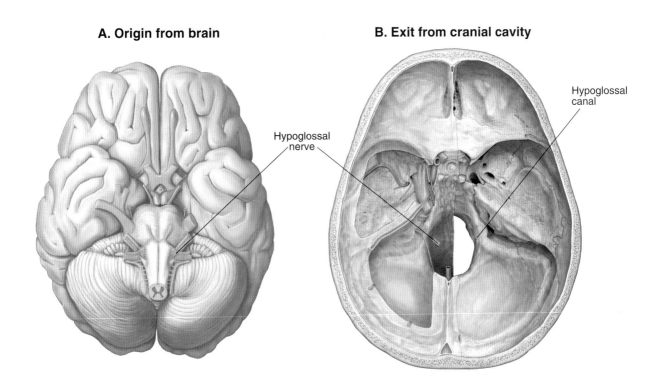

Hypoglossal nerve

Hypoglossal canal

C. Skeletal muscle innervation

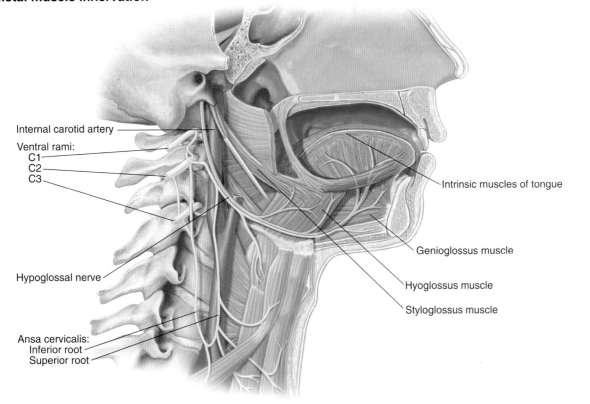

Internal carotid artery

Ventral rami:
C1
C2
C3

Hypoglossal nerve

Ansa cervicalis:
Inferior root
Superior root

Intrinsic muscles of tongue

Genioglossus muscle

Hyoglossus muscle

Styloglossus muscle

PLATE 7-95   **Summary of Head and Neck Sympathetic Innervation**

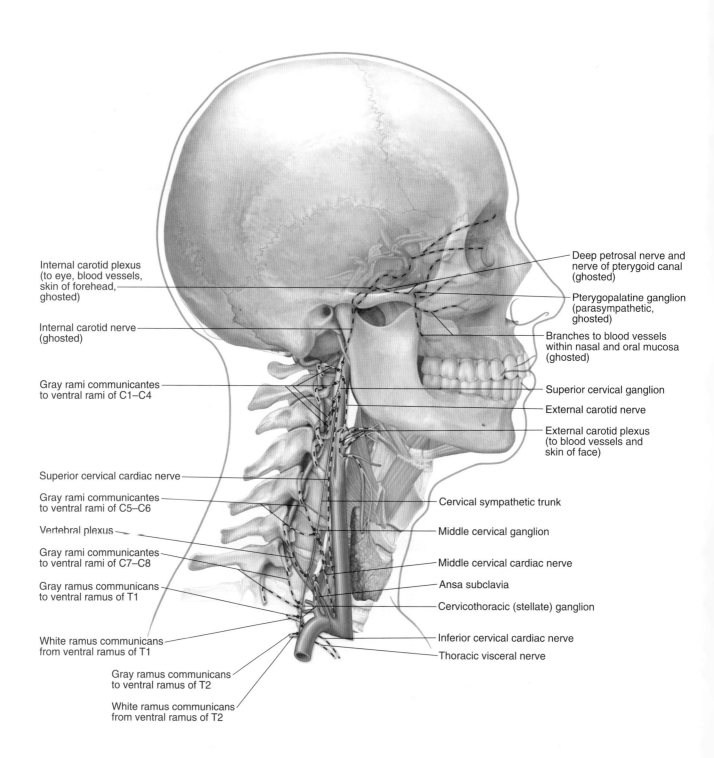

Internal carotid plexus
(to eye, blood vessels,
skin of forehead,
ghosted)

Internal carotid nerve
(ghosted)

Gray rami communicantes
to ventral rami of C1–C4

Superior cervical cardiac nerve

Gray rami communicantes
to ventral rami of C5–C6

Vertebral plexus

Gray rami communicantes
to ventral rami of C7–C8

Gray ramus communicans
to ventral ramus of T1

White ramus communicans
from ventral ramus of T1

Gray ramus communicans
to ventral ramus of T2

White ramus communicans
from ventral ramus of T2

Deep petrosal nerve and
nerve of pterygoid canal
(ghosted)

Pterygopalatine ganglion
(parasympathetic,
ghosted)

Branches to blood vessels
within nasal and oral mucosa
(ghosted)

Superior cervical ganglion

External carotid nerve

External carotid plexus
(to blood vessels and
skin of face)

Cervical sympathetic trunk

Middle cervical ganglion

Middle cervical cardiac nerve

Ansa subclavia

Cervicothoracic (stellate) ganglion

Inferior cervical cardiac nerve

Thoracic visceral nerve

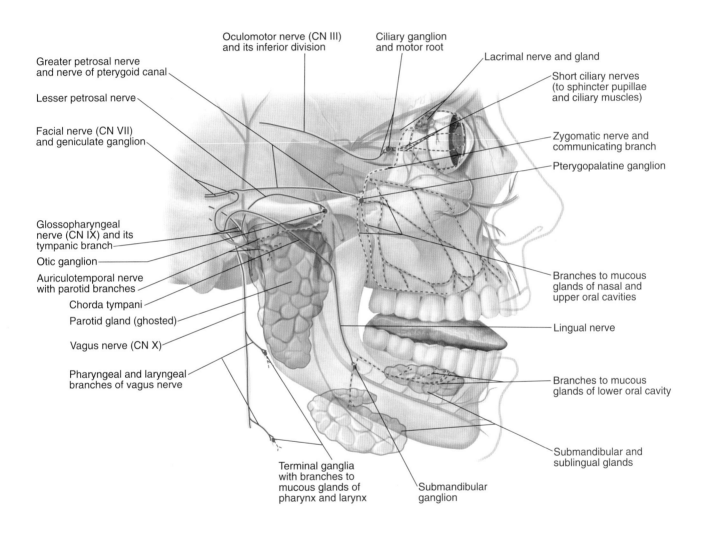

Oculomotor nerve (CN III) and its inferior division

Ciliary ganglion and motor root

Greater petrosal nerve and nerve of pterygoid canal

Lacrimal nerve and gland

Short ciliary nerves (to sphincter pupillae and ciliary muscles)

Lesser petrosal nerve

Facial nerve (CN VII) and geniculate ganglion

Zygomatic nerve and communicating branch

Pterygopalatine ganglion

Glossopharyngeal nerve (CN IX) and its tympanic branch

Otic ganglion

Auriculotemporal nerve with parotid branches

Chorda tympani

Parotid gland (ghosted)

Branches to mucous glands of nasal and upper oral cavities

Lingual nerve

Vagus nerve (CN X)

Pharyngeal and laryngeal branches of vagus nerve

Branches to mucous glands of lower oral cavity

Terminal ganglia with branches to mucous glands of pharynx and larynx

Submandibular ganglion

Submandibular and sublingual glands

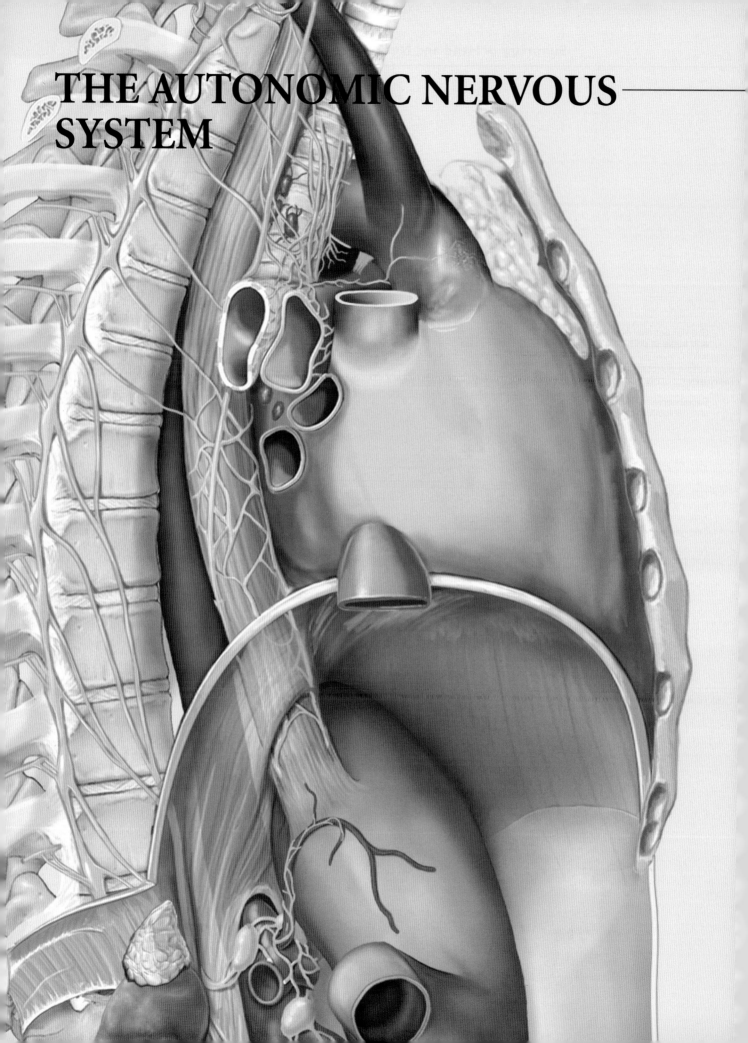

THE AUTONOMIC NERVOUS SYSTEM

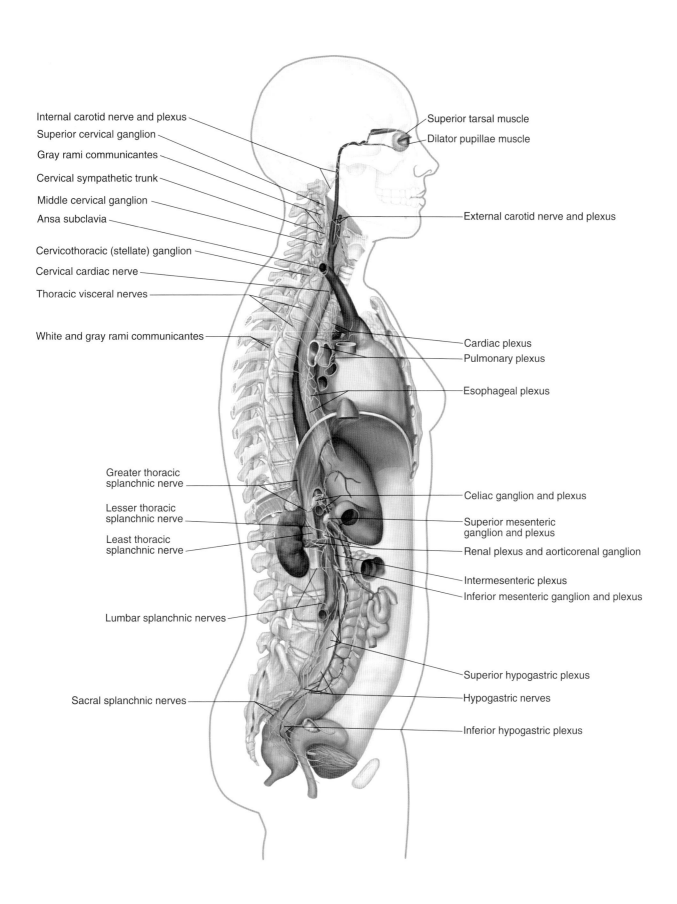

Internal carotid nerve and plexus

Superior cervical ganglion

Gray rami communicantes

Cervical sympathetic trunk

Middle cervical ganglion

Ansa subclavia

Cervicothoracic (stellate) ganglion

Cervical cardiac nerve

Thoracic visceral nerves

White and gray rami communicantes

Greater thoracic splanchnic nerve

Lesser thoracic splanchnic nerve

Least thoracic splanchnic nerve

Lumbar splanchnic nerves

Sacral splanchnic nerves

Superior tarsal muscle

Dilator pupillae muscle

External carotid nerve and plexus

Cardiac plexus

Pulmonary plexus

Esophageal plexus

Celiac ganglion and plexus

Superior mesenteric ganglion and plexus

Renal plexus and aorticorenal ganglion

Intermesenteric plexus

Inferior mesenteric ganglion and plexus

Superior hypogastric plexus

Hypogastric nerves

Inferior hypogastric plexus

PLATE 8-02 Components of the Sympathetic Nervous System I

A. Location of presynaptic cell bodies

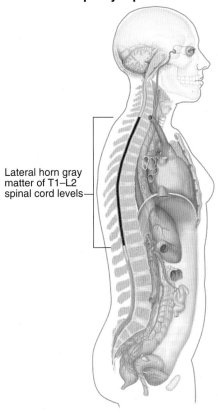

Lateral horn gray matter of T1–L2 spinal cord levels—

B. Sympathetic trunk

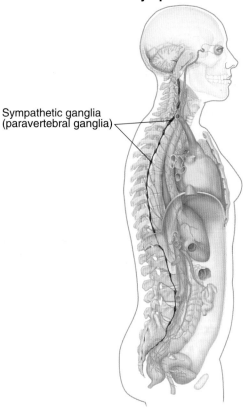

Sympathetic ganglia (paravertebral ganglia)

C. White rami communicantes

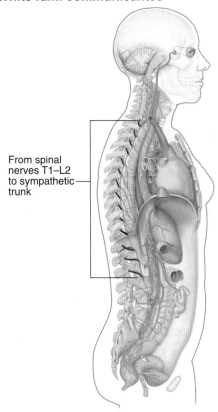

From spinal nerves T1–L2 to sympathetic trunk

D. Gray rami communicantes

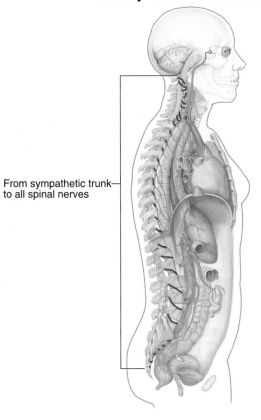

From sympathetic trunk to all spinal nerves

A. Nerves that carry sympathetic fibers

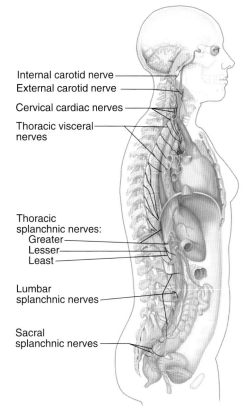

Internal carotid nerve
External carotid nerve
Cervical cardiac nerves
Thoracic visceral nerves

Thoracic splanchnic nerves:
  Greater
  Lesser
  Least

Lumbar splanchnic nerves

Sacral splanchnic nerves

B. Preaortic ganglia

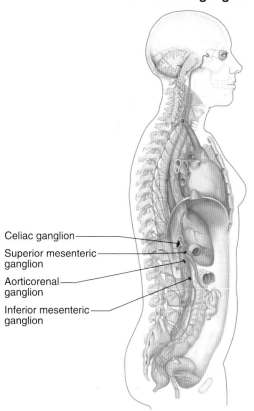

Celiac ganglion
Superior mesenteric ganglion
Aorticorenal ganglion
Inferior mesenteric ganglion

C. Plexuses that carry postsynaptic sympathetic fibers

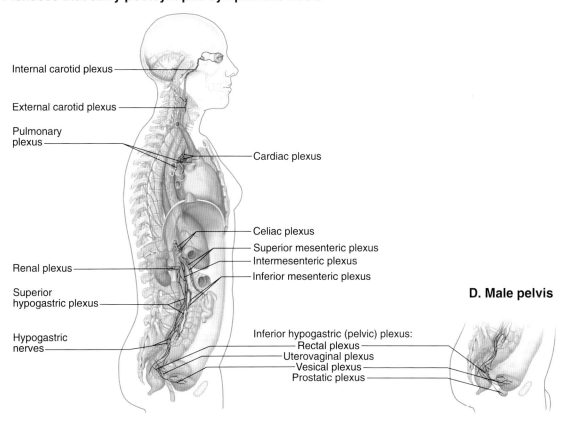

Internal carotid plexus

External carotid plexus

Pulmonary plexus

Cardiac plexus

Renal plexus

Superior hypogastric plexus

Hypogastric nerves

Celiac plexus
Superior mesenteric plexus
Intermesenteric plexus
Inferior mesenteric plexus

D. Male pelvis

Inferior hypogastric (pelvic) plexus:
  Rectal plexus
  Uterovaginal plexus
  Vesical plexus
  Prostatic plexus

PLATE 8-04 **Position of Sympathetic Trunks**

A. Lateral view

B. Anterior view

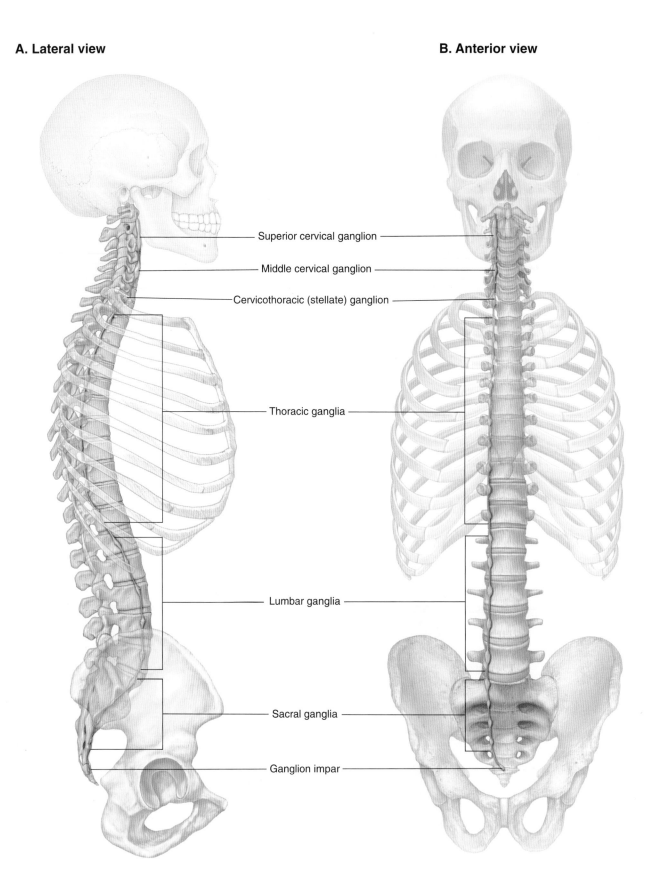

Superior cervical ganglion

Middle cervical ganglion

Cervicothoracic (stellate) ganglion

Thoracic ganglia

Lumbar ganglia

Sacral ganglia

Ganglion impar

A. C1–C8 levels

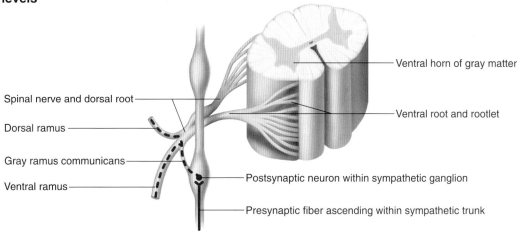

Ventral horn of gray matter

Spinal nerve and dorsal root

Dorsal ramus

Gray ramus communicans

Ventral ramus

Ventral root and rootlet

Postsynaptic neuron within sympathetic ganglion

Presynaptic fiber ascending within sympathetic trunk

B. T1–L2 levels

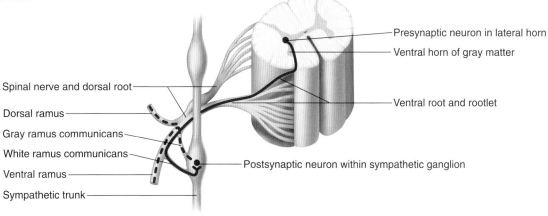

Presynaptic neuron in lateral horn

Ventral horn of gray matter

Spinal nerve and dorsal root

Dorsal ramus

Gray ramus communicans

White ramus communicans

Ventral ramus

Sympathetic trunk

Ventral root and rootlet

Postsynaptic neuron within sympathetic ganglion

C. L3–Co levels

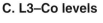
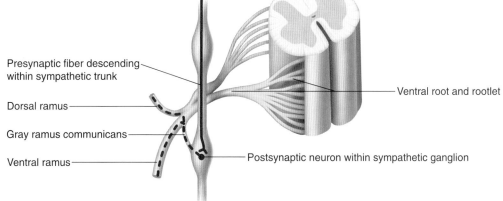

Presynaptic fiber descending within sympathetic trunk

Dorsal ramus

Gray ramus communicans

Ventral ramus

Ventral root and rootlet

Postsynaptic neuron within sympathetic ganglion

PLATE 8-06 Pathways of Sympathetic Neurons, Oblique View II

A. Cervical levels (C1–C8)

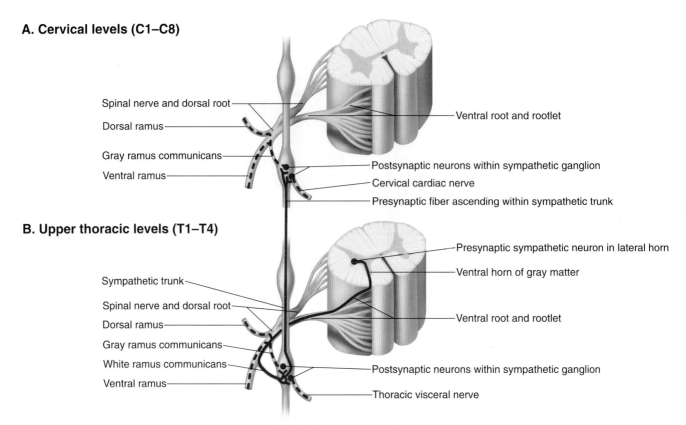

Spinal nerve and dorsal root

Dorsal ramus

Gray ramus communicans

Ventral ramus

Ventral root and rootlet

Postsynaptic neurons within sympathetic ganglion

Cervical cardiac nerve

Presynaptic fiber ascending within sympathetic trunk

B. Upper thoracic levels (T1–T4)

Sympathetic trunk

Spinal nerve and dorsal root

Dorsal ramus

Gray ramus communicans

White ramus communicans

Ventral ramus

Presynaptic sympathetic neuron in lateral horn

Ventral horn of gray matter

Ventral root and rootlet

Postsynaptic neurons within sympathetic ganglion

Thoracic visceral nerve

C. Lower thoracic or upper lumbar levels (T5–L2)

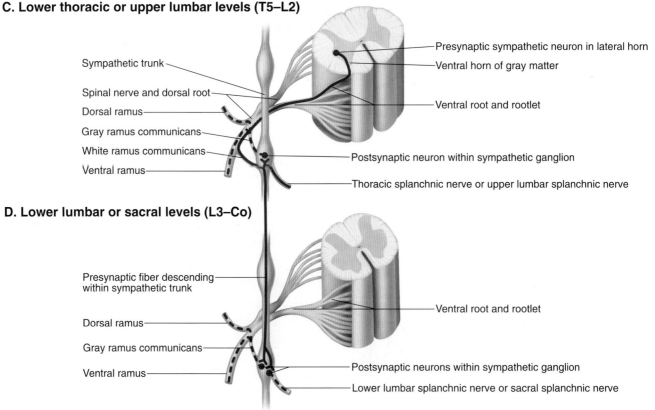

Sympathetic trunk

Spinal nerve and dorsal root

Dorsal ramus

Gray ramus communicans

White ramus communicans

Ventral ramus

Presynaptic sympathetic neuron in lateral horn

Ventral horn of gray matter

Ventral root and rootlet

Postsynaptic neuron within sympathetic ganglion

Thoracic splanchnic nerve or upper lumbar splanchnic nerve

D. Lower lumbar or sacral levels (L3–Co)

Presynaptic fiber descending within sympathetic trunk

Dorsal ramus

Gray ramus communicans

Ventral ramus

Ventral root and rootlet

Postsynaptic neurons within sympathetic ganglion

Lower lumbar splanchnic nerve or sacral splanchnic nerve

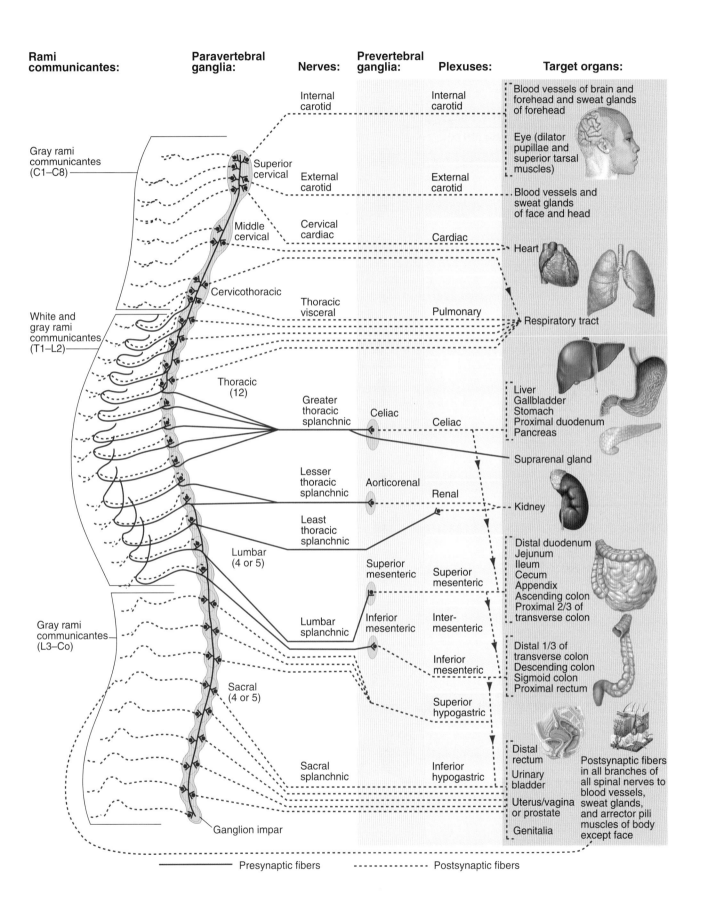

Rami communicantes:

Gray rami communicantes (C1–C8)

White and gray rami communicantes (T1–L2)

Gray rami communicantes (L3–Co)

Paravertebral ganglia:

Superior cervical

Middle cervical

Cervicothoracic

Thoracic (12)

Lumbar (4 or 5)

Sacral (4 or 5)

Ganglion impar

Nerves:

Internal carotid

External carotid

Cervical cardiac

Thoracic visceral

Greater thoracic splanchnic

Lesser thoracic splanchnic

Least thoracic splanchnic

Lumbar splanchnic

Sacral splanchnic

Prevertebral ganglia:

Celiac

Aorticorenal

Superior mesenteric

Inferior mesenteric

Plexuses:

Internal carotid

External carotid

Cardiac

Pulmonary

Celiac

Renal

Superior mesenteric

Inter-mesenteric

Inferior mesenteric

Superior hypogastric

Inferior hypogastric

Target organs:

Blood vessels of brain and forehead and sweat glands of forehead

Eye (dilator pupillae and superior tarsal muscles)

Blood vessels and sweat glands of face and head

Heart

Respiratory tract

Liver
Gallbladder
Stomach
Proximal duodenum
Pancreas

Suprarenal gland

Kidney

Distal duodenum
Jejunum
Ileum
Cecum
Appendix
Ascending colon
Proximal 2/3 of transverse colon

Distal 1/3 of transverse colon
Descending colon
Sigmoid colon
Proximal rectum

Distal rectum

Urinary bladder

Uterus/vagina or prostate

Genitalia

Postsynaptic fibers in all branches of all spinal nerves to blood vessels, sweat glands, and arrector pili muscles of body except face

———— Presynaptic fibers   - - - - - - - - Postsynaptic fibers

PLATE 8-08   Overview of the Parasympathetic Nervous System

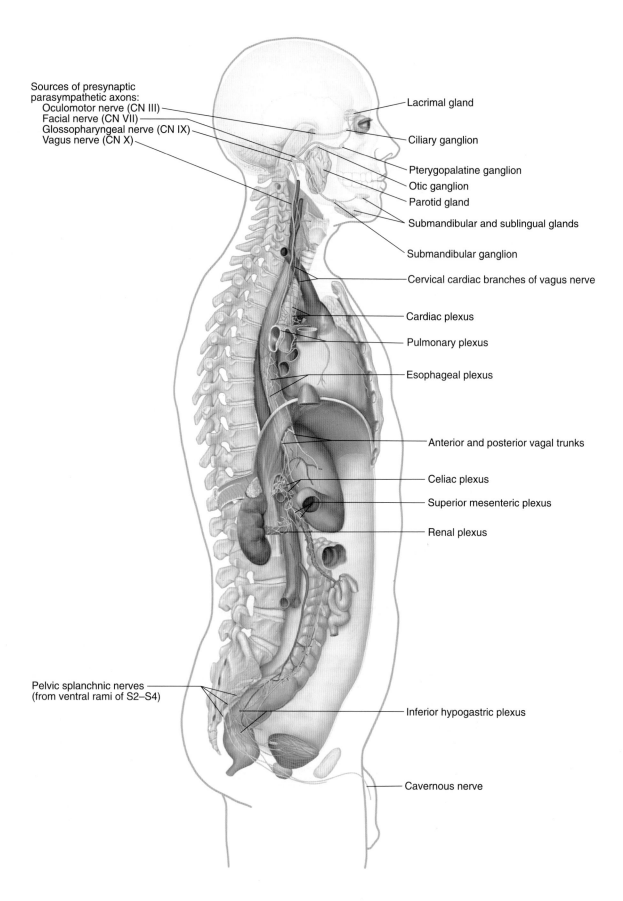

Sources of presynaptic
parasympathetic axons:
Oculomotor nerve (CN III)
Facial nerve (CN VII)
Glossopharyngeal nerve (CN IX)
Vagus nerve (CN X)

Lacrimal gland

Ciliary ganglion

Pterygopalatine ganglion
Otic ganglion
Parotid gland
Submandibular and sublingual glands

Submandibular ganglion

Cervical cardiac branches of vagus nerve

Cardiac plexus

Pulmonary plexus

Esophageal plexus

Anterior and posterior vagal trunks

Celiac plexus

Superior mesenteric plexus

Renal plexus

Pelvic splanchnic nerves
(from ventral rami of S2–S4)

Inferior hypogastric plexus

Cavernous nerve

A. Location of presynaptic parasympathetic cell bodies

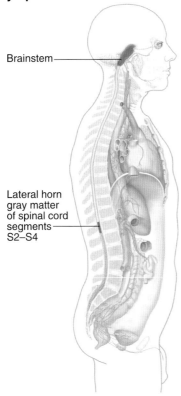

Brainstem

Lateral horn gray matter of spinal cord segments S2–S4

B. Nerves that carry presynaptic parasympathetic fibers

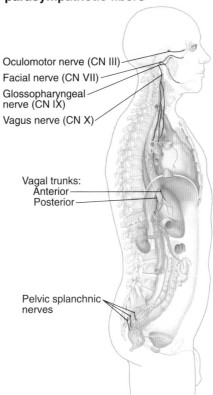

Oculomotor nerve (CN III)
Facial nerve (CN VII)
Glossopharyngeal nerve (CN IX)
Vagus nerve (CN X)

Vagal trunks:
  Anterior
  Posterior

Pelvic splanchnic nerves

C. Plexuses that carry presynaptic parasympathetic fibers

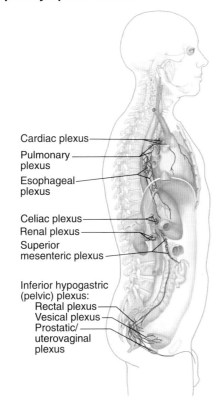

Cardiac plexus
Pulmonary plexus
Esophageal plexus
Celiac plexus
Renal plexus
Superior mesenteric plexus

Inferior hypogastric (pelvic) plexus:
  Rectal plexus
  Vesical plexus
  Prostatic/ uterovaginal plexus

D. Location of postsynaptic parasympathetic cell bodies

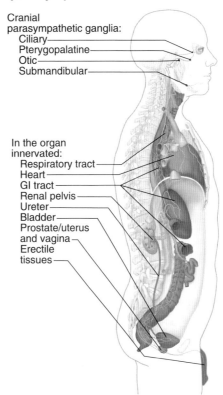

Cranial parasympathetic ganglia:
  Ciliary
  Pterygopalatine
  Otic
  Submandibular

In the organ innervated:
  Respiratory tract
  Heart
  GI tract
  Renal pelvis
  Ureter
  Bladder
  Prostate/uterus and vagina
  Erectile tissues

PLATE 8-10 **Parasympathetic Ganglia of the Head**

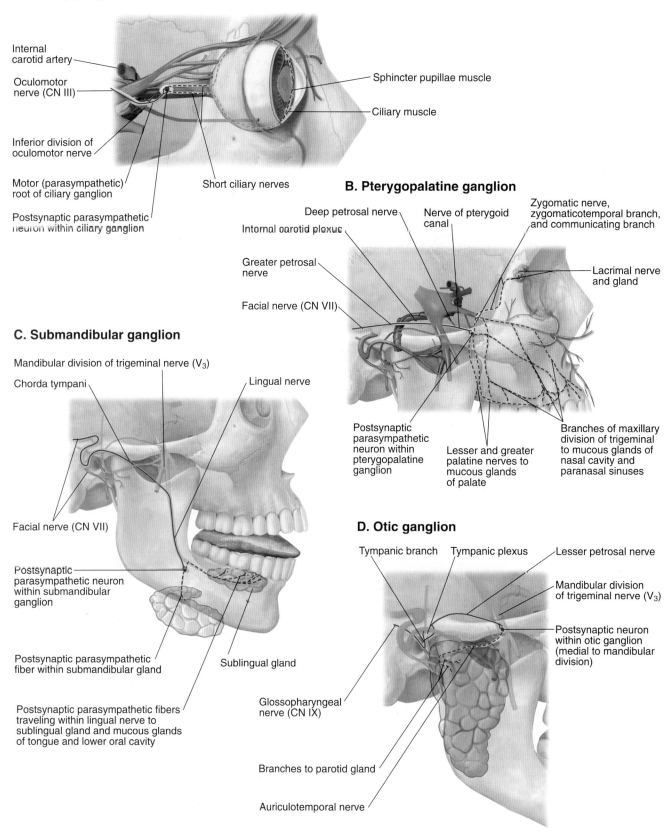

A. Ciliary ganglion

Internal carotid artery

Oculomotor nerve (CN III)

Inferior division of oculomotor nerve

Motor (parasympathetic) root of ciliary ganglion

Postsynaptic parasympathetic neuron within ciliary ganglion

Sphincter pupillae muscle

Ciliary muscle

Short ciliary nerves

B. Pterygopalatine ganglion

Deep petrosal nerve

Internal carotid plexus

Greater petrosal nerve

Facial nerve (CN VII)

Nerve of pterygoid canal

Zygomatic nerve, zygomaticotemporal branch, and communicating branch

Lacrimal nerve and gland

Postsynaptic parasympathetic neuron within pterygopalatine ganglion

Lesser and greater palatine nerves to mucous glands of palate

Branches of maxillary division of trigeminal to mucous glands of nasal cavity and paranasal sinuses

C. Submandibular ganglion

Mandibular division of trigeminal nerve (V₃)

Chorda tympani

Lingual nerve

Facial nerve (CN VII)

Postsynaptic parasympathetic neuron within submandibular ganglion

Postsynaptic parasympathetic fiber within submandibular gland

Sublingual gland

Postsynaptic parasympathetic fibers traveling within lingual nerve to sublingual gland and mucous glands of tongue and lower oral cavity

D. Otic ganglion

Tympanic branch

Tympanic plexus

Lesser petrosal nerve

Mandibular division of trigeminal nerve (V₃)

Postsynaptic neuron within otic ganglion (medial to mandibular division)

Glossopharyngeal nerve (CN IX)

Branches to parotid gland

Auriculotemporal nerve

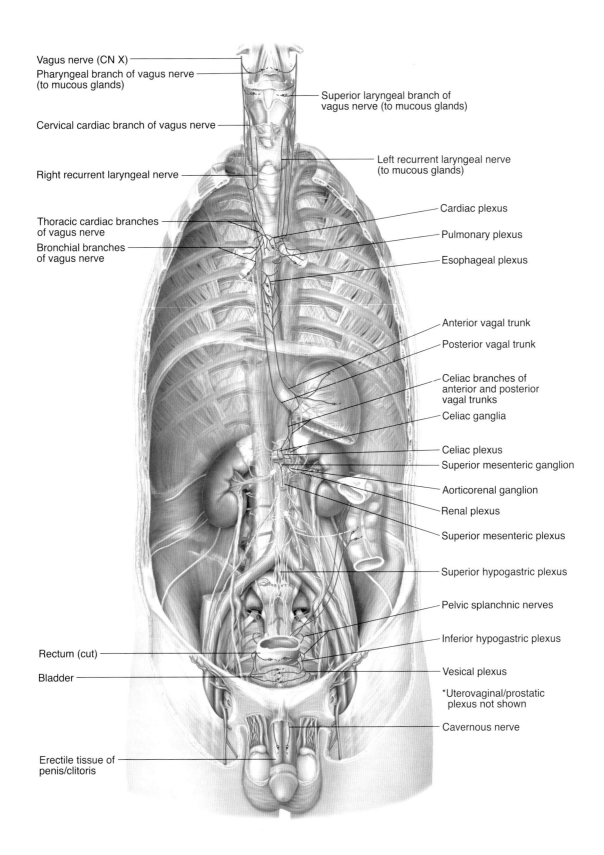

Vagus nerve (CN X)

Pharyngeal branch of vagus nerve
(to mucous glands)

Superior laryngeal branch of
vagus nerve (to mucous glands)

Cervical cardiac branch of vagus nerve

Left recurrent laryngeal nerve
(to mucous glands)

Right recurrent laryngeal nerve

Cardiac plexus

Thoracic cardiac branches
of vagus nerve

Pulmonary plexus

Bronchial branches
of vagus nerve

Esophageal plexus

Anterior vagal trunk

Posterior vagal trunk

Celiac branches of
anterior and posterior
vagal trunks

Celiac ganglia

Celiac plexus

Superior mesenteric ganglion

Aorticorenal ganglion

Renal plexus

Superior mesenteric plexus

Superior hypogastric plexus

Pelvic splanchnic nerves

Inferior hypogastric plexus

Rectum (cut)

Vesical plexus

Bladder

*Uterovaginal/prostatic
plexus not shown

Cavernous nerve

Erectile tissue of
penis/clitoris

PLATE 8-12   Pathways of the Parasympathetic Nervous System

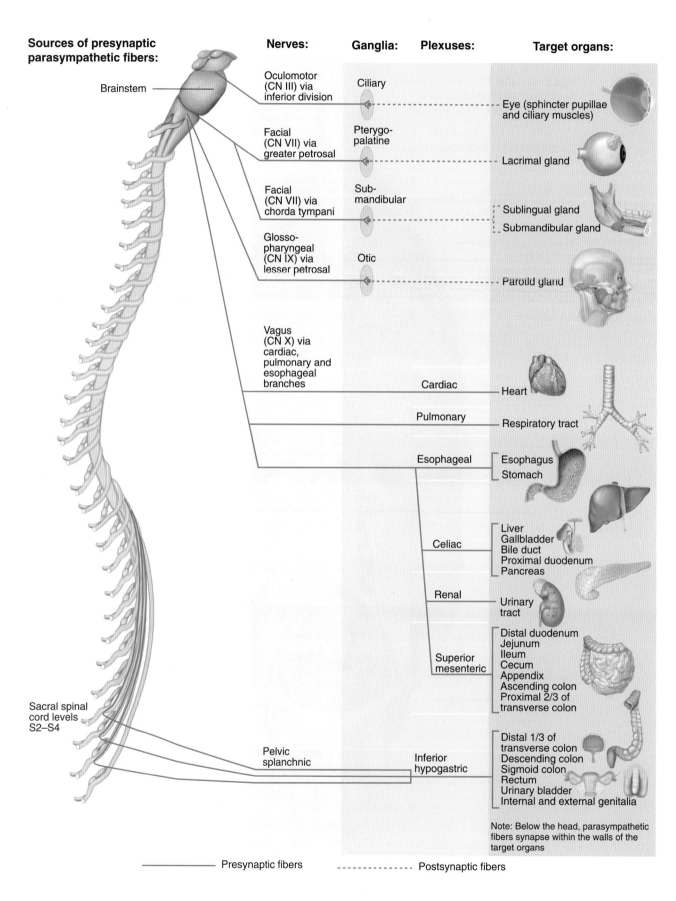

Sources of presynaptic parasympathetic fibers:

Nerves: Ganglia: Plexuses: Target organs:

Brainstem

Oculomotor (CN III) via inferior division — Ciliary — Eye (sphincter pupillae and ciliary muscles)

Facial (CN VII) via greater petrosal — Pterygo-palatine — Lacrimal gland

Facial (CN VII) via chorda tympani — Sub-mandibular — Sublingual gland / Submandibular gland

Glosso-pharyngeal (CN IX) via lesser petrosal — Otic — Parotid gland

Vagus (CN X) via cardiac, pulmonary and esophageal branches

Cardiac — Heart

Pulmonary — Respiratory tract

Esophageal — Esophagus / Stomach

Celiac — Liver / Gallbladder / Bile duct / Proximal duodenum / Pancreas

Renal — Urinary tract

Superior mesenteric — Distal duodenum / Jejunum / Ileum / Cecum / Appendix / Ascending colon / Proximal 2/3 of transverse colon

Sacral spinal cord levels S2–S4

Pelvic splanchnic — Inferior hypogastric — Distal 1/3 of transverse colon / Descending colon / Sigmoid colon / Rectum / Urinary bladder / Internal and external genitalia

Note: Below the head, parasympathetic fibers synapse within the walls of the target organs

————— Presynaptic fibers   - - - - - - - - Postsynaptic fibers

A. Nerves carrying sympathetic fibers to the limbs and body wall

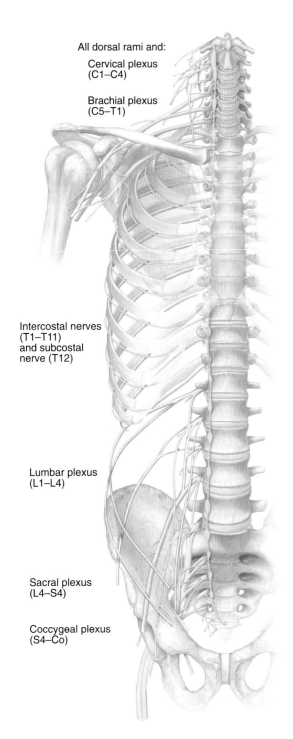

All dorsal rami and:

Cervical plexus
(C1–C4)

Brachial plexus
(C5–T1)

Intercostal nerves
(T1–T11)
and subcostal
nerve (T12)

Lumbar plexus
(L1–L4)

Sacral plexus
(L4–S4)

Coccygeal plexus
(S4–Co)

B. Sympathetic pathways at C1–C8 levels

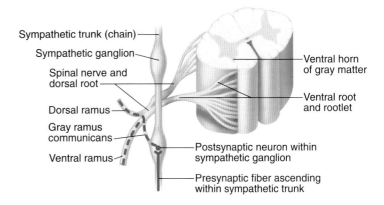

Sympathetic trunk (chain)

Sympathetic ganglion

Spinal nerve and
dorsal root

Dorsal ramus

Gray ramus
communicans

Ventral ramus

Ventral horn
of gray matter

Ventral root
and rootlet

Postsynaptic neuron within
sympathetic ganglion

Presynaptic fiber ascending
within sympathetic trunk

C. Sympathetic pathways at T1–L2 levels

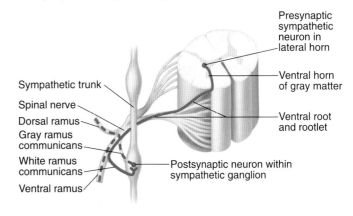

Sympathetic trunk

Spinal nerve

Dorsal ramus

Gray ramus
communicans

White ramus
communicans

Ventral ramus

Presynaptic
sympathetic
neuron in
lateral horn

Ventral horn
of gray matter

Ventral root
and rootlet

Postsynaptic neuron within
sympathetic ganglion

D. Sympathetic pathways at L3–Co levels

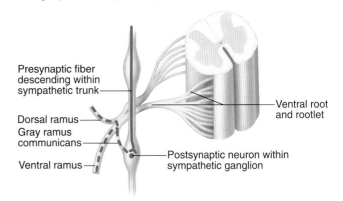

Presynaptic fiber
descending within
sympathetic trunk

Dorsal ramus

Gray ramus
communicans

Ventral ramus

Ventral root
and rootlet

Postsynaptic neuron within
sympathetic ganglion

PLATE 8-14   **Autonomics of the Thorax, Sympathetic Pathways**

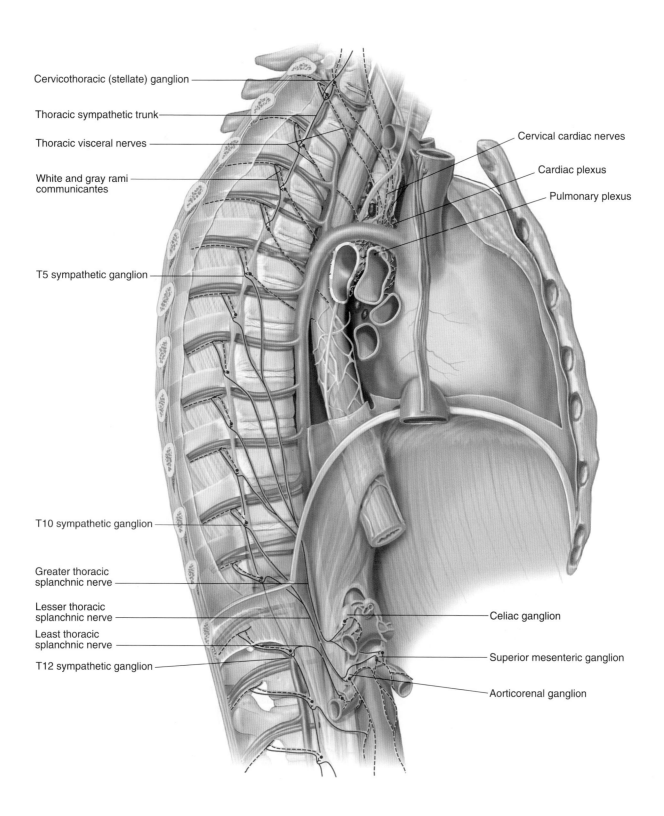

Cervicothoracic (stellate) ganglion

Thoracic sympathetic trunk

Thoracic visceral nerves

White and gray rami
communicantes

T5 sympathetic ganglion

T10 sympathetic ganglion

Greater thoracic
splanchnic nerve

Lesser thoracic
splanchnic nerve

Least thoracic
splanchnic nerve

T12 sympathetic ganglion

Cervical cardiac nerves

Cardiac plexus

Pulmonary plexus

Celiac ganglion

Superior mesenteric ganglion

Aorticorenal ganglion

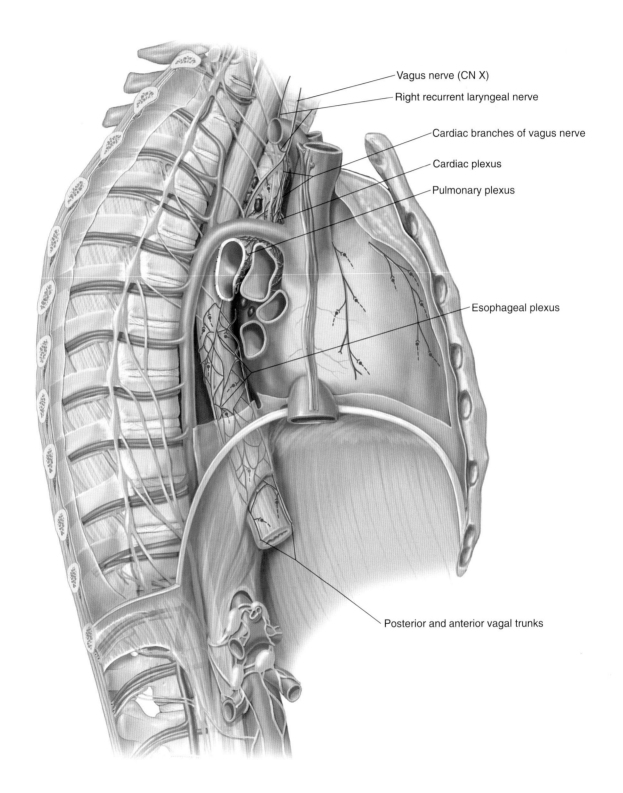

Vagus nerve (CN X)

Right recurrent laryngeal nerve

Cardiac branches of vagus nerve

Cardiac plexus

Pulmonary plexus

Esophageal plexus

Posterior and anterior vagal trunks

PLATE 8-16 **Autonomics of the Abdomen, Sympathetic Pathways**

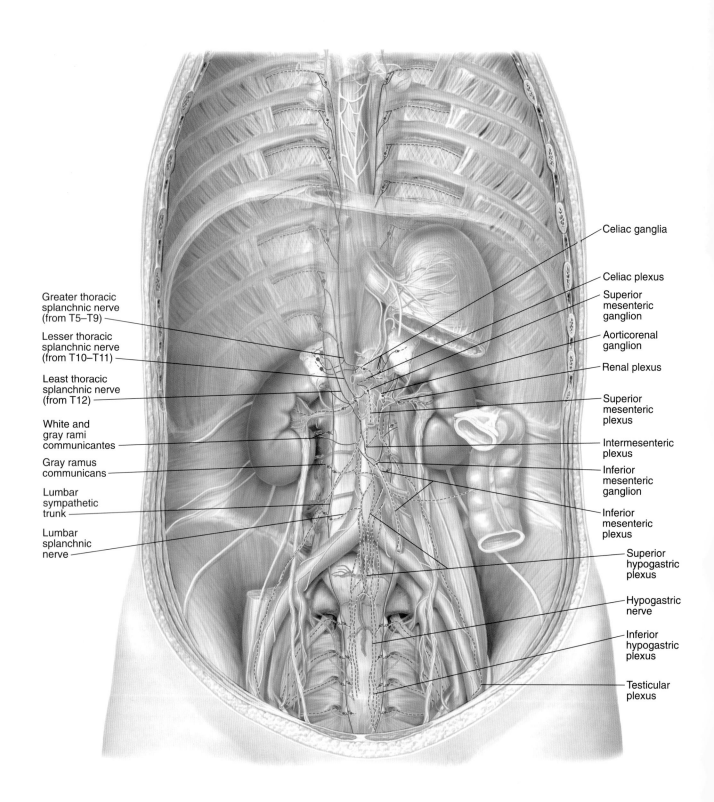

Greater thoracic
splanchnic nerve
(from T5–T9)

Lesser thoracic
splanchnic nerve
(from T10–T11)

Least thoracic
splanchnic nerve
(from T12)

White and
gray rami
communicantes

Gray ramus
communicans

Lumbar
sympathetic
trunk

Lumbar
splanchnic
nerve

Celiac ganglia

Celiac plexus

Superior
mesenteric
ganglion

Aorticorenal
ganglion

Renal plexus

Superior
mesenteric
plexus

Intermesenteric
plexus

Inferior
mesenteric
ganglion

Inferior
mesenteric
plexus

Superior
hypogastric
plexus

Hypogastric
nerve

Inferior
hypogastric
plexus

Testicular
plexus

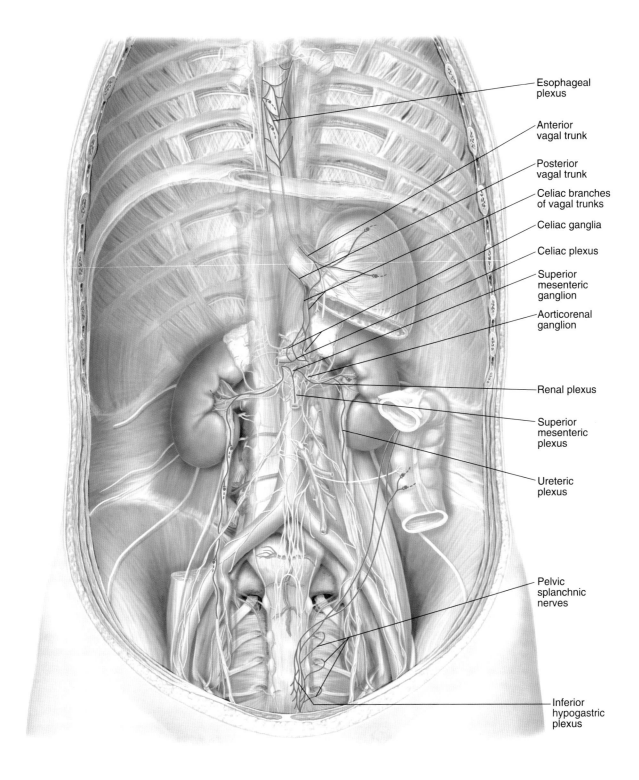

Esophageal plexus

Anterior vagal trunk

Posterior vagal trunk

Celiac branches of vagal trunks

Celiac ganglia

Celiac plexus

Superior mesenteric ganglion

Aorticorenal ganglion

Renal plexus

Superior mesenteric plexus

Ureteric plexus

Pelvic splanchnic nerves

Inferior hypogastric plexus

PLATE 8-18   **Autonomics of the Pelvis, Sympathetic Pathways, Female**

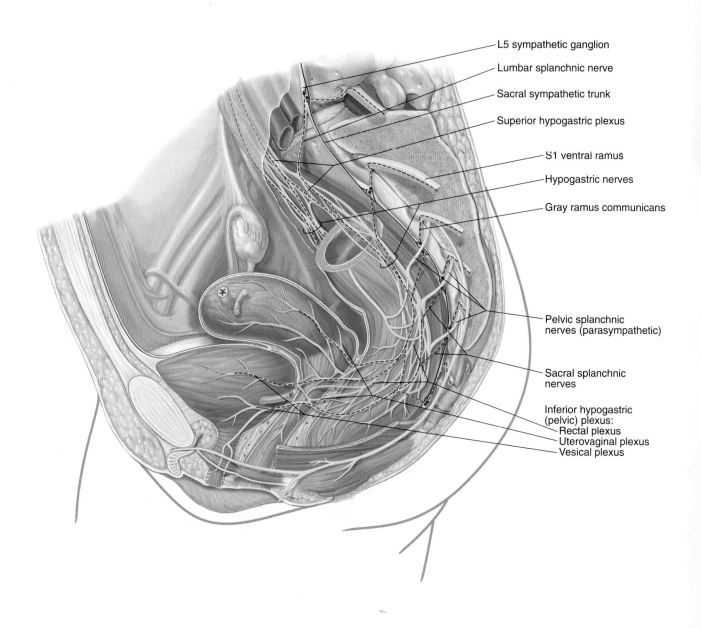

L5 sympathetic ganglion

Lumbar splanchnic nerve

Sacral sympathetic trunk

Superior hypogastric plexus

S1 ventral ramus

Hypogastric nerves

Gray ramus communicans

Pelvic splanchnic
nerves (parasympathetic)

Sacral splanchnic
nerves

Inferior hypogastric
(pelvic) plexus:
  Rectal plexus
  Uterovaginal plexus
  Vesical plexus

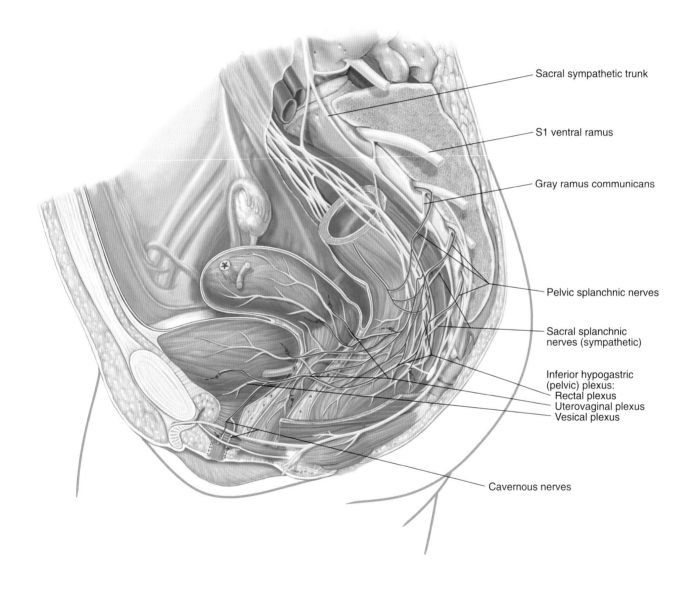

Sacral sympathetic trunk

S1 ventral ramus

Gray ramus communicans

Pelvic splanchnic nerves

Sacral splanchnic nerves (sympathetic)

Inferior hypogastric (pelvic) plexus:
Rectal plexus
Uterovaginal plexus
Vesical plexus

Cavernous nerves

PLATE 8-20 | **Autonomics of the Pelvis, Sympathetic Pathways, Male**

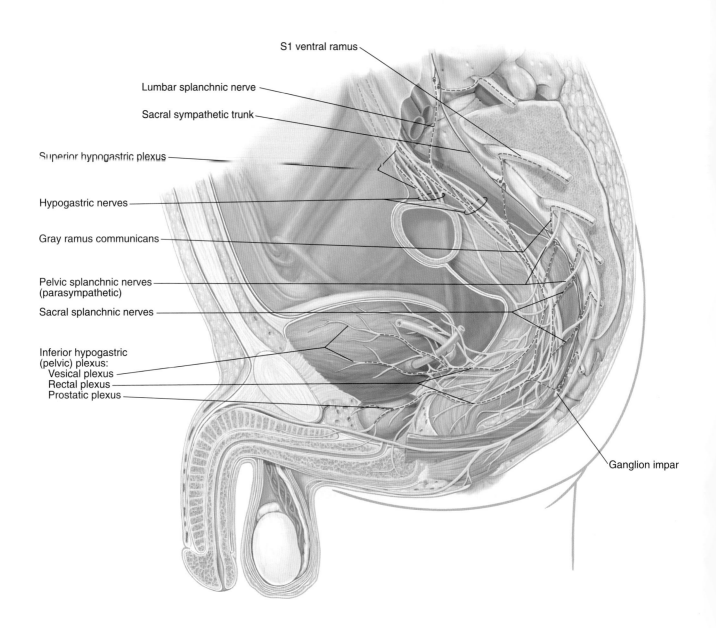

S1 ventral ramus

Lumbar splanchnic nerve

Sacral sympathetic trunk

Superior hypogastric plexus

Hypogastric nerves

Gray ramus communicans

Pelvic splanchnic nerves
(parasympathetic)

Sacral splanchnic nerves

Inferior hypogastric
(pelvic) plexus:
    Vesical plexus
    Rectal plexus
    Prostatic plexus

Ganglion impar

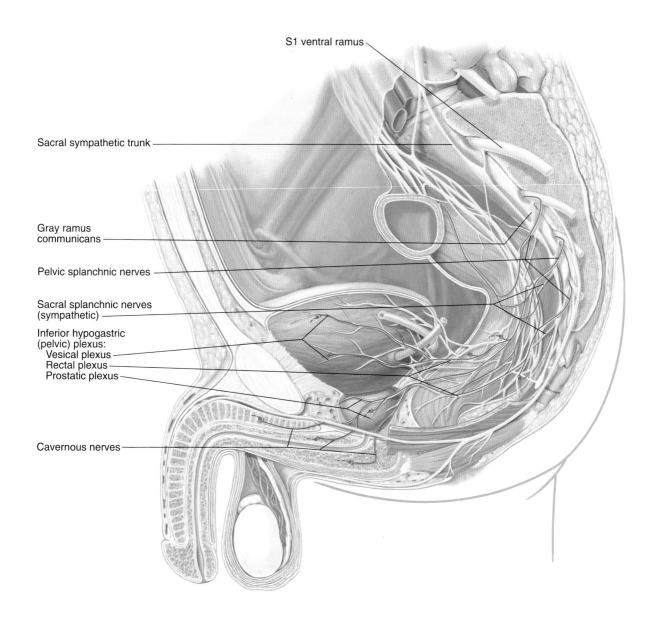

S1 ventral ramus

Sacral sympathetic trunk

Gray ramus
communicans

Pelvic splanchnic nerves

Sacral splanchnic nerves
(sympathetic)

Inferior hypogastric
(pelvic) plexus:
    Vesical plexus
    Rectal plexus
    Prostatic plexus

Cavernous nerves

PLATE 8-22   **Autonomics of the Head and Neck, Sympathetic Pathways**

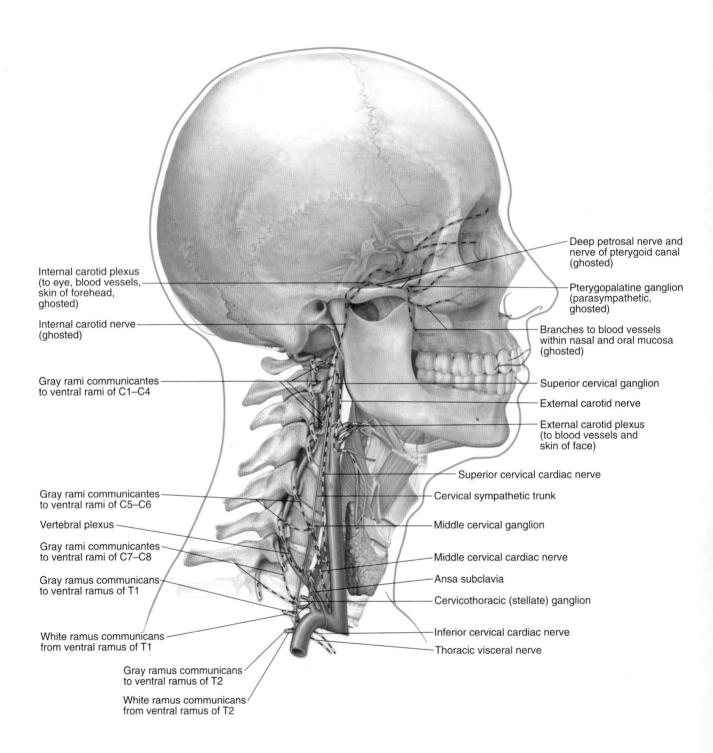

Internal carotid plexus
(to eye, blood vessels,
skin of forehead,
ghosted)

Internal carotid nerve
(ghosted)

Gray rami communicantes
to ventral rami of C1–C4

Gray rami communicantes
to ventral rami of C5–C6

Vertebral plexus

Gray rami communicantes
to ventral rami of C7–C8

Gray ramus communicans
to ventral ramus of T1

White ramus communicans
from ventral ramus of T1

Gray ramus communicans
to ventral ramus of T2

White ramus communicans
from ventral ramus of T2

Deep petrosal nerve and
nerve of pterygoid canal
(ghosted)

Pterygopalatine ganglion
(parasympathetic,
ghosted)

Branches to blood vessels
within nasal and oral mucosa
(ghosted)

Superior cervical ganglion

External carotid nerve

External carotid plexus
(to blood vessels and
skin of face)

Superior cervical cardiac nerve

Cervical sympathetic trunk

Middle cervical ganglion

Middle cervical cardiac nerve

Ansa subclavia

Cervicothoracic (stellate) ganglion

Inferior cervical cardiac nerve

Thoracic visceral nerve

Greater petrosal nerve
and nerve of pterygoid canal

Oculomotor
nerve (CN III)

Ciliary ganglion
and its motor root

Lacrimal nerve and gland

Short ciliary nerves
(to sphincter pupillae
and ciliary muscles)

Zygomatic nerve and
its communicating branch

Pterygopalatine ganglion

Facial nerve (CN VII)

Lesser petrosal nerve

Glossopharyngeal nerve (CN IX)
and tympanic branch

Chorda tympani

Otic ganglion and
auriculotemporal nerve

Branches to mucous glands
of nasal cavity and upper
oral cavity

Parotid gland

Branches to mucous glands
of lower oral cavity

Vagus nerve (CN X)
with branches to mucous glands of
viscera of neck

Submandibular and
sublingual glands

Lingual nerve

Submandibular ganglion

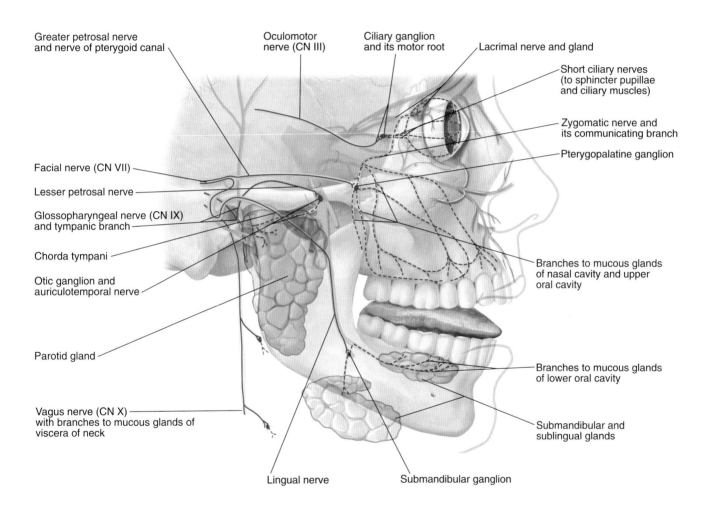